Biskon

Y0-BYK-757

Calcium and cAMP as Synarchic Messengers

CALCIUM AND cAMP as SYNARCHIC MESSENGERS

Howard Rasmussen

Departments of Medicine and Physiology
Yale University School of Medicine
New Haven, Connecticut

A WILEY-INTERSCIENCE PUBLICATION

JOHN WILEY & SONS

New York • **Chichester** • **Brisbane** • **Toronto** • **Singapore**

Copyright © 1981 by John Wiley & Sons, Inc.

All rights reserved. Published simultaneously in Canada.

Reproduction or translation of any part of this work
beyond that permitted by Sections 107 or 108 of the
1976 United States Copyright Act without the permission
of the copyright owner is unlawful. Requests for
permission or further information should be addressed to
the Permissions Department, John Wiley & Sons, Inc.

Library of Congress Cataloging in Publication Data:

Rasmussen, Howard.
    Calcium and cAMP as synarchic messengers.

    "A Wiley-Interscience publication."
    Bibliography: p.
    Includes index.
    1. Calcium—Physiological effect. 2. Cyclic adenylic acid—
Physiological effect. 3. Cellular control mechanisms. I. Title.
II. Title: Synarchic messengers. [DNLM: 1. Adenosine cyclic
monophosphate—Physiology. 2. Calcium—Physiology. QV
276 R228c]
QP535.C2R34   1981   599.01'88   81-10482
ISBN 0-471-08396-8   AACR2

Printed in the United States of America

10 9 8 7 6 5 4 3 2 1

To Maurice Pechet in recognition of his
constant friendship, support, and encouragement

Preface

The purpose of this monograph is to survey data obtained in the last 15 years concerning stimulus–response coupling in both the neural and endocrine systems. From these data, the conclusion is drawn that rather than two more or less distinct modalities of stimulus–response coupling in the neural and endocrine systems employing respectively calcium ion and cAMP as the coupling factors, there is a single modality which functions in both systems and nearly always employs the dual messengers calcium and cyclic AMP (cAMP). Furthermore, evidence is presented in support of the concept that within this system there are a number of particular variations on the universal calcium–cAMP theme. I have paid particular attention to certain endocrine and neural systems that have been intensively studied, and have excluded from consideration others because the data from their study are insufficient to either support or refute the major thesis presented. No attempt has been made to be exhaustive. Nonetheless, an attempt has been made to be comprehensive in the sense that nearly all the recognizable patterns of calcium-cAMP interactions have been discussed in the context of one type of cellular response or another.

No amount of thanks can express my debt to my teachers, students, fellows, and scientific collaborators who have participated in my scientific quest and intellectual growth. These include Fuller Albright, Alexander Leaf, Roland Westall, Lyman Craig, Irving Schwartz, George Cotzias, Lee Peachey, Maurice Pechet, Hector DeLuca, Claude Arnaud, Constantine Anast, Jan Fischer, Alan Tenenhouse, Marie Fang, Charles Hawker, Travis Littledike, George Kimmich, Etsuro Ogata, Britton Chance, James Allen, Naokazu Nagata, Kiyoshi Kurokawa, Satoshi Kimura, Joel Feinblatt, William Lake, Earl Guthrow, Jr., Francis DiBella, Eric Lein, John Harley, Arthur Balin, Stewart Lipton, Edward Max, Walter Davis, Naomi Friedmann, Pamela Jensen, Mark Haussler, Philippe Bordier, Daniel Bikle, Michael Berridge, William Prince, Craig Dise, Carol Clayberger, Michael Gustin, Jeffery Stadel, Jeffery Gimble, Olivier Fontaine, Toshito Matsumoto, Paula Barrett, Edward Puzas, David Waisman, Richard Foster, Larry Rubin, and in particular my close associate and collaborator for over 12 years, David Goodman. Each has contributed indirectly to what is set forth in the ensuing pages.

Above all, the writing of this monograph has involved the participation of my children and my wife, Jane. Without their tolerance and support it would not have been accomplished. In particular, they were of immense help in dealing with the material in the bibliography. Much of the actual writing was done in the seclusion of the house of Drs. Luigi and Elaine (Pierson) Mastroianni in Woods Hole, Massachusetts. Their generosity in allowing me to isolate myself in such a setting contributed immeasurably to the writing. These few words are inadequate to express my thanks to them.

Equally important was the willingness of my colleagues Michael Gustin, Paula Barrett, Irving Schwartz, and Alan Tenenhouse to read all or parts of this monograph and offer detailed but constructive criticism. The final product is much improved because of their efforts. Both Mrs. Nancy Canetti and Ms. Anita See provided expert secretarial assistance for which I am most grateful.

Likewise, I am indebted to Victor Bers of the Classics Department of Yale University for discussing the nature of these relationships and suggesting the term synarchic regulation to define them. I appreciate both his time and interest.

Finally, the experimental work done in my own laboratory over the past 25 years has contributed to the insights and concepts presented. This work has been supported largely by grants from The Institute for Arthritis, Metabolism and Digestive Diseases of the U.S. Public Health Service. I am grateful to the members of various review panels as well as the members of the administrative staffs of this Institute for their support and assistance.

HOWARD RASMUSSEN

New Haven, Connecticut
May 1981

Contents

CHAPTER 3
Information Flow in Stimulus–Response Coupling   60

CHAPTER 10   306
Summary and Perspective

References   319

Index   363

1

Stimulus–Response Coupling in Historical Perspective

EXCITABLE CELL

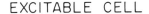

NONEXCITABLE CELL

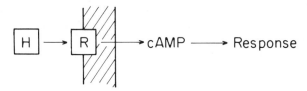

INTRODUCTION

One of the earliest attributes of cellular life was excitability, which is defined as the ability to respond in some appropriate fashion to an environmental stimulus. This heritage is evident today in the ability of bacterial cells to alter their motile behavior in response to chemical signals and in the ability of a swimming paramecium to alter its movement in response to a mechanical barrier. These examples of altered cellular behavior can be considered the prototypes of all patterns of stimulus–response coupling. This term encompasses all the events that occur between the time the cell encounters and recognizes an extracellular stimulus until it has made an appropriate response to it. The general cell property underlying this behavior is excitability. In this sense excitability means more than simply electrical excitability.

1

It includes chemical, mechanical, thermal, and photoexcitability as well. Likewise, response means any change in cellular activity—contractile, electrical, thermal, or metabolic. Coupling includes all the steps between stimulation and eventual response. The purpose of this monograph is to summarize the data in support of the hypothesis that one of the most universal coupling systems in cell activation employs calcium and cyclic AMP (cAMP) as interrelated intracellular messengers.

The experimental evidence indicates that these two modalities of coupling, chemical (nucleotide) and ionic (calcium), developed early in evolution, are shared by nearly all differentiated cells of higher organisms, and nearly always act in concert to determine the response of most cells to the particular extracellular messengers that control their specialized response. It is this latter aspect which will be emphasized. The system to be discussed involves a specific type of extracellular messenger (peptide or amine hormones, or neurotransmitters), which interact predominantly, if not exclusively, with receptors on the cell surface to initiate a flow of information into the cell. This information is of a particular type. It induces the differentiated cell to perform its specialized function, namely, contraction, secretion, or a change in a specific transport or metabolic process. In every case this function can be considered a catabolic or work function which subserves the needs of the organism.

For emphasizing the basic duality of messenger function within this universal system of stimulus–response coupling, Dr. Victor Bers of Yale University has suggested the term *synarchy*. This is based upon the Greek term *archon*. The archons were rulers or heralds of a very special status. Because of the importance of their role in disseminating information, they were often employed in pairs either to carry the same message or, under other circumstances, only part of the total message. Because an analogy exists between the functions of cAMP and calcium and those of the *archons*, the term *synarchic* regulation (*syn* meaning together) is proposed to categorize this system. By this definition, emphasis is placed on the fact that the two intracellular messengers operate together to convey the essential information to subcellular systems to direct their functions.

The process under discussion can be viewed as an information transfer sequence involving a number of discrete steps: (1) *recognition* of the external signal by specific receptors on the cell surface; (2) *transduction* of the extracellular signal within the membrane system into an intracellular message(s); (3) *transmission* of the intracellular message from cell surface to cell interior; (4) *intracellular reception* by specific receptor proteins; (5) *modulation* of the structure and activity of cell proteins by these intracellular receptor proteins; (6) *response* of one or more (response) elements within the cell leading to an alteration in cell behavior; and (7) *termination* of the message either within the cell and/or at its site of generation. The biochemical and molecular features of each of these steps are discussed in detail in Chapter 3.

In the ensuing chapters, various specific organizational modes of *synarchic regulation* in particular cell types are considered. In the remainder of this introductory chapter, the historical developments in the fields of stimulus–response coupling in the nervous system and of peptide hormone action are reviewed. Our knowledge of cellular calcium metabolism is then presented in the second chapter as a necessary prelude to the discussion of synarchic regulation in the succeeding chapters.

HISTORICAL DEVELOPMENTS

One could, of course, pick up the roots of the developments in these fields at nearly any point in human history, but for the sake of our present discussion, we will confine ourselves to two rather recent discoveries which each, in its own way, formed one of the cornerstones upon which our present-day understanding of stimulus–response coupling is built. The first of these was the discovery of bioelectricity, and the second, the concept of a hormone as a substance manufactured in one cell for the express purpose of being released by that cell into the circulation and to travel to, then interact with, a distant cell to change its function. The second of these developments is discussed first, even though historically they took place in the reverse order.

HORMONES AS CHEMICAL MESSENGERS

The concept of hormones and the endocrine glands was developed considerably later than the discovery of bioelectricity, at the beginning of this century. The discovery that a chemical compound liberated in small amounts by one cell type could bring about large changes in the activity of another cell was a significant intellectual milestone because it focused attention on the fact that cell activation could be achieved by chemical rather than electrical means.

Over the first half of the twentieth century, endocrine research was dominated by work aimed at the isolation, identification, and characterization of these amazing biological messengers. Their most remarkable attributes were their diversity of structure, their diversity of action, their high degree of target cell specificity, and the small amounts necessary to induce an appropriate response. These attributes challenged biologists to ask how such chemical messengers could recognize only particular target cells and, once arrived at these cells, induce a specific response. Their answers, not surprisingly, depended on the historical stage of development of biochemistry and cell biology.

Since the first hormones discovered were those which acted immediately on their target cells, it was only a short leap from the concept of chemical excitability to that of specific surface receptors for the particular chemical messenger or hormone. From the very onset of hormone research and the proposition of a surface receptor, one major hypothesis was that the hormone caused a change in the surface structure of the cell, and this change was somehow communicated to the cell interior to elicit the response. It seemed likely that for each hormone the surface change was unique. However, because the first major success of biochemistry was the recognition of specific proteins as the catalysts of specific metabolic reactions within the cell, the membrane theory of hormone action was superceded by the enzyme theory. This followed from the discovery that many vitamins, which are externally required trace substances, functioned as specific cofactors for particular enzyme-catalyzed reactions. From this discovery, the dictum of one enzyme–one trace substance was enunciated. Hormones, which are internally generated trace substances, were therefore thought to be coenzymes of a particular enzyme or class of enzymes. Only it did not prove to be so.

As the list of enzymes and the list of hormones grew, so did the list of effects of particular hormones on specific enzymes. However, none of these effects had the necesary specificity or sensitivity to substantiate the conclusion that this particular hormonal effect on this particular enzyme was the physiological basis of the hormone's action on the cell in question. Yet it was in wrestling with this particular problem in this context in a highly purified enzyme system that Earl Sutherland and Theodore Rall arrived at a profoundly important new insight into the nature of cell activation.

THE DISCOVERY OF CYCLIC AMP

To appreciate this new insight, the stage must be set more fully. The one enzyme–one trace substance idea had dominated research into hormone mechanisms for nearly 25 years. This hypothesis had been reinforced by the discoveries that hormones were highly diverse in chemical structure and biological effects. The small peptide adrenocorticotropin, an anterior pituitary hormone, was found to stimulate the adrenal gland to produce specific steriod hormones, whereas the even smaller peptide vasopressin, from the posterior pituitary, caused the kidney to retain H_2O and the amine hormone adrenaline (epinephrine) caused the liver to release glucose. Given these types of diversity, chemical and physiological, and the philosophical milieu of the one enzyme–one trace substance hypothesis, problems of hormone action were cast as separate, unrelated problems. It seemed unlikely that control of glucose release and H_2O retention would share similar cellular control elements (see Hechter, 1955).

One of the difficulties with the research aimed at testing the enzyme activation hypothesis was that much of the work was done with little attention to the known physiology of that particular hormone. The facts that the properties of phosphorylase enzyme in the phosphorolysis of glycogen were being worked out and the discovery that a major physiological effect of adrenaline or glucagon on the liver was to stimulate the breakdown of glycogen with the resultant release of glucose made a study of this system attractive because of the clear evidence that the hormone activated this particular enzyme complex within the cell. Using this knowledge and this enzyme (phosphorylase), Sutherland and Rall tried to demonstrate that direct addition of a purified hormone to a well-characterized and physiologically relevant enzyme system would lead to the appropriate change in activity of this system.

From the work of the Coris (Cori et al., 1938; Cori and Cori, 1945), it had become clear that in muscle and liver the enzyme phosphorylase, which catalyzes the breakdown of glycogen to glucose-1-phosphate, existed in two forms: *a* and *b*, or active and inactive. However, a considerable improvement in biochemical technology was required before Krebs and Fischer (1956) found an enzyme which catalyzed the conversion of phosphorylase *b* (inactive) to phosphorylase *a* (active). They eventually demonstrated that the conversion of Phos b → Phos a involved the phosphorylation of this enzyme and found that this conversion required the presence of ATP:

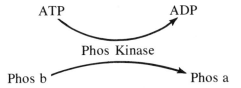

They named this enzyme phosphorylase kinase (Phos K) and showed that the phosphorylase-converting enzyme previously identified by the Coris was actually a phosphoprotein phosphatase catalyzing the reaction

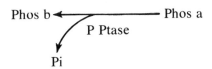

where Pi is inorganic phosphate. They named this enzyme phosphorylase phosphatase (P Ptase). They also developed ways of isolating phosphorylase *b* and *a* from tissues under conditions which prevented their interconversion during the isolation process. When resting muscle was extracted by these techniques, over 90% of the total phosphorylase was in the *b* or inactive form. But if extracted from working muscle a considerable percentage was in the *a* or active form.

From these findings, a simple theory concerning the control of phosphorylase activity and thus of glycogen breakdown was developed. This theory proposed that only phosphorylase *a* was active and that the stimulation of glycogenolysis resulted from a shift of phosphorylase *b* to phosphorylase *a* by either a stimulation of phosphorylase kinase and/or an inhibition of phosphorylase phosphatase:

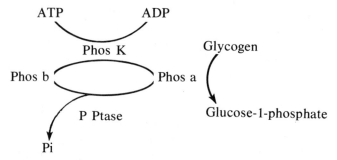

At approximately the same time, Sutherland and coworkers found that the phosphorylase system in liver was similar to that in muscle, with a kinase and a phosphatase regulating the interconversions between phosphorylase *b* and phosphorylase *a* (Sutherland, 1950). Two other facts were also known: the adrenal medullary hormone epinephrine and the pancreatic hormone glucagon caused an immediate and dramatic stimulation of hepatic glycogenolysis, and in the process phosphorylase *b* was converted to phosphorylase *a*.

Sutherland and Rall (1958) undertook to demonstrate that the addition of epinephrine directly to the phosphorylase complex *in vitro* induced the conversion of phosphorylase *b* to phosphorylase *a*. They were unable to do so. The problem was that of deciding whether the failure to show a direct

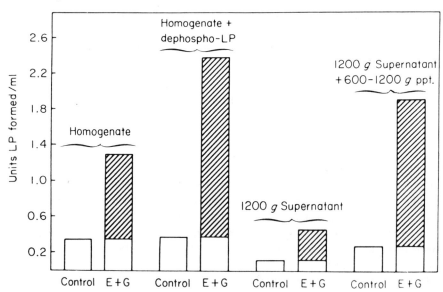

Figure 1.1   Effect of epinephrine and glucagon (E + G) on phosphorylase activation in whole and fractioned cat liver homogenates. The units of active (phosphorylated) liver phosphorylase (LP) are plotted for control homogenates and those to which inactive LP was added (left), or for the 1200 *g* supernatant plus the 600 to 120 *g* particulate fraction from fractionated homogenates (right). From Rall, Sutherland, and Berthet (1957), with permission.

hormonal effect was simply a matter of the wrong techniques, wrong environment, or wrong theory.

The crucial step was taken when addition of hormone to a broken cell preparation was found to stimulate glycogen breakdown. This was followed by the demonstration that addition of hormone to a particulate preparation containing nuclei, mitochondria, and various cell membranes induced the formation of a heat-stable factor which, when added directly to the isolated phosphorylase system, induced the conversion of phosphorylase b to phosphorylase a (Figure 1.1).

Work then centered on the isolation and identification of this factor. Sutherland and coworkers found it to be an adenine nucleotide. At the time they were attempting to determine its structure, David Lipkin was analyzing the structure of an unknown nucleotide isolated from a barium hydroxide hydrolyzate of ATP. The structure of this nucleotide was found to be cyclic 3', 5'-adenosine monophosphate (cAMP) (Lipkin et al., 1959). It was found to be identical to the nucleotide isolated from the liver system.

These discoveries were followed by three additional ones: First, the enzyme responsible for the synthesis of cAMP, adenylate cyclase, was found to be a component of the plasma membrane fraction of the cell. It could be activated in the isolated membrane by the direct addition of the hormone. Second, an enzyme, phosphodiesterase (PDE), found in the soluble fraction of the cell homogenate was found to catalyze the conversion of cAMP to 5'-AMP (5'-adenosine monophosphate):

$$cAMP \xrightarrow{\text{PDE}} 5'\text{-AMP}$$

The activity of this enzyme could be inhibited by the drugs caffeine or theophylline. Third, cAMP, adenylate cyclase, and phosphodiesterase were found in the cells of animals in all phyla and in nearly all differentiated cell types in all of these organisms. In other words, the cAMP system was universally present in animal cells (Robison et al., 1971).

THE SECOND MESSENGER MODEL

The logical step from these discoveries was to test the idea that other hormones acting on other cells might activate them by regulating cAMP synthesis. This approach was startingly successful. Within a few years, an impressive number of peptide and amine hormones were found to influence the concentration of cAMP in their respective target cells. From these data, Sutherland and coworkers propounded the second messenger hypothesis of hormone action. Their original hypothesis is presented schematically in Figure 1.2.

In this model, the first step is the interaction of the first messenger, or extracellular chemical, with its specific receptor on the cell surface. This interaction leads to the generation of the second, or intracellular, messenger,

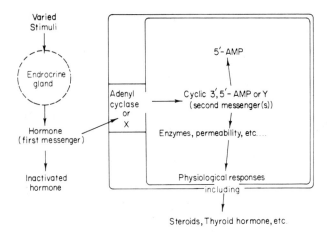

Figure 1.2 Schematic representation of the second messenger hypothesis developed by Sutherland and coworkers. From Robison, Butcher, and Sutherland (1971), with permission.

cAMP. The second messenger interacts with one or more effector elements within the cell to generate the changes that are measured as cell response. The enzyme phosphodiesterase serves to limit or terminate the message.

Recognizing that any hypothesis requires validation, Sutherland and co-workers (1968) established a set of criteria that had to be met before a particular hormone could be considered to act by this mechanism (Table 1.1). Implicit in this model are two types of specificity that help explain how hormones of different structure acting on different cells elicit such diverse responses while employing a common control mechanism. The first involves the attribute of discrimination at the plasma membrane. The adenylate cyclase in the membrane responds only to those hormones for which the particular cell possesses a specific receptor for that hormone. The second involves the presence, in specific differentiated cell types, of different effector elements that are responsive to the cAMP message.

Table 1.1   Criteria of Second Messenger Model

1. Addition of the hormone to the target cell should cause an increase in cAMP concentration.
2. Addition of methylxanthines in the presence of submaximal doses of hormone should enhance the hormonal effect.
3. Addition of exogenous cAMP should mimic the action of the hormone.
4. It should be possible to demonstrate a hormone-sensitive adenylate cycle in the plasma membrane fraction of the cell.
5. A cAMP-dependent protein kinase should be activated.[a]

[a]Added later than the other criteria.

MECHANISM OF CYCLIC AMP ACTION

Once the second messenger concept had been proposed, study after study in diverse systems validated its presence. The focus of attention then shifted to events within the cell. The question arose how an increase in cAMP concentration could in one cell cause an increase in the rate of glycogenolysis yet in another an increase in steroid hormone biosynthesis, and in a third a change in the H_2O permeability of the plasma membrane. Logic appeared to be on the side of those who considered it likely that cAMP was an allosteric modifier of a whole host of proteins, enzymes, transport carriers, and so on. This was the same logic that prevailed in the consideration of hormone action before the advent of the second messenger model. As discussed previously, it was thought that different hormones acted by different mechanisms because they varied so widely in chemical structure and in biological or cellular effects. However, just as the second messenger model changed the focus from multiple individual problems to a single general one, so did the extension of the protein kinase model of cAMP action change the focus from a consideration of multiple molecular mechanisms to a single one.

The discovery of the effect of cAMP upon the phosphorylase system spurred renewed interest in this enzyme control system. Further work demonstrated that the cAMP response element was a specific protein kinase, phosphorylase *b* kinase kinase (Walsh et al., 1968), that catalyzed the phosphorylation of phosphorylase *b* kinase from an inactive (nonphosphorylated form) to an active (phosphorylated form):

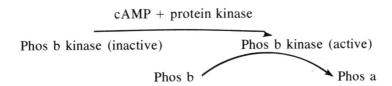

Krebs and his coworkers went on to demonstrate two features of this cAMP-dependent protein kinase: the mechanism by which cAMP exerts its effect (Beavo et al., 1975; Brostrom et al., 1971) and the fact that it also catalyzed the phosphorylation of glycogen synthetase (Soderling et al., 1970a,b), the enzyme-regulating glycogen synthesis.

The mechanism of action of cAMP upon this enzyme was found to involve the participation of a specific cAMP receptor protein (R). This protein interacts with the catalytic component (C) of the enzyme. When R and C are combined, the enzyme is inactive. Addition of cAMP leads to a dissociation of R from C, and C now is an active enzyme (see Figure 3.18).

The other discovery was to be the first step toward the development of the concept that cAMP regulates cell function by controlling the activity of a single class of enzyme, the protein kinases. Originally, it was proposed that the phosphorylase system regulated both the synthesis and degradation of glycogen. However, Leloir's discovery of a separate enzyme, glycogen synthetase, which catalyzed the synthesis of glycogen was an important step not only in defining the pathways of glycogen metabolism but also in the philosophic sense. This discovery helped point the way to the generalization that in bidirectional systems of metabolism, the forward and backward steps, at regulatory points in the system, are catalyzed by separate enzymes. Clearly, if this is the case, then some coordinated means must exist for controlling the activities of the two separate enzymes. It was this logic that led to the exploration of the idea that a cAMP-dependent protein kinase regulates the activity of the glycogen synthetase as well as the phosphorylase system. Such a kinase was found. In fact, the same cAMP-dependent protein kinase (PK) that catalyzes the phosphorylation of phosphorylase kinase and thus activates the phosphorylase cascade also stimulates the phosphorylation of glycogen synthetase (GS) and in so doing converts the active form of this enzyme to an inactive form:

$$\text{active GS} \underset{\text{cAMP-PK}}{\overset{\text{Phosphatase}}{\rightleftharpoons}} \text{inactive GS}$$
$$\text{inactive Phos b kinase} \rightleftharpoons \text{active Phos b kinase}$$

Thus, two important intracellular effects of cAMP were mediated by a common mechanism.

The extension of these findings and this concept by Kuo and Greengard (1969) was to consider the possibility that all the diverse effects of cAMP are mediated by this common mechanism. They first demonstrated that cAMP-dependent protein kinases were present in virtually all cell types. This discovery by itself was not sufficient since virtually all cells have some stores of glycogen and hence possess the enzymes of the phosphorylase system. However, it was soon shown that any number of cellular proteins, in addition to phosphorylase kinase and glycogen synthetase, were substrates for cAMP-dependent protein kinases. So just as the problem of hormone action had been transformed from multiple parochial ones to a single universal problem by the discovery of cAMP, the problem of cAMP action was transformed to a single, universal problem by the discovery of the pervasive presence of cAMP-dependent protein kinases.

The second messenger hypothesis was extended to include this attribute (Figure 1.3), and the requirements for such a system (see Table 1.1) were expanded to include as a fifth attribute that the cell should contain cAMP-dependent protein kinases. This requirement was later extended to include not only the fact of its presence, but evidence of a shift in the activity of this enzyme(s) from cAMP-dependent to cAMP-independent forms in the cell after hormone addition. Hence, in those cells in which activation by an extracellular messenger led to the generation of cAMP, the elucidation of the sequence of events from hormone–receptor interaction to cell response required the identification of the particular protein substrates for the cAMP-dependent protein kinases in different specific cell types and relating

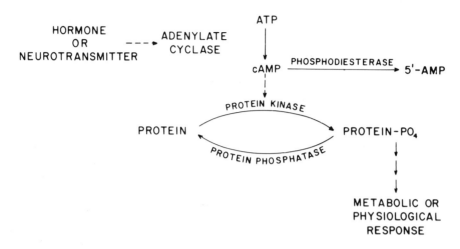

Figure 1.3 The extended second messenger model developed by Greengard and Kuo. From Greengard (1978), with permission.

their phosphorylation to changes in cell response. This continues to be an active area of research, and the ultimate effector protein has yet to be identified in many systems. On the other hand, the discovery that both cAMP-dependent protein kinases and protein substrates for these enzymes can be membrane-bound has provided a potential link between cAMP generation on the one hand and changes in membrane transport, membrane excitability, and cell secretion on the other.

LIMITATIONS OF THE SECOND MESSENGER MODEL

The appealing simplicity of the second messenger model led to its widespread adoption as a valid model of the mechanism of peptide and amine hormone action. Nonetheless, a growing literature indicates that the systems underlying cell activation are much more intricate, complex, and elegant than simply receptor–cyclase interaction and cAMP generation. From its inception, the second messenger model of hormone action possessed limitations which became more apparent as additional experimental evidence accumulated. Much of these data and their relevance to the second messenger model are discussed in later sections of his monograph. However, at this point several more general comments are in order.

Perhaps the point of greatest interest is a philosophical one. The second messenger model represents a fixed, rather stereotyped system with an either–or type of response. The fact that glycogenolysis is also a very stereotyped kind of response and was the first system in which the role of cAMP was explored undoubtedly biased opinion toward this rather rigid type of control device underlying the control of more plastic types of cellular responses. However, a consideration of physiological control systems shows that in both the endocrine and neural control systems at the organismal level there is considerable plasticity. For example, the hormonal control of glucose metabolism appears, at first glance, to be a system controlled by two opposing influences. On the one side is insulin, the glucose storage hormone, and on the other a group of counterregulatory hormones including epinephrine, glucagon, and cortisol, which are the glucose-mobilizing or glucose-producing hormones. In a stereotyped dual control system, one would logically expect that insulin acted as an anticounterregulatory hormone and/or the counterregulatory hormones acted as anti-insulins. Neither is in fact true. Consider the relationship between insulin and epinephrine, for example. They both act on liver, muscle, and adipose tissue. Insulin stimulates glucose uptake, glycogen synthesis, and lipid synthesis. Epinephrine stimulates glycogen phosphorolysis and lipid hydrolysis but does not inhibit glucose uptake; it may in fact stimulate it.

Pursuing the limitations of the second messenger model, there is an additional notable deficiency: the lack of feedback control. The *sine qua non* of control in both neural and endocrine systems is the provision of continuous and automatic feedback of information so that the cell generating the signal can constantly reassess and readjust the strength and/or duration of that signal. The same must also hold true within the responding cell. Information must flow not only from the cell surface to cell interior but also in the opposite direction. As originally proposed, the second messenger model was an open loop rather than a closed loop control system (Figure 1.4).

CONSEQUENCE OF SECOND MESSENGER MODEL

The field of hormone research changed dramatically after the discovery of the cAMP messenger system. What had been conceived as a series of parochial problems in endocrine research now became a single problem of

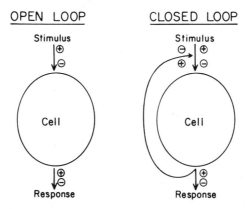

Figure 1.4. Comparison of an open vs closed loop cellular control system. An essential feature of a closed loop system is that of feedback control. This is not a feature of an open loop system such as the second messenger model.

general significance because cAMP also existed in nerve cells, exocrine secretory cells, smooth muscle cells, heart cells, and blood cells (Robison et al., 1971)—in electrically excitable as well as chemically excitable cells. So this one daring thought changed the course of our thinking about how cells are stimulated to perform their particular function; and for over a decade, research in cellular control mechanisms was dominated by cAMP and the second messenger concept. In the process, the model of chemical excitability was validated and extended. The first chemical messenger, the hormone, induced the generation of the second chemical messenger, the cyclic nucleotide (Figure 1.5). All in all, a brilliant chapter in the building of that twentieth-century cathedral, the molecular model of the fundamental unit of life—the individual cell.

Even so, this concept constituted only one cornerstone in the construction of that edifice. Another of equal elegance was also unfolding. This was the concept that in excitable cells such as nerve and muscle, an ionic extracellular message, the action potential, gives rise to an ionic intracellular message, calcium ion, which is responsible for the initiation of cell response (Figure 1.5).

BIOELECTRICITY AND THE EXCITABLE CELL

The development of our understanding of the bioelectricity from the nineteenth-century controversy between Galvani and Volta to the computer analysis of the modern electroencephalogram represents one of the greatest monuments to man's inquisitiveness. Throughout it all, a problem that fascinated generation after generation of physiologists was how an electric

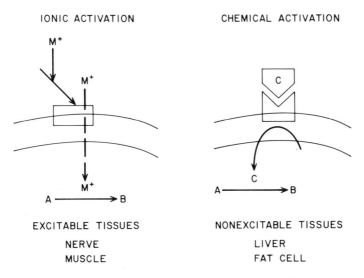

Figure 1.5 Contrast between the ionic model of activation in excitable tissues (left) and the chemical model of activation in nonexcitable tissues (right).

current applied at one point on a nerve fiber caused a propagated action potential along the length of that fiber (see Katz, 1966). The concern for understanding this process led to the recognition that electric currents in biological membranes are ionic rather than electronic as in the ordinary metal wire. In addition, it was realized that all animal cells maintain an asymmetric distribution of ions between their own fluid phase (the intracellular phase) and the fluid phase that surrounds them (the extracellular phase) and that this asymmetry is maintained by the expenditure of energy by the cell. One of the major tenets of modern neurophysiology is that excitability in nerve cells is based on transient changes in the permeability of the nerve cell membrane to small positively charged ions (cations) in a membrane across which an asymmetric distribution of these same ions is maintained by the expenditure of metabolic energy.

A second problem of equal importance was how this electrical signal traveling down a motor nerve to a muscle induced a contraction once it got to the muscle cell. For some time, it was considered possible that the electric currents themselves interacted with the contractile system. However, this simple hypothesis became untenable once the presence of neurotransmitters was demonstrated.

NEUROTRANSMITTERS—CHEMICAL MESSENGERS IN EXCITABLE CELLS

The central focus in neurophysiology was and has been the phenomenon of bioelectricity. Otto Loewi, however, added a crucially important dimension, namely, the finding that when the electrical signal in a nerve fiber is propagated to its end (the synapse) and stimulates there either another nerve, a muscle, or some other cell to activity, the signal that passes across the junction between the two cells is *chemical* and not *electrical* in nature. Yet when one analyzes the sequence of events in skeletal muscle, one finds the electric current, that is, the action potential, traveling down the nerve, reaching the nerve ending or synapse, inducing there the release of the neurotransmitter acetylcholine, which in turn acts upon the muscle cell to induce an action potential in the membrane of this cell. A chemical messenger induces an ionic current which propagates across the surface of the muscle cell. These findings meant that chemical messengers can give rise to ionic messages as well as chemical messages.

CALCIUM IN EXCITATION–CONTRACTION COUPLING

This intriguing system, the nerve–muscle preparation, became an object of intense study. Of major interest were two problems: the first, how the electrical signal in the nerve cell induces the release of the neurotransmitter, the second, how the ionic current sweeping across the muscle cell surface is translated or transduced into a mechanical response—the contraction of that same muscle cell. To fully explore these questions and define the molecular basis of these responses, it was necessary both to define the nature of the neurosecretory system and the components of the contractile apparatus and how they interact. This has only recently been accomplished. However, even before it was done, a conclusion of great significance was reached. This conclusion was that calcium ion was the coupling factor between electrical stimulation and neurotransmitter release at the synapse and between stimulus and contraction in muscle (Katz, 1966; Sandow, 1952). These conclusions were reached just before or at the time of Sutherland's discovery of cAMP. In a sense, these separate systems seemed to be distinct mechanisms by which excitable (ionic) and nonexcitable (chemical) cells were activated (Figure 1.5).

Just as the discovery of cAMP represented a turning point in our thinking about hormone action, the discovery of the coupling function of calcium ion in skeletal muscular contraction represented a crucial step in the development of our understanding of stimulus–response coupling. Hence, it is worthwhile considering in more detail the historical developments in this field.

The English physiologist Ringer discovered in 1885 that if a frog's heart was put in a calcium-free NaCl solution, it stopped beating; that when it did so, it was always in the relaxed rather than the contracted state; and that it could be reactivated to beat regularly by the readdition of calcium. Furthermore, if very high amounts of calcium were added, the heart stopped beating but always in the contracted states.

These studies were the first clear demonstration of a role of calcium ion in the regulation of cell activity. However, they did not immediately focus attention on the possibility that calcium ion served a coupling function in regulating the cardiac cycle. In part, this was so because the importance of this particular question had not been realized, the knowledge of cell structure was primitive, and the techniques to explore this question were not available. Nonetheless, another development also misled physiologists. With advances in techniques for the study of the conduction of impulses down nerve fibers, it became evident that if the calcium ion concentration surrounding a nerve fiber was reduced, the electrical properties of the nerve were dramatically altered; and if calcium were totally absent, the nerve would not conduct an electrical impulse. Hence, it was considered likely that the change in surface membrane properties induced by changes in extracellular calcium ion concentration was responsible for the effects of calcium on the frog heart.

As the classical work of Hodgkin, Huxley, Katz, and coworkers developed (see Katz, 1966), it was shown that the nerve action potential results from sequential changes in the Na^+ and K^+ permeabilities of the nerve membrane. Parenthetically it was noted that Ca^{2+} permeability also increased. However, investigate attention centered upon the dramatic effects of altered calcium ion concentrations upon the Na^+ permeability of the plasma membrane. When the calcium ion concentration was reduced, the resting Na^+ permeability increased. This response explained the effect of calcium ion on the electrical response of the nerve. The fact that calcium ion could be removed from the external medium of a skeletal muscle and that muscle could still be induced to contract by applying a sufficient electrical shock to the muscle led to the belief that calcium probably was not involved as a coupling factor in muscle. Three possible factors that were considered and, in turn, shown not to couple excitation to contraction were (1) the electric currents themselves interacting directly with the contractile system; (2) the changes in ATP concentration seen when contraction took place, and (3) the inward flow of Na^+ when the muscle cell membrane was stimulated.

At about this time, Heilbrunn (1940) was studying the response of cells to injury of their plasma membranes. He found that when a restricted injury was inflicted on the cell surface, there was a dramatic change in that portion of the cytoplasm immediately beneath the injury site. He concluded that this response to injury involved some type of sol–gel transformation of the cytoplasmic contents. In searching for a factor in the extracellular fluids that might be involved in initiating this transformation, he discovered that the response did not occur if calcium ion was removed from the bathing solution. From these discoveries, he reasoned that an influx of calcium at the injury site led to the sol–gel transformation. From this line of reasoning he was led to consider the possibility that the controlled "sol–gel" transformation of musclar contraction might also involve calcium ion as its mediator. Kamada and Kinosita (1943) tested this hypothesis and found that local contractures of skeletal muscle segments could be induced by the application of calcium but not a variety of other ions to the denuded surface of a muscle, that is, one in which the surface membrane had been removed without destroying the underlying contractile apparatus.

A few years later, in 1947, Heilbrunn and Wiercinski showed that Ca^{2+} was the only physiological substance which, when microinjected into a living cell, could induce localized contractures at the site of injection. From these results and studies on the behavior of other cells to altered ionic environments, Heilbrunn proposed that calcium ion was a general intracellular messenger and was specifically the link between excitation and contraction. Additional evidence in support of this thesis developed, and in 1952 Sandow introduced the term excitation–contraction coupling to describe this phenomenon. He reviewed additional evidence that supported the Heilbrunn theory.

However, this theory was not immediately accepted because of the discovery of a particulate relaxing factor from fractionated muscle cells (Marsh, 1952; Fujita, 1954). This fraction, when applied to glycerinated muscle cells (no longer possessing an intact membrane), caused the relaxation of the fibers and reversed the contractile effects of Ca^{2+}. This reversal required ATP. However, improvements in the techniques of microinjection, in preparing denuded muscle fibers, and in the study of muscle cell structure and biochemistry soon established clearly that calcium ions were the coupling agent between excitation and contraction. One of the features that delayed establishing this model was that Heilbrunn had originally proposed that the calcium was released from, or entered into, the cell across its surface membrane. However, simple calculations soon revealed that the rate of diffusion of calcium into the cell would be much too slow to bring about the rapid response seen in a fast skeletal muscle cell. The elucidation of the extensive membrane system that coupled cell surface to cell interior in such a cell and the discovery that the relaxing factor was actually fragments of this membrane system led to the demonstration that this sarcoplasmic reticulum stores calcium and has the capability of releasing and reaccumulating it by an energy-dependent mechanism (Ebashi, 1961; Ebashi and Lippman, 1962; Hasselbach and Makinose, 1961). These discoveries were followed by the finding that Ca^{2+}, when added directly to crude actin-myosin preparations, would induce "superprecipitation" and activate the myosin ATPase (Weber, 1959; Weber and Herz, 1962; Weber and Wenicur, 1961).

The final proof of the model came from the experiments of Ashley and Ridgeway (1968, 1970) who were able to inject the calcium-sensitive photoprotein Aqueorin into a living muscle cell and monitor directly the magnitude and time course of change in cytosolic calcium ion concentration. They showed that calcium release, as predicted, followed electrical depolarization but preceded the mechanical event of contraction (Figure 1.6).

The development of this model of calcium action in muscle was important not only because it represented the prototype of the system in which calcium

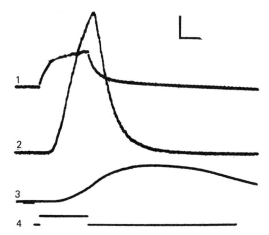

Figure 1.6 Time course of change in membrane potential (1), calcium-induced light emission (2), isometric tension (3), and period of electrical stimulation (4) of a single *Balanus* muscle fiber injected with 0.2 μ of a saturated solution of Aequorin in 100 mM TES buffer, pH 7.3. The change in trace 2 from baseline value to peak response represents a change in free Ca^{2+} concentration from approximately 0.10 to 0.45 μM. Vertical bar (upper right) represents the calibration of 20 mV for membrane potential and 5 gm wt for tension development; horizontal bar represents 100 msc. From Ashley and Ridgeway (1970), with permission.

might serve to couple stimulus to response, but also because it revealed that the intracellular calcium ion concentration is extremely low, normally 10^{-7} M; that the control concentration range over which calcium ion functions is from approximately 5×10^{-8} to 10^{-6} M; and that intracellular organelles, in addition to the plasma membrane, play a critical role in the regulation of intracellular calcium metabolism.

MECHANISM OF CALCIUM ACTION

Once it was established that Ca^{2+} was the coupling factor between excitation and contraction, it became of interest to define its mechanism of action. It was found that when purified actin interacts with myosin, it stimulates the ATPase activity of the myosin. Considerable circumstantial evidence suggested that an increase in the ATPase was a biochemical counterpart of muscle contraction. It was then shown that Ca^{2+} did not influence this isolated actin–myosin system.

However, Weber (1959) showed that crude actin–myosin preparations possessed a myosin ATPase activity which was inhibited by EDTA and stimulated by the addition of micromolar quantities of calcium or manganese (Figure 1.7). As the tropomyosin was purified, it lost its calcium sensitivity (Ebashi and Endo, 1968). These facts led Ebashi and coworkers (1966, 1968, 1969) to the discovery of a group of tropomyosin-associated proteins named

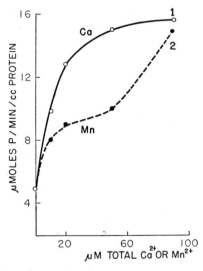

Figure 1.7 Activation of myosin ATPase, measured as release of inorganic phosphate, by micromolar concentrations of Ca^{2+} or Mn^{2+}. The reaction mixture contained crude actomyosin with the regulatory components 0.1 mM ATP, 1.1 mM Mg^{2+} and increasing amounts of either Ca^{2+} or Mn^{2+}. Note that the calcium concentration is the total concentration in the presence of EDTA, ATP, and Mg^{2+}. The free concentration is an order of magnitude lower. From Weber (1959), with permission.

troponins, one of which bound calcium ions with a very high affinity. This protein was isolated and characterized. It was found to interact both with calcium ions and with the tropomyosin complex and to confer calcium sensitivity upon the tropinin, the tropomyosin, and the actin–myosin complex. Hence, a specific calcium receptor protein was identified. It appeared not to have any enzymatic function but to act as a regulatory protein. The present concept of its function is illustrated in Figure 1.8. Interaction of calcium with this protein leads to a conformational change in the tropomyosin complex which normally inhibits the interaction between actin and myosin. In its calcium–troponin altered conformation, tropomyosin no longer blocks binding sites on the actin molecule, thus allowing actin and myosin to interact (Weber and Murray, 1973). The biochemical counterpart

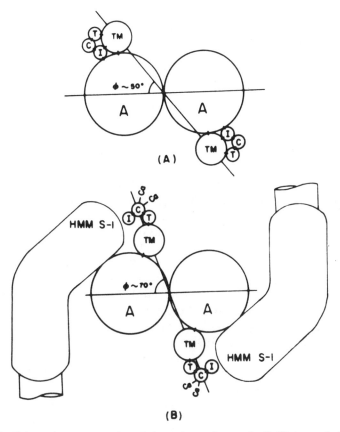

Figure 1.8 Schematic representation of the actions of troponin C (C) in regulating skeletal muscle contraction. In the absence of calcium, tropin I (I) fits in a groove between tropomyosin (TM) and actin (A), thereby blocking the interaction of A with heavy meromyosin (HMM). When calcium bonds to C, the I component of the troponin complex is displaced out of the groove and actin–myosin interaction follows. From Potter et al. (1977), with permission.

of this response is the calcium–troponin-activated ATPase activity of myosin (Figure 1.7).

CALCIUM IN SMOOTH MUSCLE

In addition to coupling excitation to contraction in skeletal muscle, calcium was found to serve a similar function in other types of muscle. In contrast to the situation in skeletal muscle, extracellular calcium was found to be required for stimuli to induce contraction in nearly all forms of smooth muscle (Bolton, 1979). This was true whether the stimulus to contraction was hormonal (e.g., oxytocin-induced myometrical contraction) or neural (e.g., parasympathetic stimulation of smooth muscle). However, estimates of the calcium needed to induce a particular response and that calculated to enter the cell often showed a discrepancy. In many smooth muscle cells, not enough calcium entered to account for the magnitude of the subsequent contractile response. This discrepancy led to a search for a sarcoplasmic reticulum in smooth muscle. This organelle was found, but in a less highly developed state than in fast striated muscle. The present consensus is that in most smooth muscles, the calcium needed to induce contraction comes both from a release of calcium from this internal store and from an increase in the influx of calcium into the cell across the plasma membrane (Bolton, 1979). It is also clear that the relative contribution of these two pools to stimulus–response coupling varies from one type of smooth muscle to another.

Smooth muscle research has also led to two other important concepts in our general understanding of calcium-mediated cell responses. Both relate to the mechanism by which calcium ion regulates the actin–myosin interaction in these muscles. Having discovered that the troponin–tropomyosin complex was the calcium receptor system in skeletal muscle, a logical question was whether this was a universal control mechanism. It was shown to operate in cardiac muscle (Chapman, 1979). However, in a variety of smooth muscles it appeared not to operate. Rather, a calcium-sensitive light chain of the myosin complex was discovered. The calcium receptor protein in this complex was shown to be structurally similar to, but not identical with, troponin C and was later identified as calmodulin (Sobieszek, 1977; Dabrowska and Hartshorne, 1978; Hathaway and Adelstein, 1979; Dabrowski et al., 1978; Barron et al., 1979). Furthermore, the binding of calcium was found to lead to a phosphorylation of a regulatory light chain of myosin, that is, there was a calcium-sensitive protein kinase as a component of the myosin complex. In contrast, in skeletal muscle when troponin C interacts with calcium, a conformational change in the troponin–tropomyosin complex takes place that does not involve protein phosphorylation but modulates the structure of actin (light chain regulation). Hence, the mechanism of calcium control in the two types of muscle appeared completely different. From the philosophical point of view, the discovery of this difference was important because it showed that calcium could serve as an activator of a class of enzymes such as protein kinases in the same way that cAMP did.

CALCIUM IN STIMULUS–SECRETION COUPLING

With the development of interest in the nature of excitation–contraction coupling, interest also developed in the question of how excitation was coupled to secretion of substances at nerve endings and from exocrine and endocrine glands. During studies on calcium influx into nerve, Hodgkin and Keynes (1957) showed that intracellular calcium was low and that upon passage of the nerve impulse there was an increased influx of calcium into the cell. They, and also Birks and MacIntosh (1957), raised the possibility that this inward calcium current might play a role in release of neuro-transmitter. This hypothesis was confirmed largely by Katz (1950, 1962) and coworkers (Katz and Miledi, 1965, 1967, 1968), who demonstrated the absolute requirement for calcium in order for a nerve impulse to release acetylcholine. They also demonstrated that the iontophoretic application of calcium to the nerve terminus resulted in the local increase in transmitter release.

Douglas and Rubin (1961) initiated a series of studies on the mechanism by which the neurotransmitter acetylcholine (Ach) induced the release of catecholamines from the adrenal medulla. They employed the technique of the perfused cat adrenal gland. They showed that omission of K^+ or marked reduction in Na^+ concentration had little effect upon Ach-mediated catecholamine secretion. However, removal of calcium ion resulted in a complete lack of secretion (Figure 1.9). They also showed that catecholamine release could be induced by raising extracellular K^+. The ability of K^+-induced depolarization to induce contraction in various forms of muscle had been noted by earlier investigators and had been attributed to a K^+-induced release of Ca^{2+}. In the case of the adrenal, the K^+-induced secretion was abolished if Ca^{2+} was removed from the perfusing solution. Also, over a considerable range of extracellular calcium concentration, the quantity of catecholamine released was a direct function of the calcium ion concentration. Finally, if a gland was perfused with a calcium-free Locke's solution for a period of time and then a calcium-containing solution was perfused through the gland, transient spontaneous secretion (without Ach) occurred. This latter observation was interpreted to mean that removal of calcium led to an increase in the permeability of the plasma membrane to calcium as well as sodium ion. Hence, when the glands were then suddenly exposed to a high ambient calcium concentration, sufficient calcium entered the cell to initiate secretion before the added calcium had interacted with ligands in the plasma membrane and reduced calcium permeability to nor-mal.

Douglas and Rubin concluded that calcium ion played the dominant role in stimulus–secretion coupling and that the source of the calcium that coupled

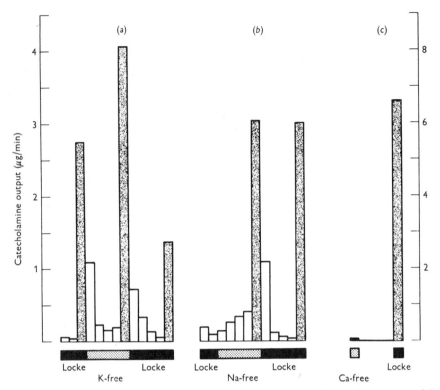

Figure 1.9   Effect of removal of different cations from the buffer solution on the response of the isolated cat adrenal medulla to stimulation of catecholamine release by acetylcholine. Each open bar represents a control period; each stippled bar represents the application of acetylcholine. Note that removal of either K^+ or Na^+ did not inhibit response, but removal of Ca^{2+} caused a complete inhibition of catecholamine release which could be restored to normal by the reintroduction of normal calcium-containing Locke's solution. From Douglas and Rubin (1961) with permission.

excitation to response after Ach addition was the calcium pool in the extracellular space. In addition to broadening the systems in which calcium seemed to play a key role in stimulus–response coupling, this work also indicated that in contrast to the situation in the skeletal muscle, where the calcium involved in excitation–response coupling came from an internal pool, in the adrenal medulla the calcium involved in excitation-response coupling came from an extracellular pool, as it did at synapses.

CALCIUM IN STIMULUS–PERMEABILITY COUPLING

To add to the complexity of initiating events, a rise in intracellular calcium affects the permeability of the plasma membrane in many different cell types (Putney, 1979). Studies in the late 1930s an early 1940s showed that when red cells were exposed to lead or fluoride, they lost K^+. In restudying this phenomenon in 1958, Gardos discovered that this K^+ loss required Ca^{2+}. Ten years later, Whittam (1969) proposed that this effect was mediated by intracellular rather than extracellular calcium. This hypothesis has been fully confirmed by subsequent studies. These have shown that micromolar concentrations of calcium are sufficient to activate the K^+ channel in the red cell membrane (Figure 1.10). Most recently, evidence has been presented in support of the concept that this effect of calcium is mediated by the calcium-receptor protein calmodulin.

Shortly after Whittam's proposal, it was found that the permeability of certain excitable cells is also determined by the intracellular calcium concentration (Meech, 1976; Putney, 1979). Injection of calcium into either motor neurons in the cat or into neurons from the invertebrate Aplysia was shown to lead to an immediate increase in the potassium conductance of the cell membrane. Similar results were described in the mammalian heart. Hence, in excitable tissues, in which Ca^{2+} entry was a consequence of the initial excitatory event, the subsequent rise in intracellular calcium could bring about additional changes in the permeability properties of the cell mem-

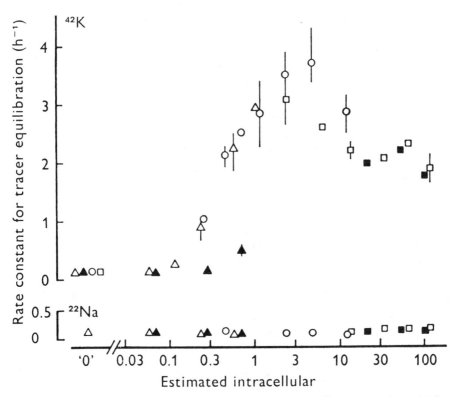

Figure 1.10   Effect of changes in estimated intracellular free Ca^{2+} concentration (μM, log scale) on the permeability of the red cell membrane to Na^+ and K^+. Open symbols indicate results in the absence of Mg^{2+}, and closed symbols, results in the presence of 2 to 2.5 mM Ma^{2+}. From Simons (1975), with permission.

brane, indicating the presence of important feedback signals at the level of the membrane.

CALCIUM AND CYCLIC AMP IN ENDOCRINE SYSTEMS

The discovery of cAMP came from a study of stimulus–metabolism coupling in the liver and specifically the hormonal excitation of the phosphorylase system. For some years, this origin led to a concentration of attention on the role of cAMP in hormone action, particularly on hormones that regulated metabolism. The concurrent discoveries of the coupling function of calcium in muscle contraction and secretion seemed to represent an exploration of a second type of control system, one in which an ionic coupling factor was responsible for regulating the activity of the final response element in the cell (Figure 1.5). However, it soon became evident that in many systems in which cAMP was found to be involved in stimulus–metabolism coupling, there was also evidence that calcium ions played a regulatory role (Rasmussen and Tenenhouse, 1968). The significance of this evidence became apparent to Nagata and me during our studies of the ionic and hormonal control of renal gluconeogenesis (Nagata and Rasmussen, 1970). Calcium ion and cAMP appeared to operate as dual second messengers in the action of the parathyroid hormone (PTH) upon glucose production in isolated rat renal tubules.

The results of an experiment that was of crucial importance are shown in Figure 1.11. The effects of PTH upon cAMP content and glucose production were measured in the presence and absence of extracellular calcium ion at both high and low pH. If the pH was reduced from 7.4 to 6.8, glucose production increased but cAMP concentration did not change, whether

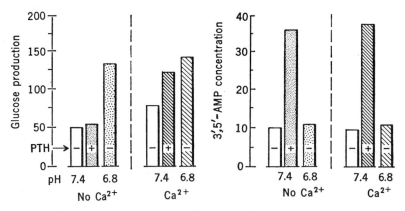

Figure 1.11 Effect of changing medium pH or of adding parathyroid hormone (PTH) to isolated rat renal tubules on the rate of glucose production and cAMP content in the absence and presence of Ca^{2+} in the incubation medium. Note that even though PTH caused a rise in cAMP content when Ca^{2+} was absent or present, it stimulated glucose formation only when Ca^{2+} was present. A shift of the pH from 7.4 to 6.8 caused an increase in glucose formation both in the presence and in the absence of Ca^{2+}. From Rasmussen (1970), with permission.

extracellular calcium was present or absent. When PTH was added to tubules incubated in the presence of calcium ion at pH 7.4, an increase in cAMP concentration and in rate of glucose production was seen. At pH 7.4 in the absence of calcium, PTH addition caused a comparable rise in cAMP content but no increase in rate of glucose production. These and other data (see Chapter 5) led to the conclusion that calcium as well as cAMP served a messenger function in this hormonally regulated metabolic response.

At approximately the same time, Namm and Mayer (1968) were studying the effect of epinephrine upon myocardial glycogenolysis. They found that if calcium ions were removed from the medium before epinephrine was added, an increase in cAMP concentration as well as an increase in the active form of phosphorylase *b* kinase were seen, indicating that cAMP had stimulated the cAMP-dependent protein kinase, but without increasing the phosphorylase *a* activity. We now know that this failure was due to the fact that phosphorylase *b* kinase is a calcium-regulated enzyme or a calcium-dependent protein kinase (see Chapter 4). However, at the time this experiment was done, the significant conclusion derived from it was that the action of cAMP in at least two metabolic systems requires the presence of calcium ion, that is, the calcium ion plays a permissive role in stimulus–metabolism coupling. Other data, however, led to the conclusion that the role of calcium ion is more than permissive. These included data from studies of stimulus–response coupling in muscle.

CALCIUM AS REGULATOR OF MUSCLE METABOLISM

The insect flight muscle, when stimulated, is one of the most metabolically active tissues known. As a consequence, there is a sustained dependence primarily on oxidative metabolism. There are stores of trehalose which can be broken down and give rise to the phosphorylated intermediates of the glycolytic sequence. However, for glycolysis to operate at high rates, there is a major need to reoxidize the reduced NADH formed at the glyceraldehyde phosphate dehydrogenase step of the glycolytic sequence existing in the muscle cell cytosol. This is achieved by an NADH shuttle that involves a specific mitochondrial glycerol dehydrogenase. It is essential for the insect that there is a mechanism by which changes in metabolic demand (flight) are coupled to changes in metabolic flux and particularly the reoxidation of cytoplasmic NADH.

Hansford and Chappell (1967) showed that a rise in cytosolic calcium ion concentration caused a marked activation of the mitochondrial glycerol phosphate dehydrogenase. Subsequent work has shown that both the substrate binding site, and the calcium binding site of the enzyme are located on the outer surface of the inner mitochondrial membrane (Klingenberg and Buchholz, 1970). Thus, the substrate does not enter the mitochondrial matrix space but is transformed into cytosolic dihydroxyacetone phosphate, with the simultaneous reduction of a specific mitochondrial flavoprotein linked directly to the electron transport chain. The dihydroxyacetone phosphate generated can then be rereduced to glycerol phosphate in the cytosol with the conversion of cytosolic NADH to NAD, thus providing NAD for maintenance of the glyceraldehyde phosphate dehydrogenase step in glycolysis. The activity of the mitochondrial enzyme is sensitive to changes in calcium ion concentration in the range of 5×10^{-8} to 5×10^{-6} M, with a K_m of activation of 10^{-7} M.

In the case of skeletal muscle, it was demonstrated that epinephrine stimulates glycogenolysis, that this stimulation appears to be due to the action of cAMP on phosphorylase b kinase kinase, and that it occurs without any activation of the contractile system. Since the contractile system is extremely sensitive to small changes in calcium ion concentration, this constituted rather good evidence that there was no significant increase in intracellular calcium ion concentration. On the other hand, glycogenolysis is also activated by repetitive neural stimulation of the same muscle. This stimulation of glycogen breakdown occurs without a measurable rise in cAMP concentration.

The clue to the nature of the coupling between electrical excitation and glycogenolysis in this tissue was provided by the discovery that the enzyme phosphorylase b kinase is a calcium-sensitive enzyme (Meyer et al., 1964; Ozawa et al., 1967). Following this discovery, the role of calcium in activating this enzyme was defined. Both the "inactive" (nonphosphorylated) and the "active" (phosphorylated) forms of the enzyme are activated by calcium ion, but the inactive form requires a higher calcium ion concentration than the active form to achieve the same rate of activity. It has since been demonstrated that phosphorylase b kinase is a multisubunit enzyme and that one of the subunits is the universal calcium receptor protein calmodulin. It is the phosphorylation of other subunits of the enzyme and not of calmodulin, the calcium-binding subunit, that alters the calcium binding properties of the holoenzyme. This means that phosphorylation of other subunits alters the conformation of calmodulin in such a way as to enhance its affinity for calcium.

Of equal interest is the fact that more recent studies (Hollosgy and Narahara, 1965; Clausen et al., 1975; Bihler, 1972; Schudt et al., 1976) have shown that a rise in the cytosolic calcium ion content leads to a stimulation of glucose entry into the muscle cell. This represents another example of the integrative effects of messenger action upon cell function.

CYCLIC AMP AND CALCIUM IN NEURAL TISSUE

Just as calcium was found to serve as counterpoint to cAMP in hormonally responsive tissues, cAMP was found to serve as counterpoint to Ca^{2+} in electrically excitable nervous tissues.

Two major discoveries relating the cAMP to the calcium messenger systems at the molecular level were made by investigators studying the properties of the cAMP control system in brain tissue. The first of these was the discovery by Cheung (1970) and Kakikuchi and Yamazki (1971) that calcium ions activated a soluble cyclic nucleotide phosphodiesterase from brain tissue (Figure 1.12). This calcium-activated enzyme was later discovered in other tissues (Wang, 1976). In attempting to define the mechanism by which calcium controls the activity of this enzyme, Teo, Wang, and Wang (1973) demonstrated the presence of a specific regulatory subunit, devoid of catalytic activity, which had a very high affinity for calcium. This protein was initially given the name of calcium-dependent regulator, or CDR. Following its identification and isolation, it was found to be universally distributed in animals cells; to be structurally related to the other calcium receptor protein, troponin; and to mediate the effect of calcium on a number of cellular response elements (Wang and Waisman, 1979; Cheung, 1980). It has since been named calmodulin (Cheung, 1980) and is recognized as a universal intracellular calcium receptor protein.

An additional effect of calmodulin, first elucidated in studies with brain tissue, is that of regulating the activity of particulate adenylate cyclase as well as soluble phosphodiesterase (Brostrom et al., 1975). This finding indicated that changes in calcium ion concentration can regulate the behavior of the cAMP messenger system both at the site of cAMP message generation (the cyclase) and message termination (the phosphodiesterase).

Even though these discoveries had profound implications in terms of defining some of the molecular aspects of the interrelationship between calcium and cAMP, they did not help immediately in defining the function of cAMP as a coupling factor or intracellular messenger in neurotransmitter action in the nervous system. Because of the complexity of neural tissue as compared to endocrine tissue, these definitions have not been as easy to achieve in the former as they have been in the latter. Nevertheless, data to be reviewed in nearly every one of the ensuing chapters have shown that cAMP plays a critically important role in modulating events in the nervous

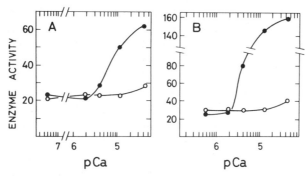

Figure 1.12 Effect of calcium on the activity of soluble brain phosphodiesterase when 1 μM cAMP (A) or 0.4 μM cGMP served as substrate. The rates were determined in the absence ($\bigcirc$) and presence ($\bullet$) of a protein-activating factor (PAF). Note that only in the presence of PAF was the enzyme activated by Ca^{2+}. From Kakiuchi et al. (1973) with permission.

system. It can function either at the level of neurosecretion from the pre-synaptic terminus or postsynaptically to regulate neural response. In doing so, one of its major functions is that of modulating the behavior of the calcium messenger system.

EXCITABLE VERSUS NONEXCITABLE CELLS

At several points throughout the preceding discussion, a distinction has been made between excitable and nonexcitable cells or tissues. This operational distinction was made years ago by nerve and muscle physiologists. According to Webster, excitable means "capable of being aroused to action" or "being responsive to a stimulus." By these definitions, all the hormonally responsive tissues under discussion as well as the neurally regulated ones are excitable. However, in the physiological sense, the term has come to have a more restricted usage. A distinction has been made between excitable and nonexcitable tissues, even though all of these "nonexcitable" tissues will respond to appropriate stimuli.

Excitability in the physiological sense has been restricted to those tissues that are electrically excitable and display action potential as a consequence of this excitation. This has meant primarily nerve and muscle. In the nerve, this propagated disturbance can carry a signal from one part of the cell (the cell body) to another (the synapse), where it initiates the synaptic events that lead to the transfer of information to another cell. In skeletal muscle, as the action potential is propagated across the cell surface, it is coupled to the underlying T system and from there to the sarcoplasmic reticulum, causing a consequent release of calcium. Clearly, then, in these two tissues the action potential serves as a rapid means of carrying a message from one part of the cell surface to another. The question is: is this a unique property of nerve and muscle? The question can be considered in two parts: The first is, do all nerve and muscle cells display action potentials when stimulated? The second is, do any other cells display action potentials when stimulated?

The answer to the first question is no; not all muscles display action potentials when stimulated to contract. A group of muscles known as slow muscles show only a stepwise shift, a depolarization, in membrane potential as the strength of stimulus increases. There are no action potentials. Furthermore, there is a nearly linear correlation between the degree of depolarization and the strength of contraction; that is, there is rather direct coupling between changes in membrane potential and calcium release. This means that excitation–contraction coupling does not require an action potential to initiate response in every kind of muscle cell.

If we analyze the difference between this type of muscle and fast skeletal muscle, the most striking difference is in the time constant of their respective responses. The skeletal muscle response takes place in milliseconds, the slow response, in seconds. Therefore, an action potential is a mechanism for initiating a rapid response and not a unique device for initiating muscle cell response.

In considering these two types of muscle cells, it is worth pointing out that in both the change in electrical behavior of the membrane is an indication of a change in ion currents across the membrane. It is these ion currents which, each in their own way, initiate cellular response. It would appear arbitrary to classify the fast muscle cells as excitable and the slow muscle cells as nonexcitable when, in fact, both are excited by a similar type of extracellular signal, both respond with a similar change in activity, and both employ the same intracellular signals to couple stimulus to response.

The answer to the second question is yes; cells other than nerve and muscle display action potentials. One such cell is the beta cell of the Islets of Langerhans (Dean and Matthews, 1970a). This cell secretes insulin in response to changes in blood glucose. When glucose concentration is increased, membrane potential changes, but in addition, a series of action potentials are entrained in the cell membrane (see Chapter 6). The current carrier of these spikes is calcium ion, coupling membrane excitation to cellular response. Hence, by the classic restricted definition of excitability, the beta cell of the pancreas is excitable and the slow muscle fiber is nonexcitable.

Even though the beta cells are excitable in the classic physiological sense, most secretory cells display electrical characteristics similar to those of slow muscle cells. Characteristically, both exocrine and endocrine secretory cells respond to stimulation with changes in membrane potential. This means that one of the characteristic responses to chemical or electrical excitation is a change in ion currents across the membrane. Nor is this situation confined to secretory and contractile cells. Changes in the membrane potential are seen in osteoclasts after stimulation with hormones. These cells respond to two hormones with opposing effects. Parathyroid hormones stimulate these cells to resorb bone. Calcitonin inhibits their bone resorptive action. Parathyroid hormone causes a depolarization of the membrane, and calcitonin causes a hyperpolarization (Mears, 1971). It is not yet known how these changes are produced, namely, what ionic fluxes are increased, or what their roles are in coupling stimulus to response. Nonetheless, hormones with opposing effects have opposite influences on these ion currents, leading logically to the hypothesis that such changes are an intimate component of the response of these cells to chemical or hormonal stimulation.

CONCLUSION

Over the past 15 years, two broad lines of biological research, those concerned with stimulus–response coupling in nerve and muscle and with peptide hormone action, have converged. It has become apparent that these two apparently quite different mechanisms of cell-to-cell communication share a similar dual system of intracellular messengers, cAMP and calcium, to couple stimulus to response. This universal system is given the name synarchy.

2

Cellular Calcium Metabolism

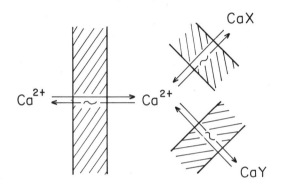

INTRODUCTION

Our knowledge of cellular calcium metabolism has advanced rapidly in the past decade (Baker, 1973, 1976, 1978; Borle and Anderson, 1976; Blaustein, 1974; Brinley, 1978; Carafoli and Crompton, 1976; Borle, 1973; Foreman et al., 1976; Scarpa, 1979; Rasmussen and Goodman, 1977; Lehninger, 1970; Berridge, 1976b; Moore and Pastan, 1978; Lehinger et al., 1967, 1978; Martonosi et al., 1978; Blaustein et al., 1978; Carafoli and Crompton, 1978; Loewenstein and Rose, 1978; Ashley, 1978; Schatzmann and Burgin, 1978; Rasmussen and Gustin, 1978; Ebashi et al., 1978; Stephenson and Podolsky, 1978; Carafoli, 1979; Randle et al., 1979; Matthews, 1970, 1979; Blinks et al., 1976; Kretsinger, 1979). A variety of experimental approaches have provided the information upon which to construct a fairly detailed model of cellular calcium homeostasis. These approaches include (1) the kinetic analysis of calcium metabolism in whole cells or tissues using radioisotopes of calcium; (2) the study of calcium uptake by isolated fragments of cell membranes or endoplasmic reticulum, or by intact mitochondria; (3) the behavior of calcium-sensitive enzymes; (4) the use of calcium-sensitive intracellular indicators in large cells such as barnacle muscle and squid axons; (5) the study of calcium content and exchange in the extruded axoplasm from the squid axon; and (6) the use of labeled drugs that bind specifically to calcium receptor proteins.

Rather than describe the data derived from these separate approaches, a model of cellular calcium metabolism based on these data will be presented. This will serve as a basis for the discussion of the significance of each cellular component in cellular calcium homeostasis and of some of the unresolved questions relating to the role of specific cellular pools of calcium in stimulus–response coupling.

CALCIUM METABOLISM IN AN IDEALIZED CELL

The pathways of calcium metabolism in an idealized cell are shown schematically in Figure 2.1. From the point of view of the informational role of calcium ion in cell function, the critically important compartment is the free calcium ion concentration in the cell cytosol. This is normally in the range of 0.05 to 0.5 μM in resting cells. Yet the total cytosolic calcium content is in the range of 70 to 300 μM. This means that a cytosalic calcium buffer system is present. The capacity of this system to bind calcium has been most clearly demonstrated in the case of extruded axoplasm from the squid axon (Figure 2.2). The nature of this cytosolic buffer is not known. In addition to the total cytosolic pool, there are significant pools of calcium in the endoplasmic reticulum (CaR), in the mitochondria (CaM), and in some cells in secretory vesicles (CaV). Although the exchange ability of the latter pool is a point of continuing debate, much of the calcium contained in the mitochondria and

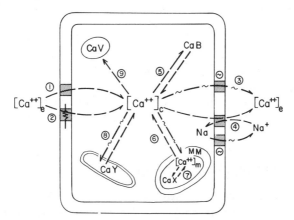

Figure 2.1 Schematic representation of calcium metabolism in an idealized mammalian cell. The symbol $[Ca^{2+}]_c$ represents the free Ca^{2+} concentration in the cell cytosol. This pool is in rapid exchange with a buffer pool in the cytosol (CaB), with a pool in the mitochondria (CaX lower right), another in the microsomes (CaY lower left), and with the extracellular pool $[Ca^{2+}]_e$. Entry of calcium into the cell may take place by either a voltage-independent (1) or voltage-dependent (2) pathway. Efflux from the cell is an energy-requiring process that may be driven by an ATP-dependent calcium pump (3) or by the Na^+ gradient (4) and Na^+–Ca^{2+} exchange. Buffering of an unknown cytosolic component (5) is supplemented by active, energy-dependent uptake of Ca^{2+} by both mitochondria (6) and microsomes (8). The calcium in the mitochondrial matrix space exists in both ionic $[Ca^{2+}]$ and nonionic (CaX) pools. The mechanism of exchange (7) between them is thought to be controlled primarily by intramitochondrial pH and phosphate concentration. Uptake (9) into secretory vesicles (CaV) appears to be unidirectional.

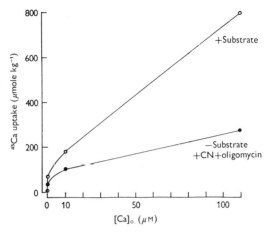

Figure 2.2 Uptake of radiocalcium by isolated axoplasm. The uptake in the absence of substrate and presence of oligomycin and cyanide (CN) is presumed to represent cytosolic buffering. This component had a calcium-binding capacity of 20 to 40 μmol / kg axoplasm and was half-saturated at a calcium concentration of 0.5 μM. From Baker (1976), with permission.

the endoplasmic reticulum is rapidly exchangeable. If all this calcium were ionized, the concentrations within these organelles would be in the millimolar range. As it is, a significant percentage of the calcium in each organelle is nonionic; nonetheless, our best estimates of the free or ionic calcium in these two subcellular compartments are in the range of 10^{-5} to 10^{-4} M, that is, 100 to 1000 times greater than that in the cytosol. To maintain these calcium gradients, both organelles possess calcium pumps oriented so as to pump calcium out of the cytosol into the respective subcellular pool. Likewise, a leak of calcium back into the cytosolic pool from these compartments occurs. The activities of these pump–leak systems as well as those in the plasma membrane determine the steady state level of ionized calcium in the cell cytosol.

EVENTS AT THE PLASMA MEMBRANE

The difference in calcium concentration between cytosol and extracellular fluid is approximately 10,000-fold. It is maintained by two features of the plasma membrane. First, under resting conditions the calcium permeability of the membrane is quite low. Second, there are active, energy-dependent mechanisms for extruding calcium from cell interior to the extracellular space. The first of these is a specific Ca^{2+}/Mg^{2+} ATPase or calcium pump, which has been most thoroughly studied in the human red cell (Schatzmann, and Burgen, 1978; Vincenzi, 1978; Schatzmann and Vincenzi, 1969; Bond and Clough, 1973; Farrance and Vincenzi, 1977a,b; Gopenath and Vincenzi, 1977; Niggli et al., 1979; Hinds et al., 1978; Waisman et al., 1981). The concentration of calcium that is required to cause a half-maximal rate of pump activity is in the range of 1 μM (Figure 2.3). The pump is activated by the calcium receptor protein calmodulin. The second is a $Na^+–Ca^{2+}$ ex-

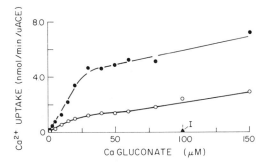

Figure 2.3 Uptake of radiocalcium into inside-out vesicles from human erythrocytes in the presence of ATP. The plotted data are calcium uptake vs the calculated free Ca^{2+} concentration using calcium–EGTA buffer systems in the presence ($\bullet$) and absence ($\bigcirc$) of calmodulin. From Waisman et al. (1981), with permission.

change mechanism (Figure 2.4) which depends upon the fact that there is an asymmetric distribution of Na^+ across the plasma membrane with a high Na^+ concentration outside and a low Na^+ concentration inside (Baker, 1976; Blaustein et al., 1978). This is maintained at the expense of metabolic energy by the action of a specific Na^+ pump or Na^+/K^+ ATPase. This Na^+ gradient represents an electrochemical gradient which can serve to drive a variety of other transport reactions. For example, the Na^+ gradient is the immediate energy source for the concentrative uptake of amino acids, glucose, phosphate, and other substances by cells. It is also a driving force, via $Na^+–Ca^{2+}$ exchange, for the energy-dependent efflux of calcium from the cell. The concentration of internal calcium required for half-maximal activation is in the range of 0.7 to 1.0 μM. This exchange is also dependent on the internal ATP concentration.

   The relative importance of these two energy-dependent mechanisms for

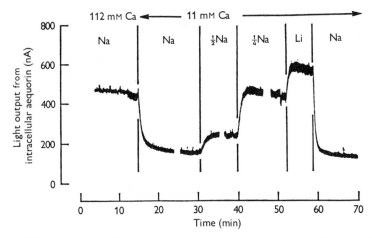

Figure 2.4 Changes in intracellular ionized calcium (as measured by light output from the luminescent protein aequorin) when a squid axon was immersed in media of different sodium and calcium contents. From Baker (1976), with permission.

regulating calcium efflux are not known for most cells. However, the Na^+–Ca^{2+} exchange system has been found in nerve axons, at presynaptic termini, in smooth muscle cells, in endocrine cells, and in renal tubule cells. There are indications that it probably exists in many other cells. Conversely, the Ca^{2+}/Mg^{2+} ATPase has been found in red cell, nerve, kidney, and enterocytes but is probably more widely distributed.

The best estimates of the relative importance of these two mechanisms in the same tissue have been made by Baker (1978) and Dipolo et al. (1976) from studies of calcium fluxes in the squid axon. Baker estimates are that under basal conditions each pathway contributes upward of 50% of the total efflux. Dipolo showed that a Na^+-dependent efflux was dominant at relatively high cytosolic calcium concentration ($[Ca^{2+}]_c$), whereas ATP-dependent Ca^{2+} extrusion was more important at lower $[Ca^{2+}]_c$.

One feature of the pattern of influx and efflux in the resting cell is the influence of calcium upon both fluxes. The permeability of the membrane to calcium is an inverse function of the extracellular calcium ion concentration. The available evidence shows that a lack of calcium in the external medium leads to an increase in both Na^+ and Ca^{2+} permeability. This can be viewed as a rather simple control mechanism making the rate of calcium influx into the cell more or less independent of the external calcium ion concentration. Conversely, the rate of efflux is a complex function of the internal calcium ion concentration. When this concentration is below 0.2 μM, the Ca^{2+}/Mg^{2+} ATPase is shifted to a high K_m form, which means that the rate of efflux decreases automatically. When calcium ion concentration increases, the calcium ions bind to the calcium receptor protein calmodulin, and the calcium–calmodulin complex interacts with the high K_m form of the Ca^{2+}/Mg^{2+} ATPase and causes it to shift to a low K_m form. The precise mechanism by which calcium–calmodulin brings about this change is not known. The consequences, however, are clear. A rise in cytosolic calcium ion concentration acts as a stimulus to markedly enhance the efflux of calcium from the cell and thus to maintain cellular calcium homeostasis. Thus, changes in the concentration of either external or internal calcium ion lead to immediate adjustments at the plasma membrane so that cytosolic calcium ion concentration is maintained at an operational level. If such a mechanism did not operate and the cell employed calcium ion to couple stimulus to response, then a severe depletion of calcium would lead to an unexcitable cell even though the extracellular signal induced the influx of some calcium.

If an influx of calcium across the cell membrane often serves to couple stimulus to response, a significant change in calcium influx must occur after cell activation. Three- to fivefold changes in calcium entry rate have been described after cell activation. At least three separate mechanisms have been identified by which an increase in calcium entry occurs in response to cell activation. The first, seen in excitable tissues, is an early entry of Ca^{2+} concurrent with the onset of the action potential (Baker, 1973, 1976). This calcium entry is blocked by the same agents that block Na^+ entry; it has the same time course as Na^+ entry. These data indicate that calcium is entering via the Na^+ channel. The second, seen in a variety of tissues including nerve, smooth muscle, cardiac muscle, beta cells in pancreatic islets, and chromaffin cells, is a voltage-dependent calcium channel which is relatively specific for calcium ion and is blocked by certain heavy metals and by Verapamil. The third is a non-voltage-dependent calcium entry after hormone–receptor interaction (the so-called receptor operated channel) in mammalian and fly salivary gland, liver cells, smooth muscle cells, mast cells, and probably a variety of other tissues (Borle, 1973). There may also be a fourth mechanism, because a calcium-dependent calcium entry has also been described; that is, an increase in calcium influx in response to a rise in internal (cytosolic) calcium ion concentration has been described, but the characteristics of this calcium control system have not been analyzed.

An important feature of the voltage-dependent channel is that in most tissues it becomes inactivated by prolonged depolarization. The question of greatest importance is whether the voltage-dependent channel in tissues like the nerve axon and the voltage-independent channel in the mast cell or smooth muscle are actually similar in terms of the molecular basis for the change in calcium permeability. Present evidence suggests they may have common attributes.

EVENTS IN THE ENDOPLASMIC RETICULUM

An intracellular calcium pool that has a well-characterized messenger function is that contained in the endoplasmic or sarcoplasmic reticulum. This membrane system is must highly developed in fast skeletal muscle, somewhat less well developed in cardiac muscle, and even less developed but obviously present in smooth muscle and in a variety of secretory cells. Its importance in stimulus–response coupling in skeletal and cardiac muscle is generally accepted. Its role in various forms of smooth muscle and in nonmuscle cells and tissues continues to be a matter of debate. One of the most completely characterized calcium pump systems is that found in the sarcoplasmic reticulum of mammalian skeletal muscle (Figure 2.5). The active uptake of calcium is stoichometrically linked to the hydrolysis of ATP. For each mole of ATP hydrolyzed, 2 atoms of Ca^{2+} are transferred across the membrane. The transfer of calcium is associated with a phosphorylation and dephosphorylation of an aspartic acid residue in the protein (Hasselback and Makinose, 1961, 1963; Martonosi et al., 1978). In biochemical terms, the pump works via the following reaction sequence:

$$E + ATP \rightleftharpoons E \cdot ATP \qquad (1)$$

$$E \cdot ATP + 2Ca^{2+} \rightleftharpoons E \overset{\nearrow ATP}{\underset{\searrow 2Ca}{}} \qquad (2)$$

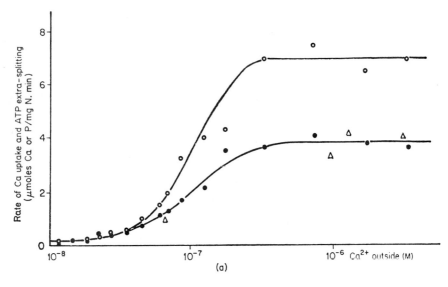

Figure 2.5   Rates of calcium accumulation ($\bigcirc$) and ATP hydrolysis ($\bullet$,$\triangle$) as function of free Ca^{2+} concentration by vesicles prepared from the sarcoplasmic reticulum of mammalian skeletal muscle. From Hasselbach et al. (1970), with permission.

$$E \overset{ATP}{\underset{2Ca}{\diagdown}} \rightleftharpoons E \overset{\sim P}{\underset{2Ca}{\diagdown}} + ADP \qquad (3)$$

$$E \overset{\sim P}{\underset{2Ca}{\diagdown}} \rightleftharpoons E^* \overset{\sim P}{\underset{2Ca}{\diagdown}} \qquad (4)$$

$$E^* \overset{\sim P}{\underset{2Ca}{\diagdown}} \rightleftharpoons E^* \overset{\sim P}{} \quad + 2Ca^{2+} \qquad (5)$$

$$E^* \overset{\sim P}{} \rightleftharpoons E^* + Pi \qquad (6)$$

$$E^* \rightleftharpoons E \qquad (7)$$

According to this scheme, formation of the phosphoprotein (steps 1 through 3) takes place on the outer surface of microsomal membrane. Step 4 involves a conformation change resulting in the transfer of calcium to the inner face of the membrane. Dissociation of calcium from the complex (step 5) is followed by the hydrolysis of the phosphoprotein (step 6), and then the enzyme returns to its original conformation (step 7). Kinetic data indicate that step 6, phosphoprotein hydrolysis, is the rate-limiting step in the overall process. The exact mechanism of calcium translocation (step 4) is not known, but in analogy with other transport ATPase some type of a gated pore is considered likely.

The fate of the calcium once it enters the membrane space is not completely established. The ATPase can establish a calcium gradient of approximately 10^3. If the external (cytosolic) calcium concentration $[Ca^{2+}]_c$ is 10^{-7}, then the calcium ion concentration within the reticulum is 10^{-4}. However, *in situ* the total calcium content of the sarcoplasmic reticulum (SR) is in the millimolar range. Most of this calcium is bound in some readily releasable form. Two possibilities are (1) that the calcium is complexed with phosphate, and (2) the calcium is bound to the internal surface of the membrane. A specific acid protein with a high capacity (43 moles Ca^{2+} per M.W. of 46,000) but relatively high dissociation constant, K_d, for calcium (K_d of 8×10^{-4} M), calsequestrin, has been shown to be an extrinsic membrane protein existing on the inner surface of the microsomal membrane. It represents approximately 7% of the total protein of skeletal muscle sarcoplasmic reticulum. It could account for approximately 90 nmol calcium per mg vesicle protein, which is probably sufficient to bind all the calcium accumulated by the SR.

The K_m for ATP-dependent calcium accumulation has been found to vary in various preparations of isolated SR from 0.1 to 1.0 μM. The value of the intact SR is probably closer to the lower value. This value is of interest in terms of the threshold concentration of calcium needed to initiate contraction, which is in the range of 1.0 μM.

A point of considerable concern has been the fact that measured values of the maximal rate of calcium accumulation in isolated vesicles from sarcoplasmic reticulum are too slow by an order of magnitude to account for the rate of relaxation. However, estimation of this rate in skinned muscle fibers in which the SR is intact indicate that rates of accumulation are sufficiently rapid to account for the measured rates of relaxation.

Although not as completely studied, microsomal preparations from cardiac and smooth muscle also accumulate calcium by a similar ATP-dependent process. The maximal rates observed in the cardiac preparations are an order of magnitude lower than those measured in skeletal muscle preparations. These rates of calcium uptake can be enhanced by either cAMP-dependent or calcium-dependent (calmodulin regulated) protein kinases (see chapter 9). These enzymes catalyze the phosphorylation of a specific membrane protein, phospholamban, and this phosphorylation leads to an increase in calcium transport and ATPase activity. The effect appears to be that of increasing the rate of dephosphorylation of the aspartylphosphate enzyme intermediate. The calcium uptake in smooth muscle microsomes is also stimulated by cAMP. Hence, one apparently widespread and common effect of cAMP on cellular calcium metabolism is that of stimulating microsomal calcium uptake.

Similar ATP-dependent calcium uptake systems have been described for the endoplasmic reticulum-containing microsomes from liver, kidney, brain, salivary gland, and platelets. Most of these preparations are impure. Nonetheless, their maximal capacities for calcium accumulation are considerably lower than those of vesicles from skeletal muscle (liver ~ 400 nmol/mg protein: skeletal muscle ~ 1800 nmol/mg protein). Also the K_m values have ranged from 4 to 100 μM, in contrast to 0.1 to 1.0 μM in skeletal muscle. Some of this marked difference is probably attributable to technical problems, so it is not yet possible to determine whether the K_m for calcium of this membrane pump system actually varies so widely from tissue to tissue.

If the sarcoplasmic reticulum is to serve as the source of calcium in stimulus–response coupling, then a mechanism for the rapid release of its stored calcium must exist. In spite of considerable experimental effort, the mechanism responsible for release from the sarcoplasmic reticulum of skeletal muscle is still not completely defined. Two major mechanisms have been proposed: (1) calcium-dependent calcium release; and (2) depolarization-induced release of calcium. Present evidence strongly favors the view that in skeletal muscle, depolarization is the primary mechanism inducing calcium release. However, in skinned muscle fibers, Stephenson and Podolsky (1978) have shown that the chloride-induced depolarization of SR is calcium dependent. This raises the possibility that the primary signal is a depolarization leading to an initial release of calcium which then, in turn, causes a further release. These authors suggest that depolarization not only induces calcium release but also inhibits its ATP-dependent uptake. The combination of these changes leads to an amplification of the initial depolarizing signal.

In the case of cardiac muscle, Fabiato and Fabiato (1978) have presented convincing evidence that small physiologically appropriate amounts of free calcium ion cause the release of calcium stored in the SR. These authors argue that in this muscle, the major factor regulating release of stored calcium is this calcium-dependent calcium release. In this view, the initial or "trigger" calcium needed to stimulate SR release is calcium that enters the cell across the sarcolemma (plasma membrane) during the plateau of the action potential.

This model represents another instance of calcium serving to couple excitation to a change in membrane permeability. The unique aspects of this situation are two. The first is that in contrast to the other cases discussed previously which involved the plasma membrane, this case involves a change in the permeability of a subcellular membrane. The second is that calcium induces a change in the permeability of a membrane to calcium rather than, as in other cases, to monovalent cations (K^+ and/or N^+) or anions (Cl^-).

Nothing is yet known about the mechanisms by which calcium may be released from the endoplasmic reticulum in other cell types such as secretory cells, presynaptic nerve termini, and liver cells. It seems likely that calcium exchange between cytosol and endoplasmic reticulum may be of importance in stimulus–response coupling in some, if not in many, of these cells, and that mechanisms similar to those operating in muscle cells function to couple events at the plasma membrane, that is, hormone–receptor interaction, with release of calcium from the endoplasmic reticulum.

EVENTS IN THE MITOCHONDRIA

Mitochondria isolated from nearly any mammalian tissue and from tissue of lower forms when studied in isolation are able to accumulate large quantities of calcium from the medium. Accumulation is energy dependent and may be driven either by substrate oxidation or ATP hydrolysis (Chance, 1965; Rasmussen, 1966; Bygrave, 1978; Carafoli and Crompton, 1978; Scarpa, 1979). In either case, the primary driving force for calcium entry is the electrical component (ΔE) of the total electrochemical gradient, Δu_{H^+} generated either by substrate oxidation or ATP hydrolysis: $\Delta u_{H^+} = \Delta E - 60 \Delta pH$ (Mitchell, 1969; Hinkle and Mitchell, 1970; Mitchell, 1976; Rottenberg and Scarpa, 1974). In this view, calcium is driven electrophoretically into the matrix space via a calcium uniport (Nicholls, 1978a,b). If this takes place in the absence of a permeant anion, respiration and calcium uptake soon cease because the mitochondrial matrix space becomes alkaline. Addition of permeant anion which can donate H^+ within the matrix space leads to an uptake of the anion, to the generation of protons within the matrix space,

$$HA + Ca \cdot X \rightleftharpoons H^+ + CaA$$

and to release of calcium from the inner surface of the inner membrane. These anions stimulate calcium uptake. Under physiological conditions, the major anion is phosphate, which upon entering the matrix space interacts with calcium to form a nonionic calcium phosphate complex which is osmotically inactive. Formation and/or stabilization of this complex requires the presence of ATP, and the complex appears to have the following stoichiometry: $Ca_{15}P_{10}ATP$. Because of its formation, extremely large quantities of calcium can be taken up by isolated mitochondria. Up to 3 μmol/mg mitochondrial protein can be accumulated. Given that 1 mg mitochondrial protein is equivalent to approximately 1 μl mitochondrial volume, this would give an internal calcium ion concentration in the molar range, if it were all ionized. However, the calcium content of freshly isolated rat liver mitochondria is in the range of 15 to 20 nmoles/mg protein. Even so, this would represent a calcium ion concentration in the 20 mM range if it were all ionized. Although the exact calcium ion concentration in mitochondrial matrix space is not known, estimates range from 10^{-6} to 10^{-4} M, which means that the bulk of the calcium in the mitochondrial matrix space is in some nonionic form. Nonetheless, a significant percentage (20 to 60%) is rapidly exchangeable with extramitochondrial pools. The efflux component of this exchange occurs by a separate pathway (Pushkin et al., 1976; Nicholls, 1978a,b; Carafoli and Crompton, 1978).

Considerable controversy surrounds the question of the K_m of the mitochondrial transport system. Most recent results place the value at 2 to 10 μM (Reed and Bygrave, 1975; Scarpa, 1979). However, the lower values have been obtained with a medium in which Mg^{2+} is absent. In the presence of magnesium in the 0.5 mM range (close to the intracellular magnesium ion concentration), the K_m k for calcium is in the 10 to 20 μM range. Given this high value, considerable doubt has been raised as to the physiological significance of mitochondrial calcium accumulation *in situ*. On the other hand, Borle (1973) in his studies of calcium isotope kinetics in intact cells has shown quite clearly that an intracellular calcium pool having the characteristics expected of the mitochondrial pool is in rapid exchange with the cytosolic and extracellular calcium compartment.

The recent elegant experiments of Nicholls (1978a,b) and Nicholls and Scott (1980) have clarified the calcium buffering function of rat liver and brain mitochondria. Nicholls showed that liver mitochondria incubated in the presence of an external calcium buffer (NTA) are able to maintain an extracellular pCa^{2+} (negative log of the free calcium concentration) of 6.1 or a free calcium of 0.8 μM, and brain mitochondria are able to maintain a free calcium concentration in the range of 0.3 μM. If the extramitochondrial calcium ion concentration falls below this value, the mitochondria release calcium; if it rises above this value, the mitochondria take it up. Also as long as phosphate or a permeant weak anion is present, the pCa^{2+} changes very little even though the intramitochondrial content of total calcium increases. In terms of total calcium accumulated, these data indicate that a threefold increase in total mitochondrial calcium content can occur without a significant change in pCa$_o^{2+}$ in the cytosol. Based on the data concerning the effect of permeant anions, it is likely that in the presence of physiologically relevant phosphate concentration this capacity is significantly greater.

Under the conditions where the ΔE is above 130 mV, the rate of calcium efflux is constant, but the rate of influx varies as a direct logarithmic function of the extramitochondrial calcium concentration (Figure 2.6). The efflux rate is 5 nmol/min/mg protein, and a similar rate of influx is achieved when the extramitochondrial calcium reaches 0.8 μM (pCa$_o^{2+}$ = 6.1). At this pCa$_o^{2+}$ there is a continual recycling of calcium. The energy dissipated by this cycling is 2 nmol O_2/min/mg protein which is a small percentage of the basal rate of mitochondrial respiration.

A number of features of the mitochondrial calcium system have been

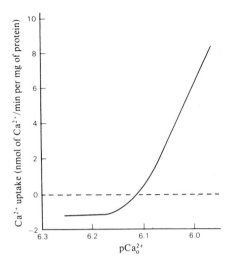

Figure 2.6 Net rate of calcium uptake into isolated rat liver mitochondria as function of the pCa_0^{2+} of the medium. Dotted line represents the fixed rate of calcium efflux. When pCa_0^{2+} falls below 6.1, there is a net release of calcium; and when it rises above 6.1, there is a net uptake. From Nicholls (1978a), with permission.

reexplored. First, Nicholls (1978a) has shown that the addition of 0.3 mM Mg^{2+} causes only a slight change in pCa_0^{2+} (6.1 to 5.95) primarily by displacing the calcium activation of the calcium uniport to the right. Conversely, an increase in extramitochondrial pH (fall in [H^+]) led to a fall in pCa_0^{2+} from 6.1 at pH 6.6 to approximately 6.5 at pH 7.4. The change in pH also seems to act by shifting the calcium dependence of the activity of the calcium uniport.

As pointed out by Nicholls, a fine control of pCa_0^{2+} could be obtained by regulating the activity of the efflux pathway. A doubling of efflux rate would lead to a fall of 0.12 in pCa_0^{2+}, that is, a rise in free Ca^{2+} from 0.8 to 1.1 μM. A tenfold rise would lead to a pCa_0^{2+} in the range of 5.6 or a free calcium ion concentration of approximately 4 μM.

A question yet to be answered is the factor determining the fixed value of the efflux pathway. Two possibilities can be considered: (1) the K_m of this pathway for internal ionized calcium is quite low so that under the conditions defined above, the calcium ion content of the matrix space is saturating and 5 nmol/min/mg protein represents the V_{max} of the efflux pathway; or (2) the matrix buffering system is such under these conditions that the calcium ion content of the matrix space is held nearly constant.

An approach to these questions has been made by Becker and coworkers (1980). Using a calcium electrode, they measured the calcium ion concentration that was maintained either by suspensions of liver mitochondria incubated in the presence of a microsomal fraction or by isolated hepatocytes incubated in sufficient digitonin to render their plasma membranes permeable to Ca^{2+}. When the K^+, ATP^{2-}, and Mg^{2+} concentrations were in the physiological range, the steady state calcium concentration was 0.5 μM in the presence of respiring mitochondria alone. Addition of microsomes led to a fall of this value to 0.2 μM. A similar concentration (0.2 μM) was maintained by suspensions of hepatocytes made permeable by digitonin treatment.

These data extend those of Nicholls (1978a) but add the important point that when microsomes were added to the respiring mitochondria and the level of free calcium fell from 0.5 to 0.2 μM, the mitochondria lost approximately 40% of their calcium and then lost no more even when more microsomes were added. Thus, the mitochondria in the presence of microsomes reached a new steady state in which efflux balanced influx even with an external calcium ion concentration of 0.2 μM, well below the "equilibrium value" reported by Nicholls (1978a). The most likely explanation is that under these conditions the free calcium concentration in the matrix fell, and hence the efflux rate fell.

The second aspect of the studies by Becker et al. (1980) was that when small increments of calcium were added to the systems of combined mitochondria and microsomes, the microsomes had a limited capacity to sequester calcium and the mitochondria were the major sequestering system.

The technique of making the cell membrane permeable to calcium (and other ions) by the incubation of liver cells with digitonin has been exploited by Murphy et al. (1980) to assess the free calcium concentration of the cell cytosol. These workers monitored the free calcium in the system by adding the calcium-sensitive dye Arsenazo III and then incubated the digitonin-treated cells with calcium–EGTA buffer containing different free calcium concentrations. The free calcium concentration of the buffer system in which there was neither uptake of calcium into or efflux of calcium from the cells was taken as the null point, or the cytosolic calcium ion concentration $[Ca^{2+}]_c$. This was found to be between 0.1 and 0.2 μM, which compares favorably with the value reported by Becker et al. (1980). When these cells were treated with glucagon, there was no change in $[Ca^{2+}]_c$. However, phenylephrine treatment caused a two to threefold increase in $[Ca^{2+}]_c$ and a net efflux of calcium from the mitochondria. This small change in $[Ca^{2+}]_c$ was associated with the conversion of phosphorylase b to phosphorylase a; that is, the rise was sufficient to cause a calcium-dependent activation of glycogenolysis. *In toto,* these data argue that mitochondria serve as important intracellular calcium buffers and may serve as a source of calcium for stimulus–response coupling in some cells.

Another question to be addressed is whether or not these rates of calcium efflux are sufficiently fast to account for the shifts in calcium metabolism seen in the intact tissue. Nicholls has calculated that a small 0.1 μM shift in cytosol pCa_o^{2+} would lead to an increase in rate of calcium uptake in the liver in the range of 1 to 5 mmol/s/gm wet weight. These values can be contrasted to those obtained by Claret-Berthon et al. (1977) studying calcium fluxes in perfused rat liver. They obtained a value of 0.5 nmoles/s/gm wet weight as the exchange rate of a kinetic pool thought to represent the mitochondrial calcium pool. Calculation by Borle (1973) in isolated kidney cells give a value of approximately 0.01 nmoles/s/gm, and this increases 40-fold to 0.4 after parathyroid hormone (PTH) addition to the cell culture. These data indicate that the rates of mitochondrial calcium exchange are sufficiently rapid to play a significant role in cellular calcium homeostasis.

PLASMA VERSUS MITOCHONDRIAL MEMBRANE AS REGULATOR OF CYTOSOLIC CALCIUM

Based on studies of the kinetics of calcium exchange in intact kidney cells, Borle (1973) has proposed that mitochondria play a major role in regulating cellular calcium metabolism. On the other hand, Rink and Baker (1974) and Brinley (1978), analyzing data obtained from the study of calcium uptake into stimulated squid axon and from an analysis of calcium content and exchange in extruded axoplasm, have concluded under most physiological circumstances the mitochondria play a minor role in cellular calcium homeostasis.

In considering these different conclusions, it is important to point out that the requirements for a messenger function in the two tissues are quite different. In nerve, a sudden calcium influx is the signal for neurotransmitter release. In this situation the calcium signal must be brief with both a rapid rise and fall. Furthermore, the major calcium response element is situated just beneath the plasma membrane, hence a rise of calcium ion concentration in this restricted cellular domain is probably sufficient to activate neurotransmitter release. This means the domain in which a change in calcium ion concentration takes place is restricted in both time and space. In contrast, in a cell such as the kidney or liver cell, a change in hormone status leads to a sustained change in metabolic response, and the response elements are throughout the cytoplasmic compartment. Under these circumstances, the domain of calcium is extended both spacially and temporally. This must require a different organization of the mechanisms regulating cellular calcium metabolism. It is also evident that in the case of the squid axon, mitochondria are sparse, hence the ratio of surface area of the mitochondrial membrane to that of the plasma membrane is quite low, that is, the plasma membrane may account for as much as 40 to 50% of the total calcium transport membrane surface. In contrast, it is estimated that in the liver, the surface area of the plasma membrane is only one-fifth of the area of the inner mitochondrial membrane.

The experimental approaches to this problem in nervous and nonnervous tissues have differed, making comparison difficult. Comparable data using the same techniques are not available. Nonetheless, if one recalculates the data from various authors (Baker, 1978; Blaustein et al., 1978; Borle and Uchikawa, 1978; Foden and Randle, 1978; Claret-Berthon et al., 1977;

Dipolo et al., 1976; Brinley, 1978) concerning cellular calcium pools, there is a surprising uniformity of results (Table 2.1). The exchangeable cell calcium is in the range of 450 ± 100 μg-atom/kg cell H_2O in all the tissues except the squid axon. Likewise, the exchangeable cytosolic compartment is in the range of 150 ± 50 ug atoms/kg in all the tissues but squid axon. The question is whether these differences between squid axon and mammalian tissues are real or are entirely due to differences in experimental techniques.

The data for squid axon were obtained by an analysis of the calcium content of extruded axon and of its calcium buffering capacity. In fresh axons, the total calcium content may be as low as 50 μg-atom/kg H2O with approximately 15 μg-atom/kg located in the cytosol and 35 μg-atom/kg in the mitochondria (Brinley, 1978). In the cytosolic compartment there are non-energy-dependent calcium binding systems one of high affinity ($K_m = 0.1$ to 0.5 M) and low capacity 20 to 40 μg-atom capacity, and another with a low affinity that does not saturate at 500 μM (Baker, 1978). The free ionized calcium concentration in this compartment is close to 0.1 μg-atom/l.

In intact axons stimulated electrically at low rates, there is an increased entry of calcium into the cell, a small rise in ionized calcium ($0.1 \rightarrow 0.3$ μg-atom) representing only a small percentage (less 2%) of the calcium entering the cell. This rise is not altered by addition of FCCP (carbonyl-cyanide, p-trifluoromethoxyphenyl hydrazone) or CN^- (uncouplers or inhibitors of oxidative phosphorylation). These data mean that in the normal axon under physiological circumstances, the cytosolic buffering system and the plasma membrane pumps provide the necessary "buffering" capacity to modulate a small, controlled rise in cytosolic calcium ion concentration. On the other hand, if "massive" calcium loading of the axon is carried out by stimulating at high rates (100/s) in high-calcium seawater, the cytosolic

Table 2.1   Cellular Calcium Pools. The Various Cellular Calcium Pools in Different Tissues, Estimated in Different Ways by Different Investigators.

Calcium Pool	Calcium Concentration (μg-atom/kg cell H_2O)				
	Squid Axon[b]	Synapto-somes[b]	Kidney[b]	Liver-1	Liver-2
Total cell	—	2000	4950	2700	2200
Exchangeable cell	60	450	340	550	385
Total mitochondrial	100	650	200 (600)	2000	660
Exchangeable mitochondrial	20	300	140	450	115
Exchangeable cytosol	15	150	200	100	270

[a]The data has been recalculated so that the same units apply (μg-atom/kg cell H_2O).
[b]The data for the squid axon are from Dipolo et al. (1976), Brinley (1978), and Baker (1978); those for synaptosomes, from Blaustein et al. (1978); those for kidney, from Borle and Uchikawa (1978); those for liver-1, from Foden and Randle (1978) using isolated liver cells; and those for liver-2, from Claret-Berthon et al. (1977) using the perfused liver.

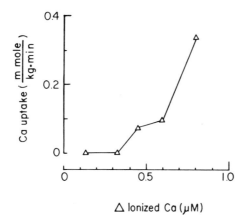

Figure 2.7   Plot of the estimated rate of uptake of Ca^{2+} by squid axons mitochondria *in situ* as function of the cytosolic Ca^{2+} concentration. From Brinley et al. (1978), with permission.

calcium ion concentration rises higher. This rise is approximately 0.3 ng-atom per μg-atom total calcium taken up by the cell. If the mitochondria are poisoned by FCCP, this rate increases to 30 ng-atom per μg-atom. These data indicate that the mitochondria play an intracellular buffering role under conditions of high calcium load. The data show that a high-capacity "non-energy-dependent" buffer system also operates. It is difficult to define the latter, but it may in part still represent mitochondrial binding. Brinley et al. (1978) have also studied the kinetics of calcium accumulation into axonal mitochondria *in situ* by studying the rate of calcium uptake into mitochondria by increasing the cytosolic pool of calcium by repetitive nerve stimulation. The calcium-sensitive dye arsenazo III was employed to monitor free calcium (Scarpa et al., 1978). After stimulation, the axon was immersed in a Ca^{+2}-free choline solution to prevent further entry of calcium and to block Na^{+}–Ca^{+2} exchange. When this was done, it was possible to calculate the rates of calcium uptake by the mitochondria as a function of the change in free calcium concentration. There was little uptake by mitochondria if the $[Ca^{+2}]_c$ was below 0.4 μM (Figure 2.7). As the calcium increased, the rate of uptake went up dramatically, so that when the calcium increased from 0.5 to 10 μM (a 20-fold increase), the rate increases by a factor of 120. Although it is not possible to make a strict comparison of these data with those of Nicholls (1978), it is nevertheless of considerable interest that the studies both suggest that the mitochondria serve to buffer cytosolic calcium in the range of 0.5 to 8.0 μM.

Another way of approaching the question of mitochondrial function is to examine the characteristics of mitochondrial calcium uptake in the axoplasm *in situ*. Such studies have revealed that the apparent K_m for such uptake is of the order of 10 μM, that is, similar to that seen in isolated mitochondria. More significant, the threshold for calcium accumulation by mitochondria was in the range of 0.2 to 0.4 μg-atom/l. These data would imply that in the resting cell, the rate of calcium exchange into and out of mitochondria are very low—that when a two-to threefold rise in ionic calcium occurs, there is little increase in mitochondrial exchange; but that at values above 0.3 μg-atom/l, the mitochondria play an increasingly important role in buffering changes in cell calcium (Brinley, 1978). Clearly, in this tissue in which the spatial and time domain of calcium is restricted, the need is for efficient mechanisms for limiting the rise in calcium in both domains. The systems operating to accomplish this are (1) a high affinity–low capacity buffering system in the cell cytosol; (2) a high-affinity pump system on the plasma membrane; (3) a low affinity–high capacity buffering system in the cytosol (and possibly mitochondria); and (4) a relatively low-affinity but very high-capacity mitochondrial pump system.

If we next compare the data on calcium exchange and content in synaptosomes from mammalian brain with that from the squid axon (Table 2.1), several differences are immediately obvious. The total calcium content and the various pools of exchangeable calcium are much larger. The cytosolic pool, for example, is approximately ten times larger. However, the major part of this pool is characterized as a high-affinity pool that is ATP dependent. The K_m for calcium uptake is 0.35 μg-atom/l, and it has all characteristics of a pool in the endoplasmic reticulum. Also, even though the mitochondrial calcium pool is ten times greater than the axon calcium pool, this is primarily due to a ten times greater content of mitochondria per unit volume, hence the amount of calcium per mg mitochondrial protein is similar. Just as in the axon, so in the nerve endings the mitochondria can accumulate calcium with a K_m in the range of 10 μg-atom/l and a threshold of 0.3 to 0.4 μg-atom/l. These studies suggest that under conditions of small increments in rate of calcium entry, the endoplasmic reticulum plays a major buffering role and that the mitochondrial are relatively unimportant, but that under conditions of higher calcium loading these organelles play a buffering role. Thus, the system for calcium homeostasis here has all the components of the squid axon plus the additional component of a high-affinity ($K = 0.35$ μA) and low-capacity (125 μg-atom) energy-dependent calcium uptake system in the endoplasmic reticulum.

A comparison of the data obtained in brain synaptosomes with those from kinetic studies of calcium exchange in liver and kidney shows surprisingly good agreement (Table 2.1). The respective sizes of the different subcellular pools are comparable. Although the cytosolic pools estimated by Borle and Uchikawa (1978) on the one hand and by Claret-Berthon et al. (1977) on the other are larger (200 to 270) than that in the synaptosomes, the former are likely to be an overestimation of the true pool because of a contribution from slowly exchangeable calcium on the cell surface. Also, the size of the total mitochondrial pool estimated by Borle and Uchikawa (1978) in the kidney is based upon the calculation that mitochondrial protein is 5% of the cell protein, whereas Foden and Randle (1978) found 50% in liver based upon total citrate synthase activity. Hence, a more reasonable value for total mitochondrial calcium in the kidney is 600 μg-atom/kg cell H_2O. On the other hand, the content of mitochondrial calcium (660 μg-atom/kg H_2O) found by Claret-Berthon et al. (1977) in perfused liver is considerably smaller than that reported by Foden and Randle (1978) in isolated liver cells (2000 μg-atom). It is likely that the higher values in these cells, isolated by enzymatic digestion in calcium-free media, are due to an increase in the calcium permeability of their plasma membrane so that upon exposure to calcium-containing media, extra calcium was taken up and largely sequestered in the mitochondria.

CYCLIC AMP AND MITOCHONDRIAL CALCIUM EXCHANGE

In terms of the major theme of this monograph, that of the interrelated roles of cAMP and calcium as synarchic messengers in stimulus–response coupling, a question of great importance is the possible role of cAMP as a regulator of mitochondrial calcium exchange. This question can be addressed by considering the larger question of the possible messenger role of calcium in three tissues—mammalian liver, mammalian kidney, and fly salivary gland, each of which responds to a particular hormone (glucagon, parathyroid hormone, and 5-hydroxytryptamine, respectively) with a rise in cAMP content (see Chapter 5 for a more detailed consideration of each of these systems). In each case, the rise in cAMP is followed by a prompt efflux of calcium from the particular cell or tissue. Since in all three tissues the efflux of calcium is also promoted by addition of exogenous cAMP (Figure 2.8), the presumption is that it is this nucleotide which mediates the hormon-

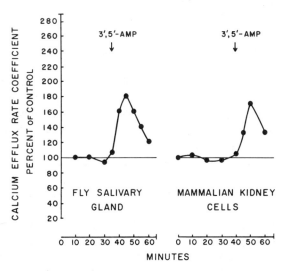

Figure 2.8 Effect of the addition of exogenous cAMP on the rate coefficient for calcium efflux in the isolated fly salivary gland and isolated mammalian kidney cells.

ally induced release of calcium. Furthermore, there is evidence in all three tissues that cAMP causes the mobilization of calcium from the mitochondrial pool.

The most direct method of analyzing this problem is that of studying the effect of cAMP addition upon calcium exchange in isolated mitochondria. This has been done. Borle (1974) reported a striking effect of cAMP on calcium efflux, but others (Scarpa et al., 1976) have been unable to reproduce these effects. Part of the difficulty is technical in that most studies have examined the effect of cAMP either on calcium uptake when rather "massive" calcium loading was taking place or calcium efflux under conditions where a reversal of the normal calcium uptake pathway contributed significantly to the total efflux.

One of the possibilities as to why no cAMP-mediated efflux is observed with isolated mitochondria is that it has been examined under the wrong experimental conditions. Juzu and Holdswork (1980) have examined one aspect of this question by exploring the effect of cAMP on calcium exchange in isolated mitochondria in which the oxidative substrate was palmitoyl CoA rather than one of the usual substrates, namely, Krebs cycle intermediate. The rationale for this approach was the observation by Lehinger et al. (1978a,b) that the redox state of the pyridine nucleotides in the mitochondria control Ca^{2+} release from these organelles. Juzu and Holdsworth (1980) reported that addition of 38 to 85 μM cAMP caused a significant release of calcium from isolated liver mitochondria incubated with palmitoyl CoA as substrate, but not from similar mitochondria incubated with succinate as substrate. These findings are of considerable interest, but their physiological significance is still not clear because of the high concentrations of cAMP required to produce these effects.

A reexamination of this question and the new observations using the approach pioneered by Nicholls are needed before it can be concluded that cAMP has no effect on mitochondrial calcium exchanges in the isolated organelle. This is particularly the case since careful studies of calcium exchange in isolated tissues or tissue culture cells provide strong evidence that cAMP does, in fact, alter mitochondrial calcium exchange (Foden and Randle, 1978; Borle and Uchikawa, 1978). The most detailed of these studies has been conducted by Borle and Uchikawa (1978) employing isolated mammalian kidney cells grown in tissue culture. These cells retain their responsiveness to the peptide parathyroid hormone (PTH).

Borle and Uchikawa (1978) have shown that addition of either PTH or cAMP leads to marked increase in the rate of calcium efflux from both mitochondrial and cytosolic pools of these cells. A comparison of their data with those summarized by Brinley (Table 2.1) reveals a number of interesting differences. First, the calcium content of the naked (glycocalyx removed) kidney cell is 500 μmol/kg, compared to 50 mol/kg in the squid axon. In the kidney cell, the mitochondrial pool represents 40% rather than 20% of total intracellular calcium. After addition of PTH, there is a threefold increase in total cell calcium, a fourfold increase in cytosolic-exchangeable pool, and a 40-fold increase in the exchangeable pool of the mitochondria. Similarly, after 10^{-7} M cAMP, there is a 1.2-fold increase in total cell calcium, a 1.5-fold increase in the cytosolic exchangeable pool, and a fourfold increase in the mitochondrial exchangeable pool. Furthermore, if cells are prelabeled with ^{45}Ca and then either PTH or cAMP is added, an increase is seen in the rate of calcium efflux into an EGTA-containing, no-calcium medium—a situation under which an enhanced entry of calcium into the cell cannot contribute to the increase in the mobilization of labeled calcium from the cell.

The point of interest is that after hormone or cAMP addition, there is an increase in calcium exchange across the mitochondrial membrane and an increase in the exchangeable pool within the mitochondria. These data leave little doubt that cAMP influences mitochondrial calcium exchange. The problem is that of defining the nature and significance of this effect. One can envision at least four possibilities: (1) the effect of cAMP is mediated at the level of the plasma membrane; (2) cAMP influences the calcium binding properties of a component in the cytosol; (3) cAMP influences calcium exchange across the mitochondrial membrane; or (4) cAMP alters the distribution of calcium between an ionic and nonionic compartment within the mitochondrial matrix space (Figure 2.9).

In considering the first possibility, the kinetic data are consistent with cAMP stimulating calcium efflux at the plasma membrane. However, if this were the case one would expect a fall in total cell calcium not a rise. Furthermore, in isolated renal tubules, when cAMP is added there is a calcium-dependent increase in gluconeogenesis and not the inhibition one would expect if cytosolic calcium ion concentration fell (see chapter 5).

In considering the second possibility, the difficulty is that of defining the nature of this rapidly exchangeable cytosolic pool. It is not possible at present to know whether or not this pool also includes the endoplasmic reticulum (ER), but it is probable that it does, in analogy with the situation in synaptosomes (Table 2.1). The endoplasmic reticulum in kidney has been shown capable of accumulating calcium, but the capacity of this system is not known. If we assume that it represents 80% of the total cytosolic pool in the resting kidney cell, the content of this pool is 150 μg-atom. Hence, the

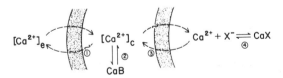

Figure 2.9   Possible sites at which an increase in the cAMP content of the cell could cause an increase in the efflux of calcium from the cell: (1) by stimulating the calcium pump in the plasma membrane; (2) by altering the properties of a cytosolic calcium buffering system; (3) by increasing the efflux of calcium from the mitochondrial matrix space; or (4) by changing the properties of the intramitochondrial buffer system.

"true" cytosolic pool in the resting cell would be of the order of 70 μmol/kg, and in the hormonally activated cell it would be in the range of 150 μmol/kg. If we further assume that this is nearly all normally bound to ligands in two buffer systems (in analogy with the situation in the squid axons), that the high-affinity system is the one of major importance, and that its total binding capacity is in the range of 150 μmol/kg, then its K_D would be approximately 0.11 μM if the concentration of the ionic calcium in the resting cell was 0.1 μM ($Ca^{2+} + B \rightleftharpoons CaB$). If cAMP influenced this system so that the K_D of B for calcium was increased to 1.1 μM, then the cytosolic calcium ion content would rise to approximately 1.0 μM. If this occurred, then the rate of calcium uptake into the mitochondria and the rate of calcium efflux across the plasma membrane would both increase. These changes would tend to cause cytosolic calcium ion to fall, but it has been shown that a rise in cytosolic calcium ion concentration *per se* increases the influx of calcium into the cell. If this calcium-dependent calcium influx occurred, it might be sufficient to compensate for the increase in cellular efflux, and thus maintain a new higher steady state calcium ion concentration in the cell cytosol with an increased cycling of mitochondrial calcium. However, because the mitochondria represent such a major calcium sink, it is not at all clear how a new steady state with a higher free calcium ion concentration could be maintained by this mechanism alone.

The third possibility would involve the net movement of calcium from the mitochondria to the cell cytosol. If there was a net movement of 70 μmol of the calcium out of the mitochondria and the K_D of the cytosol buffer did not change, then the calcium ion content of the cell cytosol would rise from 0.1 to 1.54 μM. Hence, a relatively major shift in calcium out of the mitochondria would be necessary in order to influence cytosolic calcium ion concentration. Even if we assume that the cytosolic buffer sysytem is half the above values, the net mitochondrial calcium efflux would be in the order of 35 μmol/kg. This should lead to a reduction in mitochondrial pool size rather than the expected increase. However, as noted previously, it has been shown in several cells that a rise in cytosolic calcium ion concentration *per se increases* the rate of calcium influx into the cell. Hence, a small release of mitochondrial calcium may trigger calcium entry and lead to a sustained entry of calcium into the cell. It is important to emphasize that the data of Borle and Uchikawa (1978) are from cells studied in steady state. In contrast, Foden and Randle (1978) measured the magnitude of the shift of calcium out of the mitochondria after glucagon administration under non-steady state conditions and found a shift of from 100 to 500 μmol depending upon which of two methods was used to measure the shift. Clearly, a shift of this magnitude would be sufficient to raise the cytosolic calcium ion concentration sufficiently to be of physiological significance. If other changes in cellular calcium metabolism took place as a consequence, it is possible that when this new steady state is achieved, the exchangeable calcium pool in the mitochondria would be increased rather than decreased.

The fourth possibility to be considered is that cAMP causes a shift of nonionic to ionic calcium in the mitochondrial matrix space. This would be operationally equivalent to the second possibility and would confront one with the same problems of mobilizing enough calcium to influence the calcium ion content of the cytosolic pool.

At present, there is an unresolved discrepancy between studies of the effect of cAMP on calcium exchange in isolated mitochondria and the effect of cAMP upon mitochondrial calcium exchange assessed indirectly by kinetic analyses of this event in the intact cell. The cellular data are impressive, and supporting data from other cellular systems are discussed in subsequent sections of this monograph. The logic of these data is that cAMP influences calcium exchange between cytosol and mitochondria in many cells, but the mechanism of its action remains unknown.

SODIUM ION AND MITOCHONDRIAL CALCIUM EXCHANGE

Any discussion of the role of the factors that are involved in coupling excitation to possible release of mitochondrial or intracellular calcium would be incomplete without a discussion of the possible role of sodium ion. This is particularly relevant to a discussion of the calcium coupling function in the secretory response of the exocrine pancrease (see Chapter 6). Two points about this system are worth noting. First, calcium derived largely from an intracellular pool is the factor coupling excitation to response. Second, the mobilization of calcium from this pool is *not* brought about by a change in the cAMP content of the cell.

The nature of this pool, whether mitochondrial or microsomal, is not known. Several possibilities exist. If it were microsomal, then some type of coupling between the changes in ionic currents of the plasma membrane and a depolarization of the endoplasmic reticulum could lead to a release of calcium, that is, in analogy with the situation in muscle. In pancreatic cells, the addition of veratridine leads to an increase in Na^+ permeability which in turn enhances secretion. Based upon the observation that Na^+ stimulates Ca^{2+} efflux from mitochondria in certain tissues, these data have been taken as evidence that the mitochondrial pool is the one involved.

This interpretation has to be questioned because Blaustein (1978) has shown that the uptake of Ca^{2+} by the presumed microsomal system in the synaptosomes is also Na^+ sensitive. Therefore, the effect of Na^+ might equally well be to increase release of Ca^{2+} from the microsomal as from the mitochondrial pool. Nevertheless, Crompton et al. (1978), Nicholls (1978b), and Nicholls and Stone (1980) have shown that in certain types of mitochondria (adipocyte, heart, pancreatic exocrine cell, but not liver), a small rise in Na^+ concentration increases the efflux rate of Ca^{2+} considerably (Figure 2.10). At present, it is not possible to decide whether the change in the

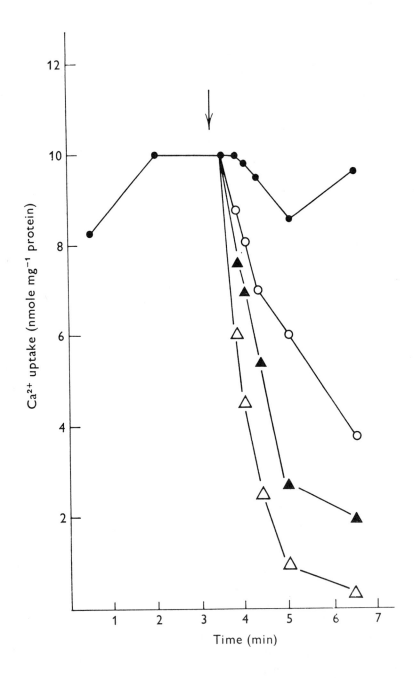

Figure 2.10 Release of accumulated calcium in rat heart mitochondria by the addition of Na⁺. At the time indicated by the arrow, ruthenium red was added to block further calcium uptake and then either 0 (●), 0.005 (0), 0.01 (▲), or 0.05 *M* (△) NaCl was added. From Carafoli and Crompton (1976), with permission.

intracellular Na⁺ concentration after cell stimulation in a cell such as cardiac muscle is sufficient to alter Ca²⁺ efflux from mitochondria.

THE CONTROL RANGE OF CALCIUM

Based on the foregoing discussion, it is evident that there is a very narrow range of calcium ion concentration in the cell cytosol over which this ion functions in information transfer. One way to place limits on this range is that of plotting the activities of the various membrane pumps as a function of $p\text{Ca}^{2+}$ (Figure 2.11). This plot shows that, given any reasonable capacity of these pumps, the concentration range over which cytosolic calcium ion operates is probably at most from a $p\text{Ca}^{2+}$ of 7 to 5 (0.1 to 10 μM). It is likely that only under extreme circumstances does the concentration rise above this value, and it is likely that under most circumstances the range is from 0.2 to 1.2 μM, that is, no more than a sixfold change in concentration. A plot of known calcium-activated processes as a function of the calcium ion concentration shows that most fall within this range. Furthermore, all go from essentially inactive to fully active over a five- to eightfold change in calcium ion concentration. From these data one could predict that a concentration of 0.5 to 0.8 μM is probably achieved in most cells when activated under physiological circumstances. This means that under physiological circumstances the control range in most cells involves no more than a fivefold change in calcium ion concentration.

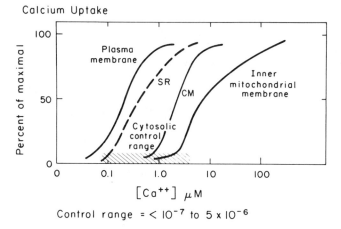

Figure 2.11 Definition of the calcium control range. The rates of calcium uptake by the plasma membrane, the sarcoplasmic reticulum (SR), and the inner mitochondrial membrane as a function of the free Ca²⁺ concentration in the cytosol. In metabolically active tissues the capacity of the mitochondrial uptake system is large so the properties of this membrane transport system and that in the plasma membrane define the control range within which cytosolic calcium can regulate cell function. Also plotted is the calcium binding curve for calmodulin (CM). Note that this falls within the cytosolic control range (the shaded bar).

CELLULAR CALCIUM HOMEOSTASIS AND
CALCIUM TOXICITY

Considerable attention has been given to the question of why calcium has become the universal messenger in eukaryote cells. Some arguments have been advanced in support of the concept that it is the unique atomic and chemical properties of this cation which explain its role (Gillard, 1970). However, if one views the problem from an evolutionary perspective, it would seem most unlikely that purely structural or chemical properties are of primary importance. A compound or agent that is to serve a messenger function need have only four attributes: (1) its concentration can be regulated rather precisely; (2) it is capable of interacting with functional groups on proteins; (3) mechanisms exist for causing both its increase and decrease within the cellular compartment in which it functions; and (4) during evolution, the potential existed for any given protein or family of proteins to develop specific binding sites for the simplest of ions to the most complex of macromolecules.

Seen from this perspective, the important historical fact is that when living organisms first developed, the calcium content of the primordial sea was quite low. Life developed in a sea rich in Mg^{2+} and K^+. Our legacy from this original sea is the high K^+ and Mg^{2+} content of our intracellular fluids. As time passed, the calcium content of this sea increased. At some point this content was sufficient to disrupt the primitive metabolic pathways which had evolved by employing various phosphate esters, including ATP, as the basis for chemical group transfer. The challenge was that of either adopting an entirely new set of metabolic chemistry other than the phosphate bond or of excluding calcium from the intracellular domain. The latter was the chosen solution. The threat of calcium toxicity was met by the evolution of mechanisms for keeping the calcium ion content of the cellular fluids quite low. The mechanisms for achieving this included the development of plasma membranes that were relatively impermeable to calcium ion, so that the rate of entry into the cell interior was slow, and had one or more systems for actively extruding calcium from the cell.

One can imagine that initially these primitive mechanisms were not perfect, so that with time some cells accumulated toxic and eventually lethal amounts of calcium. Therefore, a cell more efficient in excluding and/or extruding calcium obtained a selective advantage, survived longer, and reproduced more often.

Each major adaptive step in evolution represented not only a challenge to be met but an opportunity to be exploited. The calcium survival system was no exception. This system, which evolved to protect the cell, led eventually to the establishment of a large calcium gradient across the plasma membrane. A gradient could be and was utilized as a means of transmitting information from the cell surface to the cell interior in response to external stimuli. We recognize as one of the most primitive of these systems the calcium-mediated avoidance response of the unicellular paramecium to a mechanical stimulus. During the fashioning of this coupling system, the calcium-sensitive receptor proteins, the intracellular receiver of the calcium message, appeared. The elements of a universal system for coupling stimulus to response were born. They have survived to be exploited again and again in one fashion or another so as to couple a particular stimulus in a specific cell to the unique response of that cell.

It is this universal system which is presently under discussion. However, the demands of this system on the mechanisms for maintaining cellular calcium homeostasis have not yet been fully considered. These demands are, on the one hand, that calcium ions can be employed to couple stimulus to response and in the process allow larger quantities of calcium to enter the cell and, on the other hand, that the cell must protect itself from the toxic or detrimental effects of taking up this additional calcium.

The dimensions of this problem can be illustrated by considering the mammalian heart and its response to β-adrenergic agonists. These compounds, when acting on the heart, induce both an increase in rate and in strength of contraction—a chronotropic and an inotropic response (Tsein, 1977).

Most attention has been directed to the events underlying the inotropic response (see Chapter 9). Two possibilities as to its mechanism can be considered based on our present understanding of the contractile cycle. Upon initiation of a cardiac action potential, there is an influx of a small amount of calcium into the cell. This "trigger" calcium in some way causes the release of additional calcium from the sarcoplasmic reticulum. It is this latter pool of calcium which provides the bulk of the calcium that interacts with troponin C and provokes the contractile response. In order for an increase in strength of contraction to occur, one of two mechanisms must operate: (1) the calcium sensitivity of the troponin–tropomyosin–actinomyosin complex must increase so that the same calcium signal causes a greater response; (2) there is an increased amount of calcium released per beat in the stimulated heart. Present evidence favors the latter view. Of particular importance is a net increase in total calcium content of the heart muscle cell after hormone administration. This means that the hormone induces a net increase in calcium uptake into the cell. Part of this is taken up into the sarcoplasmic reticulum where it is released at the time of the next systole and is therefore the proximate cause of the increased strength of contraction. A portion of the calcium is also taken up by the mitochondria where, as far as we know, it does not serve in the control of the cardiac contractile cycle. The striking observation is that within a few minutes of the removal of the β-agonist from a stimulated heart, the heart rate and force of contraction return to the pretreatment values, but the total calcium content of the cell remains elevated for several hours before returning gradually to pretreatment values. During this period, the excess calcium is probably located largely within the mitochondrial compartment.

The key point is that in a heart containing two to three times its normal content of calcium, a calcium-regulated, cyclic process functions in the same way as it does in a heart containing far less total calcium. Yet with time, this calcium-loaded, normally functioning cell is able to divest itself of a significant amount of calcium without interfering with the calcium-dependent contractile cycle. Finally, if one analyzes the heart several hours after hormone treatment, its calcium has returned to precisely its basal value.

A key question to which there is no answer yet is how this precise control of calcium homeostasis is achieved. Exactly how does the cell monitor total intracellular calcium so that it is constant even though it exists in several separate subcellular compartments and exists in both ionic and nonionic forms within each of these compartments.

The importance of this question is evident if we consider what happens in the heart of a rat exposed to high concentrations of isoproterenol (Fleckenstein, 1971, 1974, 1977; Hanforth, 1962; Rona et al., 1959). In this case, there is a marked increase in the calcium content of the heart cell and a positive inotropic response. For some time, the heart continues to operate in this new physiological steady state even though there is a progressive increase in intracellular calcium, a large part of which is found within the mitochondria. Eventually, the capacity of these organelles to sequester this calcium burden is exceeded. Cell dysfunction supervenes, and the animal dies from heart failure due to a calcified heart. This sequence can be prevented by preventing the β-agonist-induced increase in cardiac calcium accumulation with drugs such as Verapamil or D-600 (α-isopropyl-α[(N-methyl-N-homo-renatryl)-α-aminopropyl]3,4,5-trimethoxyphenyl acetonitrile hydrochloride) that block the voltage-dependent calcium channel in the plasma membranes of the heart cells.

Clearly, too much calcium is lethal to the heart cell. Equally clearly, the mitochondria play an essential role in protecting these cells from calcium overload, whether on a short-term or long-term basis. So together, plasma membrane and inner mitochondrial membrane define the limits of cytosolic calcium ion concentration but, in addition, coordinate their activities to maintain cellular calcium homeostasis and with this accomplishment allow the calcium messenger system to function regardless of the total calcium load of the cell over a wide range of total calcium content.

The more general question raised by these data is the role of calcium accumulation in cell death and aging. It appears likely that a common mechanism of cell death is calcium intoxication (Schanne et al., 1979). For example, in the case of patients with Duchenne's muscular dystrophy, the universal finding is that of a marked increase in the calcium content of the muscle. At this point in our knowledge, it is not possible to decide whether this is the initial disorder of cellular function or a consequence of some other initial event. But as the disease progresses, the calcium content of muscle increases, as does the degree of muscle dysfunction. Likewise, in the case of carbon tetrachloride poisoning, a most dramatic change in the cellular content of calcium is found associated with the dramatic changes in hepatocyte function and number.

These various lines of recent evidence all emphasize three features of cellular calcium metabolism. The first is that normally not only the individual fluxes but their integration and balance control total cellular calcium content. The second is that a breakdown of cellular calcium homeostasis leads to a progressive increase in cellular calcium content and eventually to cell dysfunction or death. Third, the mitochondria play a major role as the calcium sink not only in modulating the short-term changes in cytosolic calcium ion concentration that take place during the usual events of stimulus–response coupling but also in protecting the cell during periods of sustained calcium accumulation.

In examining the possibility that calcium serves a second messenger function in stimulus–response coupling, it would be useful to establish a set of criteria similar to those developed by Sutherland and coworkers in the case of cAMP. These should include (1) an increase in calcium ion content within the cell cytosol; (2) addition of other less specific agents known to cause an increase in cell calcium to mimic the first messenger's actions; (3) agents known to inhibit uptake of calcium by intracellular organelles to enhance the response to submaximal concentrations of hormone; (4) a direct effect of hormone on calcium gating in the plasma membrane demonstrable at least in those tissues in which extracellular calcium appears to be the source of the calcium message; (5) the presence of calmodulin and/or calcium calmodulin-mediated effects on isolated membranes or enzymes.

Unfortunately, it is difficult to fulfill all of these criteria in most systems. Aside from studies in a few large cells, direct measurement of cytosolic calcium ion concentration has not yet been possible. Indirect estimates have been obtained by changes in the activity of calcium-sensitive enzymes; in the calcium-sensitive changes in membrane resistance; or by measuring the uptake of ^{3}H-Stelazine (trifluoperazine dihydrochloride) and equating this to an increase in Ca·calmodulin concentration and thus indirectly to a rise in calcium ion concentration. Two nonspecific ways of increasing calcium uptake by cells are (1) a depolarization of the membrane produced by high K^+ which increases Ca^{2+} entry into many different cells and (2) addition of a divalent ionophore. Of the various ionophores employed, A23187 has been used most successfully (Reed and Lardy, 1972). Its use is not, however, without problems. Three at least are of significance. First, the ionophore does not localize exclusively in the plasma membrane but is also taken up into intracellular membrane so that the Ca^+ fluxes into and out of various subcellular compartments are altered to different degrees in different cell types. This characteristic plus the fact that these agents may bring about marked changes in Ca^{2+} concentrations within the cell lead to the second problem—that of the changes in cytosolic calcium ion exceeding the control range of calcium and leading thereby to many deleterious effects on cell function. The third problem also relates to the first. Even if one obtains evidence using the ionophore—that calcium may play a messenger role in a particular response—one can conclude very little about the physiological source of calcium in stimulus–response coupling.

One of the greatest needs in the study of cellular calcium metabolism is for better tools to dissect out, within an intact cell, the respective roles of different subcellular compartments in the overall regulation of calcium metabolism in different functional states of the cell. This includes, in particular, methods for assessing the respective contribution of different cellular and the extracellular Ca^{2+} pools to the change in the concentration of calcium ion within the cytosol of a stimulated cell. No specific agents have yet been found that will inhibit either the influx or efflux pathways of Ca^{2+} in either microsomes or mitochondria *in situ*. The group of drugs of which Verapamil is the prototype have some usefulness as relatively specific blockers of voltage-dependent Ca^{2+} channels (Fleckenstein, 1974) in a variety of cell types, but they are not universally specific in blocking plasma membrane Ca^{2+} channels (Jensen and Rasmussen, 1977).

This problem is further complicated by the fact that an experimental manipulation, such as addition of the calcium ionophore A23187, may cause a calcium-dependent stimulation of cell function, and thus confirm the results from less direct methods concerning a messenger role of calcium in that particular cellular response, but provide no meaningful information concerning the source of calcium for stimulus–response coupling under physiological circumstances. Conversely, there are systems in which physiological data indicate that Ca^{2+} serves a messenger function in stimulus–response coupling but that do not respond when A23187 is applied to the cell, probably because in these cases specific intracellular Ca^{2+} domains are involved in coupling and A23187 addition leads to a general increase in cytosolic Ca^{2+} content.

Another approach is that of defining some biochemical counterpart of the process of Ca^{2+} flux. There is some evidence relating calcium entry across the plasma membrane in many tissues to a change in phosphoinositide turnover (see Chapter 3). However, the evidence is still far from complete, which means there is no simple marker relating changes in Ca^{2+} permeability to biochemical events in the plasma membrane as there is in the case of hormone-sensitive adenylate cyclases in the cAMP system. The only biochemical criterion that is relatively easy to fulfill is establishing the presence of calmodulin in various tissues. However, this helps only in the sense that to date it has been discovered in every tissue examined.

The difficulties outlined above are a major reason why the unraveling of the messenger function of Ca^{2+} has not been developed with the rapidity that has characterized the sequence of defining the messenger function of cAMP. However, using indirect methods such as those mentioned plus studies of calcium kinetics in intact cells and isolated organelles, the redistribution of calcium as measured by cell fractionation methods, and a variety of markers of a change in Ca^{2+} activity (*e.g.*, an increase in K^+ permeability of the plasma membrane), it has been possible to deduce the relative changes in Ca^{2+} activity within the cell cytosol. These qualitative assessments of changes in cytosolic Ca^{2+} have proved to be quite accurate when verified by more direct measurement in tissues where that has proven possible.

CONCLUSION

The recent advances in our understanding of cellular calcium metabolism have been of considerable importance in advancing our understanding of the complex way in which Ca^{2+} serves its messenger function in a given cell. Much of the information discussed in this chapter is rediscussed and reevaluated during the analysis of the role of calcium in coupling specific extracellular stimuli to particular cellular responses.

3

Information Flow in Stimulus–Response Coupling

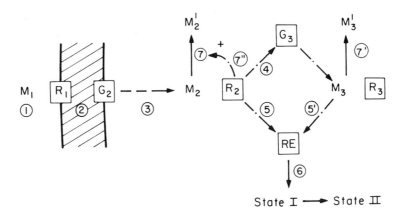

State I ⟶ State II

INTRODUCTION

A particularly instructive approach to an analysis of the properties of the cellular control systems under discussion is that of considering them primarily as systems that convey information. The focus of discussion are those hormones and neurotransmitters that alter cell function by a primary interaction with the plasma membrane and induce the cell to perform its specialized function. These agents operate as initiators of an information transfer system in which information flows from the cell surface to the cell interior and therby alters cell behavior. Viewed in this context, one can identify at least seven steps in the information transfer process: (1) *recognition* of the external signal by a receptor on the cell surface and its *coupling* to a transducing element; (2) *transduction* of this signal within the membrane into a new intracellular signal; (3) *transmission* and propagation of this signal within the cell cytosol; (4) *intracellular reception* by specific receptor proteins; (5) *modulation* of the activity of cell proteins by the signal receptor element; (6)

response of one or more elements or systems within the cell achieved as a consequence of step 5; and (7) *termination* of the signal so as to limit either its temporal and/or spacial domains (Rasmussen and Clayberger, 1979).

In the following discussion, the known aspects of each of these seven components for each of the major signaling systems are discussed. A summary of their main features is given in Table 3.1.

RECOGNITION AND RECEPTOR COUPLING

Within the first step, recognition, one can distinguish two aspects: the site on the cell surface, the *receptor,* with which the extracellular messenger interacts; and the other components within the membrane to which this receptor is *coupled.* How this coupling leads to the generation of the intracellular

Table 3.1   Characteristics of the Cyclic AMP and Calcium Information Transfer Systems

Step	Calcium System	cAMP System
1a. Recognition	Membrane receptor	Membrane receptor
1b. Coupling	Direct via coupling to Ca channel	Direct intramembrane coupling to cyclase.
	Indirect via in membrane potential	Indirect via calcium activation
2. Transduction	Calcium gate-Pi turnover; unknown second messenger	Adenylate cyclase
3. Transmission	Diffusion of message and/or receptor protein	Diffusion of message and/or receptor protein
4. Receptor	Calmodulin Troponin C Leiotonin Parvalbumin Synexin	cAMP receptor proteins
5. Modulation	Association Regulatory subunit for multi-subunit enzyme	Dissociation
6. Response	Protein kinases Ca/Mg ATPase Ion channels Microtubule assembly Actomyosin contraction	Protein kinases
7. Termination	Calcium pump Plasma membrane ER Mitochondria Vesicles	PDE Cytosolic I II Membrane bound

messenger is covered under the term *transduction,* to be discussed subsequently.

The concept of a surface receptor was introduced by Paul Erlich near the turn of the century to explain cellular events in the immune system. As employed by him, the major focus was upon the receptors as sites of recognition on the cell surface. The term has come to mean structures in or on the cell surface that have the capacity of recognize specific chemical signals and to initiate a chain of events that leads to a change in cell function. Specific recognition is not sufficient to define a receptor, because specific recognition is also involved in the case of surface enzymes such as acetylcholine esterase whose function is to degrade acetylocholine without generating an intracellular message.

In the case of hormones, it was not until 1937 that Clark presented a theory of hormone action which included the concept of a hormone receptor as that part of the cell with which the hormone interacted. Although not excluding intracellular receptor sites, Clark's view was that in many cases the hormone receptor was located on the cell surface, a view which, in the case of peptide and amine hormones, has only recently been substantiated.

As noted previously, the common mode of synaptic transmission is chemical. A small class of substances—acetylcholine, adrenaline, noradrenaline, dopamine, serotonin, and a few other small molecules—are recognized as neurotransmitters. These substances are released from presynaptic termini and diffuse across the synaptic cleft to interact with specific receptors on the plasma membrane of the postsynaptic neuron. Similarly, in hormonal control systems, the hormone, whether amine, small peptide, or complex glycoprotein, interacts with a specific receptor on the plasma membrane of its target cell. In both cases there is an extremely high degree of molecular complementarity between hormone and receptor.

In actuality, there are two kinds of surface recognition sites for many of these agents: one a true receptor involved in coupling stimulus to response, the other an acceptor site involved in the inactivation of the hormone or neurotransmitter. The latter is, in fact, the first mechanism involved in terminating the response (see below).

In considering the receptors for the common neurotransmitters acetylcholine and epinephrine, two specific types of true receptors have been discovered for each of these transmitters. In the case of acetylcholine, these are known as the nicotinic and muscarinic receptors; in the case of epinephrine, they are known as alpha and beta receptors. In both cases, in addition to exhibiting recognition sites for different parts of the neurotransmitter molecule, the two types of receptors are generally coupled to different transducing elements within the membrane or have opposing effects on the same transducing element.

Acetylcholine Receptor (Nicotinic Type)

Given the high degree of specificity and sensitivity exhibited by receptors, there is only one class of macromolecule—proteins—that is likely to serve in this capacity. As yet, a hormone receptor protein has not been completely characterized, but the nicotinic acid type of acetylcholine receptor has been (Menez et al., 1971; Weill et al., 1974; Nichel and Potter, 1973; Broches et al., 1976; Changeux et al., 1967, 1969, 1970, 1971, 1976; Chang, 1974; Barrantes 1975, 1979; Eldefraw et al., 1971; Fambrough and Hartzell, 1972; Hazelbaser and Changeux, 1974; Karlin, 1974; Meunier et al., 1974; Michaelson and Raftery, 1974; Patrick and Lindstrom, 1973; Reed et al., 1975; Schmidt and Raftery, 1973). The acetylcholine receptor is an oligomeic protein of M.W. approximately 100,000. It is an integral membrane protein and is coupled to a Na^+ channel. This channel is normally closed; but when acetylcholine interacts with the channel, it opens for a short time, that is, the complex shifts from the resting state to the active state (Figure 3.1). However, by a slower reaction, acetylcholine induces a shift of the complex to a desensitized state in which agonist binds but does not cause channel opening. It seems likely that two molecules of acetylcholine are necessary to activate one channel. The most interesting attribute of these receptor–channel complexes is that under physiological circumstances with maximal concentrations of neurotransmitters being released, only about 0.4% of the total number of ion channels in the synapses is open at any one time.

In confirmation of Langley's earlier conclusion, the distribution of acetylcholine receptors on muscle cells is nonuniform (Changeux et al., 1976; Barrantes, 1979). There are an estimated 20,000 to 30,000 receptors/μm^2 at the neuromuscular junction and 50/μm^2 on the cell surface a few (15) micrometers away. Of interest is that after denervation of the muscle cell, this nonuniform distribution disappears and the number of receptors per unit

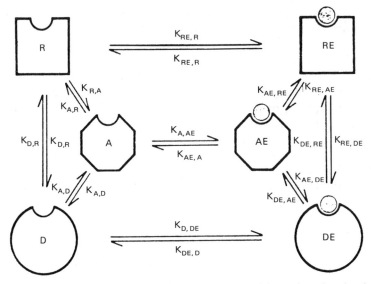

Figure 3.1 Schematic model of the acetylcholine receptor and its various functional states. From Changeux et al. (1976), with permission.

area increases and is rather uniform over the entire cell surface (Bourgeois et al., 1973). This finding implies that receptor distribution is controlled by the nerve endings of the afferent nerve cell.

This feature of receptor physiology is only one aspect of the dynamic nature of these macromolecules. Another is that the average lifetime of extrajunctional receptors in the membrane is on the order of 20 hours (Broches et al., 1976). Hence, approximately once each day a total contingent of receptor molecules on the cell surface is replaced. This turnover of receptors involves some type of internalization of the old receptors and *de novo* synthesis of new ones rather than a recycling of the same proteins.

Although it is assumed that other receptors for acetylcholine (muscarinic type) and receptors for other neurotransmitters are of similar nature much less work has been done to isolate and characterize them. The only other one in which considerable progress has been made is in the case of the β-adrenergic receptor, but because this compound can be considered as a hormone and because it is universally coupled to adenylate cyclase, its properties are discussed in the succeeding section.

In terms of our major interest, the question is whether either type of acetylcholine receptor is *coupled* to either adenylate cyclase and/or the calcium messenger systems. In nearly all cases the activation of the nicotinic type of receptor leads to a change in ion transport across the plasma membrane. There is no substantial evidence that a direct coupling of nicotininc receptors to adenylate cyclase exists. However, under special circumstances an indirect coupling may be seen. This is the case in the adrenal medulla, in which acetylcholine leads to a stimulation of catecholamine release mediated by an entry of calcium into the cell. A secondary consequence of acetylcholine action is a rise in cAMP. It is probable that this results from a calcium–calmodulin activation of cyclase secondary to the acetylcholine-induced entry of calcium into the cell. The adenylate cyclase in many neural tissues, in the endocrine pancreas, and in the adrenal cortex is a calcium–calmodulin-activated enzyme. In some of these cases, the primary messenger is the entry of calcium into the cell. This, in turn, raises the content of the calcium–calmodulin complex leading to the activation of the cyclase. Hence, in every sense, cAMP is a third (or even fourth, see below) rather than second messenger in this type of system. In other cases, the situation may be even more complex, with the calcium (or some other ionic messenger) giving rise to the release of adenosine from the cell which, in turn, interacts with a surface receptor to activate the cyclase.

The acetylcholine receptor (nicotinic type) is commonly, if not universally, associated with the calcium messenger systems, although in nearly all cases the coupling is indirect. Two examples will suffice to validate this statement: the release of catecholamines from the adrenal medulla and the initiation of an action potential in a motor neuron.

In the case of the adrenal medullary chromaffin cells, the neurotransmitter that evokes a secretory response is acetylcholine (see Chapter 9). Interaction of acetylcholine with its receptor leads to an influx of Na^+. As a consequence, the membrane is depolarized. This leads to a change in the rate of calcium entry into the cell through a relatively specific calcium channel in the plasma membrane. Other manipulations, for example, an increase in extracellular K^+ also evokes secretion independent of Ach. This K^+-evoked secretion, just like Ach-evoked secretion, is due to a membrane depolarization and a voltage-dependent increase in Ca^{2+} influx into the cell. Presently, there is no evidence for a direct relationship between the Ach receptors and this calcium channel. Yet in an operational sense, Ach initiates the flow of information in the calcium messenger system in this cell.

The situation in the motor neuron is similar. In this case, release of acetylcholine at the presynaptic terminus of a synapse leads to the generation of an action potential initiated by the same Na^+ influx and depolarization (Ulbricht, 1977) of the plasma membrane of a motor neuron. However, in the motor neuron, this depolarization leads to the generation of an action potential which passes down the axon and causes a depolarization of the membrane of the presynaptic terminus. This depolarization leads to the opening of the same type of calcium channel in the membrane of this presynaptic terminus as occurs in the chromaffin cell and initiates secretion of neurotransmitter at this site. Hence, again, even though there is a considerable spatial separation between the location of the Ach receptor and the calcium channels responsible for controlling neurotransmitter release, the Ach serves to initiate the flow of information in the calcium messenger system in this cell just as in the chromaffin cell.

Although a general feature of chemical synapses, this indirect means of activating the calcium messenger system is not confined to the action of neurotransmitters in the nervous system. A similar voltage-dependent calcium channel is seen in other tissues such as the β-cells of the endocrine pancreas and the osteoclasts, and in smooth and cardiac muscle. In the case of the pancreas, a metabolite of glucose activates this channel indirectly by causing an initial change in membrane K^+ permeability (see Chapter 6).

In the heart, epinephrine is believed to enhance the effect of membrane depolarization on the voltage-dependent calcium channel. This enhancement is not a result of direct coupling of receptor to this channel, nor does it occur indirectly as a consequence of a membrane depolarization. Rather, it appears to result from a cAMP-dependent phosphorylation of a component of this calcium channel which leads to the channel remaining open for a longer period of during following membrane depolarization. Similarly, cAMP modifies the behavioral of this channel in certain presynaptic termini (see Chapter 6). These results mean that the properties of this channel, in different cell types, can be regulated both by ionic (electrical) and chemical means.

Acetylcholine receptors of the muscarinic type are common in smooth muscle. Their activation, just as that of the nicotinic type, usually leads to a change in the ion permeabilities of the plasma membrane (Bolton, 1979), and to an increased entry of calcium into the cell. This may occur by one of several mechanisms. The first is by a voltage-dependent calcium channel as described above; the second is by a decrease in Na^+_0–Ca^{2+}_i exchange secondary to an increase in Na^+ entry; and the third is by a receptor-operated ion channel (ROC) which may be relatively specific for Ca^{2+} or be less selective and allow Na^+ and K^+ fluxes as well. In cells in which ROCs operate, contraction occurs without a change in membrane potential. Furthermore, the ROC can be shown to be voltage-independent.

This type of ROC appears common in nonmuscle cells but has not been well characterized. In the case of the parotid gland, α-adrenergic agonists, acetylcholine (muscarinic receptor), and substance P all induce an uptake of calcium into the tissue with little change in membrane potential. It appears that in this tissue there is a direct coupling of three different types of receptors to a relatively specific calcium channel (ROC) which is voltage independent.

Hormone Receptors

Much less is known concerning the structure of hormone receptors (Roth, 1973; Kahn, 1976; Levitzki, 1978; Catt et al., 1979). Two difficulties have hampered advances in this field. The first is that the number of receptor molecules per unit surface of target cells is small (10 to 200/μm^2); the second, that all high-affinity binding sites do not represent competent receptors. Nevertheless, the work that has been done (Kahn, 1976) indicates that hormone receptors are proteins and have the following characteristics: (1) they are integral membrane proteins; (2) they are separate from the adenylate cyclase molecule; (3) they can be coupled either to adenylate cyclase or to ion channels; (4) they may occur in patches on the cell surface; (5) their density on the cell surface varies under different physiological circumstances; (6) they are internalized; and (7) they may exist in several states.

One approach to defining receptor populations has been a pharmacological one. It involves the synthesis of a large number of structural analogs of the particular neurotransmitter or hormone and then an analysis of the effects of these analogs either as direct agonists or antagonists in the wide variety of cells responsive to the particular agonist. This type of approach has been most thoroughly developed in the case of the catecholamines.

Two distinct types of catecholamine receptors have been identified, alpha and beta. Recently the β-receptors have been subdivided into two subclasses (beta$_1$ and beta$_2$). The two major classes are distinct. There are relatively "pure" α - and β-agonists and antagonists. Thus, phenylephrine is an agonist which interacts almost exclusively with α-receptors, and phentolamine is an antagonist which interacts only with α-receptors. Conversely, isoproterenol is a nearly pure β-agonist, and propranolol is a pure β-antagonist.

With these pharmacological tools, it has been possible to explore the question of whether each class of receptors is always coupled to the same transducing system regardless of the cell type on which this receptor is found. In the case of the β-receptor, the available information would seem to provide an unequivocal answer. Occupied β-receptors always appear to couple to adenylate cyclase, and in no case is there substantial evidence that they can or do couple to a calcium gating system in the plasma membrane. On the other hand, the situation with the α-receptor is not so clear. In many tissues there is considerable circumstantial evidence showing that this receptor is coupled to the calcium channel in the plasma membrane. However, there are three major difficulties in assessing calcium channels as opposed to adenylate cyclase coupling with surface receptors.

The first is that the receptor–cyclase coupling can and has been widely studied in isolated membrane fragments. This is not yet possible with the receptor–calcium channel coupling. The second is that the sole cellular site of adenylate cyclase is the plasma membrane; hence, in studies in intact cells a rise in cAMP content can usually be considered a direct consequence of events taking place at the plasma membrane (unless, of course, the change is due to an alteration in phosphodiesterase activity, which can usually be easily determined). Conversely, in the case of calcium, a rise in intracellular (cytosolic) calcium ion content may reflect a change in net calcium flux across any of three cellular membranes: plasma membrane, inner mitochondrial membrane, and endoplasmic reticulum. The third difficulty is that there is no universally accepted biochemical correlate of calcium channel opening in the plasma membrane, so that one is restricted to a purely operational definition of this coupling in terms of an increase in calcium influx. However, since this influx may be voltage dependent in some cells and cAMP dependent in others, an influx of calcium may not be a direct but an indirect consequence of hormone–receptor interaction.

Recent studies of the interaction of phenylephrine with its receptor in the rat liver point up an additional problem. First, it is clear that under normal circumstances phenylephrine is a "pure" α-agonist. However, in isolated liver cells incubated in the absence of extracellular calcium, the interaction of phenylephrine with an α-receptor leads to an increase in cellular cAMP concentration (Chan and Exton, 1977). A similar situation has been described in both the adrenal medulla (Peach, 1972) and the exocrine pancreas with the acetylcholine receptor (Rasmussen et al., 1972). Under normal circumstances, acetylcholine causes a secretory response in each of these tissues without provoking any immediate increase in their cAMP content. However, if the tissues are incubated in calcium-free media and then exposed to acetylcholine, a significant rise in their cAMP content is seen. It has been concluded that this rise is secondary to a stimulation of adenylate cyclase. In the case of the liver, this conclusion is supported by the demonstration of a phenylephrine-induced stimulation of adenylate cyclase.

In a number of tissues, α-receptor activation appears to lead to an increase in the cytosolic calcium ion concentration. The original data suggested that this was due to an increase in the rate of calcium uptake by the tissue across the plasma membrane. However, there is now evidence that α-receptor activation may lead to a calcium-dependent activation of cytosolic processes and the mobilization of calcium from intracellular pools, even if there is little or no extracellular calcium ion. Some unidentified signal or second messenger is apparently generated at the plasma membrane and enters the cell to trigger calcium release. Hence, in some of the cells in which α-receptor activation generates an intracellular calcium signal, the situation is similar to that in different types of muscle cells. In some α-receptor-responsive cells, the major source of calcium for stimulus–response coupling is extracellular; in others, it is intracellular; and in many, it is both.

It would help simplify a complex situation if one would conclude that all α-receptors are coupled to the calcium signaling system. Unfortunately, this does not appear to be the case. A striking example is the α-receptor on the Islet of Langerhans. A large body of data (see Chapter 6) supports the concept that in the glucose-induced release of insulin from the pancreatic islet β-cell, a rise in cytosolic calcium ion concentration is the initial and primary stimulus. Under many circumstances, a rise in cytosolic cAMP acts as a supplementary stimulus. If the activation of catecholamine α-receptors on these cells were coupled positively to the calcium signaling system, then one would expect that hormone–receptor interaction would lead to a stimulation of insulin release. However, the contrary is observed. The α-agonist norepinephrine acts to inhibit glucose-induced insulin secretion. This inhibition is reversed by phentolamine but not by propranolol, which clearly establishes that the receptor mediating this effect as an α-receptor.

Furthermore, if the hormone epinephrine is added in the presence of phentolamine, then a β-effect, the activation of adenylate cyclase, is seen and insulin secretion is enhanced. There is no demonstrable direct effect of α-agonists upon calcium metabolism in this tissue. The inhibitory effect of α-agonists leads to a concomitant fall in the tissue cAMP content and in the rate of insulin secretion. The magnitude of the fall in insulin secretion correlates with the fall in cAMP content. Using cell homogenates, it is possible to demonstrate a direct inhibition of a particulate adenylate cyclase by α-agonists. These data are consistent with the concept that in this tissue the α- and β-receptors for catecholamines are both present, and both are coupled to the adenylate cyclase: one, the α-receptor, as a negative modifier; and the other, the β-receptor, as a positive modifier of the activity of this enzyme. In view of the interrelated roles of calcium and cAMP in the regulation of insulin secretion (see Chapter 6), the data are most consistent with the fact that the α-receptor is coupled only to the cyclase system and does not directly control the calcium signaling system. This is in direct contrast to the evidence in liver and other tissues where the α-receptor is coupled to the calcium signaling system and does not affect the adenylate cyclase.

Fain and Garcia-Sainz (1980) suggest a resolution to the apparent paradox that α-receptors are coupled to calcium channels in some tissues and to the adenylate cyclase in others. A large number of pharmacological studies have shown that α-adrenergic receptors can be subdivided into two groups: alpha$_1$ (α_1) and alpha$_2$ (α_2). Fain and Garcia-Sainz (1980) propose that α_1-receptors are coupled to the calcium ion channels in the plasma membrane, and that when these receptors are activated phosphoionositide turnover is increased (see below—transduction in the calcium messenger system) and that this turnover is coupled in some way to both a release of calcium from the internal surface of the plasma membrane and an increase in the calcium permeability of this membrane so that extracellular Ca^{2+} enters the cell. In contrast, α_2-receptors, when activated, are coupled to the adenylate cyclase system in the membrane, and serve to inhibit the activity of this system, thereby decreasing intracellular [cAMP]. Thus, depending upon the type of α-receptors and the absence or presence of β-receptors catecholamines can cause either an increase in intracellular $[Ca^{2+}]$ (α_1) an increase in intracellular [cAMP] (β), and/or a decrease in [cAMP] (α_2). Similar possibilities must exist for other amine hormones such as serotonin and histamine as well as for peptide hormones. No specific receptor coupled to an inhibition of plasma membrane calcium gating has been described, but one can predict that such a receptor type will be found.

Another question is whether the activation of a specific hormonal receptor has a single consequence in terms of a change in membrane function, for example, altering adenylate cyclase activity or opening a calcium channel, or whether it can bring about changes simultaneously in several membrane transducing systems.

Clearly, a number of changes in membrane function, in addition to adenylate cyclase activation, occur after glucagon or epinephrine action in the liver or other cells. These include changes in membrane potential, a change in cation permeability, an alteration in NADH dehydrogenase activity, and an alteration in phosphatidylethanolamine methyl transferases. The problem is to decide whether these are direct consequences of hormone–receptor interaction or whether they result from one of the direct effects. For example, since exogenous cAMP increases membrane potential as does glucagon in liver cells, it seems quite likely that this effect of glucagon on membrane function is not a direct one but is mediated by the induced rise in cAMP (Friedmann and Dambach, 1980). Likewise, the hormone phenylephrine brings about an increase in the membrane potential of the hepatocyte without causing an increase in cAMP; but again, this response is probably not direct but indirect, being mediated by a phenylephrine-induced increase in calcium entry into the cell (see Chapter 7).

However, at least three consequences of β-agonist–receptor interaction have been described that do not appear to be secondary to the rise in cellular cAMP concentration but must be considered as likely direct consequences of hormone receptor interaction. The first of these is a release of plasma membrane Ca^{2+} and a change in membrane fluidity and permeability of the human red cell (Allen and Rasmussen, 1971; Kury et al., 1974; Rasmussen et al., 1975; Levitzki et al., 1974). The second is a synthesis of phosphati-dyl-*N*-monomethylethanolamine and phosphatidylcholine from phosphati-dylethanolamine in the erythrocyte membrane (Hirata et al., 1970). The third is an inhibition of Mg^{2+} accumulation in intact 549 lymphoma cells (Maguire and Erdos, 1980). These observations indicate that even in this single well-characterized receptor, transduction of extracellular message into intracellular response may involve more than one membrane trans-ducer.

In the context of our present discussion, the point at issue can be more clearly defined and related strictly to the question of the generation of the calcium and cAMP messages in specific cells. There are in reality two related questions. The first is: does a hormone, for example, serotonin, acting on a tissue, for example, the fly salivary gland, in which there is clear evidence for a simultaneous stimulation of adenylate cyclase, and the opening of a calcium channel, bring about these two effects upon membrane function by interacting with one or two specific surface receptors? The second is: does the interaction of a hormone, for example, epinephrine, with a specific type of well-defined receptor, for example, alpha or beta, always bring about the same change in membrane function and hence the generation of the same second messenger in every cell type in which this particular receptor is found?

The answer to either of these questions is made difficult by the state of the art in identifying specific receptor populations. There are at present two basic approaches to this problem. The first is by an analysis of the specific binding sites on isolated membranes or intact cells with labeled hormone. The problem in defining whether there is more than one class of binding sites is twofold. First, there is always significant nonspecific binding as a compo-nent of total binding, and this component is subtracted from the total to obtain the derived parameters, namely, specific binding (Figure 3.2). This nonspecific component may represent 10 to 20% of total binding; and if, as often appears to be the case, there is a class of high-affinity, low-capacity binding sites on the cell surface, these may be obscured because of the "noise" in the system of analysis. Second, a favorite method of analyzing the binding data is the method first introduced by Scatchard and now known as a Scatchard plot.

A typical plot from studies on ACTH binding to isolated adrenal cells is shown in Figure 3.3. The data show a curvilinear distribution which can be resolved into two apparently linear components, leading to the conclusion that there are two classes of receptors for this hormone—one with a high affinity ($K_d = 2.5 \times 10^{-10}$ mol/l) and low capacity (3000 sites/cell), and the other of lower affinity ($K_d = 1 \times 10^{-8}$ mol/l). Unfortunately, the interpreta-tion of these data is not unambiguous. DeMetys et al. (1976) have shown that similar plots of binding vs bound/free sites display negative cooperativity, that is, receptor–receptor interaction; and as more and more receptors are occupied, they decrease the affinity of the remaining unoccupied receptor

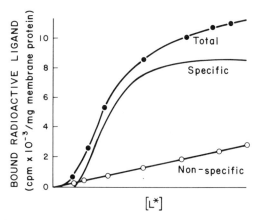

Figure 3.2   Plot of binding of labeled agonist or antagonist in the absence (●) and presence (○) of a large excess of nonlabeled agonist or antagonist as function of labeled ligand concentration [L*]. Specific binding is taken as the difference between total binding in the absence of excess cold ligand minus the nonspecific binding seen in the presence of excess cold ligand.

for hormone. These latter authors have presented methods for attempting to distinguish between the case of two distinct receptor classes vs a single class displaying negative cooperativity, but these methods have not been widely applied in the analysis of hormone binding data.

Just as was found to be true of the acetylcholine receptor (nicotinic type), so in the case of hormone receptors there is a turnover of plasma membrane

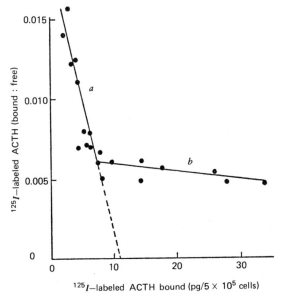

Figure 3.3   Ratio of bound (B) over free (F) labeled ACTH as function of bound hormone showing a sharp break in the curve. From McIlhinney and Schulster (1975), with permission.

receptors. In the case of the insulin receptors, progress has been made in elucidating the process of internalization (Carpentier et al., 1978; Goldfine et al., 1977; Gordon et al., 1978; Schlessinger et al., 1978; Terris and Steiner, 1975). Initially, insulin distributes rather uniformly over the cell surface; but within a short time, the aggregates appear at discrete sites on the membrane. These appear as coated pits when viewed by electron microscopy. These pits become internalized as small coated vesicles within the cytosol and migrate to the Golgi region where they appear to fuse with components of that membrane system. The exact fate of the contained insulin is not known other than the fact that it is eventually catabolized by lysomal enzymes.

A question of considerable interest is whether or not this internalized receptor–hormone complex plays a role in stimulus–response coupling. For example, when insulin acts upon a muscle cell, there are both short-term effects, for example, an increase in amino acid and glucose transport, and long-term effects, for example, increases in both glycogen and protein synthesis. Likewise, in a variety of cell systems insulin promotes cell growth and/or cell division. Logically, one might consider that the early effects of insulin are induced by binding to the receptor on the cell surface and that the long-term growth effects are induced by the internalized hormone–receptor complex.

This possibility has been tested to a limited extent in the case of insulin. It has been found that certain substituted amines when applied to the intact, insulin-responsive cell block the internalization of receptor-bound insulin but do not block the effects of insulin on glucose transport. Likewise, the methylamines enhance rather than inhibit the growth-promoting effects of insulin. On the basis of this evidence, the internalization process would not appear to be a mechanism for transferring information from cell surface to cell interior, but would appear to be concerned with the turnover and catabolism of surface-bound receptors.

The regulation of receptor number is also seen with those hormones that act on the cAMP messenger system. The most thoroughly studied is the β-adrenergic receptor for catecholamines on the nucleated erythrocyte (Lefkowitz, 1975; Lefkowitz et al., 1976; Lefkowitz and Williams, 1977; Mickey et al., 1976; Lefkowitz and Williams, 1978; Limbird and Lefkowitz, 1977, 1978; Puchwein et al., 1974). Exposure to high concentrations of isoproterenol leads to a decrease in specific hormone binding (Figure 3.4a) and to a diminution in the production of cAMP (Figure 3.4b).

These results show that the decrease in receptor number has the functional consequences of decreasing cell response as measured by cAMP production. This change in receptor number is not instantaneous but develops over several hours. Its reversal takes several hours. The change in receptor number is not associated with a decrease in the number of cyclase molecules in the membrane, as shown by the fact that fluoride-stimulated cyclase is the same in normal and desensitized cells and by the fact that in cells in which the cyclase is activated by several agonists, desensitization is confined to only the agonists used to induce the change in receptor number.

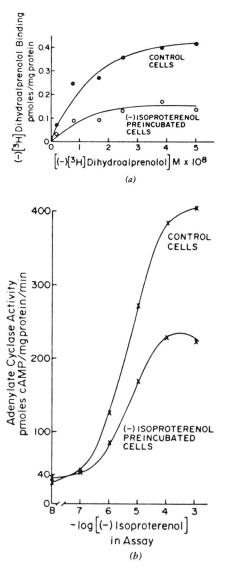

Figure 3.4 Effect of the prior exposure of frog erythrocytes to isoproterenol on their subsequent ability to bind $(-)$-$[^3H]$dihydroalprenolol (a) and to undergo adenylate cyclase activation (b) upon reexposure to isoproterenol. From Mickey et al. (1976), with permission.

Similar changes in the number of LH receptors in the ovary are seen after *in vivo* administration of a similar hormone, namely, human chorionic gonadotropin (hCG). In this case, both receptor number and total cyclase activity decreases (Catt et al., 1979). In some situations, this has been reported to lead to a decrease in steroidogenic response; in other cases, it has not been altered significantly. A number of other examples of down-regulation have been described for hormones which activate adenylate cyclase (Catt, 1979). However, down regulation does not uniformly happen. In the case of angiotensin acting on the zona glomerulosa of the adrenal cortex (Catt et al., 1979), chronic exposure to increased levels of circulating hormone induced by Na^+ deprivation leads to an increase in the number of angiotensin receptors on the cell surface (Figure 3.5). This change appears to be of functional significance because the adrenal gland becomes more sensitive and can produce more aldosterone in response to this hormone. It is of particular interest that under the same conditions there is a decline in receptor number in other angiotensin-responsive tissues such as vascular smooth muscle. This indicates that changes in receptor number can be in either direction in response to a rise in hormone concentration and must reflect adaptive advantages to the organism and not specifically those of the target tissue.

Finally, it is worth noting that in many tissues, the receptor number can be regulated by agents other than the direct agonists (Catt et al., 1979). Thus, FSH can control the LH receptor number, and thyroxine can control the number of catecholamine β-receptors. Of particular interest is that incubation of rat cerebral cortical slices with β-adrenergic agonists causes an increase in α_2-adrenergic binding in addition to inducing the expected decrease in β-adrenergic binding (Maggi et al., 1980).

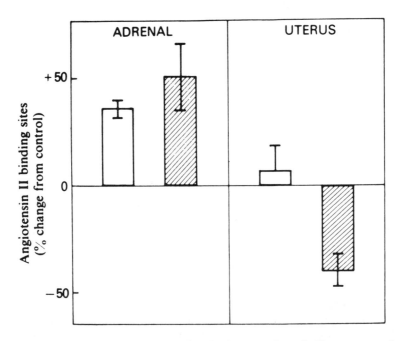

Figure 3.5 Reciprocal effects of a low sodium intake on angiotensin II receptor number in adrenal glomerulosa cells and uterine smooth muscle. Open column, 36 hours of low Na^+ intake; hatched column, seven days of low Na^+ intake, a condition in which circulating angiotensin II is chronically high. From Catt et al. (1979), with permission.

In closing this discussion of receptors and receptor coupling, it is worthwhile reviewing these processes in the context of one of our major themes. Previous evidence has been cited in support of the theme that the two messenger systems involving calcium and cAMP, respectively, act in an integrated way to regulate the response of most cells to a specific class of extracellular stimuli. This contrasts with currently held views that link the calcium system primarily to the nervous system and the cAMP system to the endocrine system (Figure 1.5). In this latter view, hormone action leads primarily to the generation of the chemical messenger cAMP and neuronal activation leads primarily to the generation of the calcium signal. However, more and more hormonal systems have been discussed in which the primary message is calcium, that is, this specific ionic message is generated by a direct coupling of hormone receptor to calcium gating. Conversely, in the nervous system, cAMP is generated in response to electrical stimulation. It is not yet clear whether this is a direct action of electrical depolarization or an indirect one mediated by calcium–calmodulin activation. If the latter, the situation with both the calcium and cAMP messenger systems in the nervous system is comparable: the message in each is generated by indirect rather than direct coupling.

TRANSDUCTION

The second step in the flow of information from cell surface to cell interior is the generation of the intracellular messenger as a consequence of hormone-receptor or neurotransmitter–receptor interaction. A great deal is known about this transducing event in the cAMP messenger system. Very little in the case of the calcium messenger system.

Transduction in the Cyclic AMP System

The transduction step in this system takes place by the interaction of the occupied hormone receptor with one or more components of the adenylate cyclase system and involves the subsequent generation of cAMP from ATP by the catalytic subunit of this system.

Work by several investigators has led to the elucidation of the components of the cyclase system and their interactions (Rodbell et al., 1971a,b; Rodbell et al., 1975; Rodbell, 1980; Pfeuffer, 1977, 1979; Cassel et al., 1977; Cassel and Selinger, 1977a,b,c, 1978; Schramm and Nairn, 1970; Oily and Schramm, 1976; Schramm et al., 1977; Schramm, 1979; Haga et al., 1977a,b; Caron et al., 1979; Dufau et al., 1973, 1975; Limbird and Lefkowitz, 1976, 1978; Schlegel et al., 1979; Ross et al., 1978; Ross and Gilman, 1977; Londos et al., 1979; Haga et al., 1977; Rimon et al., 1978; Hanski et al., 1979; Houslay et al., 1976; Maguire et al., 1977; Lin et al., 1977; Lefkowitz et al., 1971; Tolkovsky and Levitzki, 1978a,b; Catt et al., 1979; Rodbell, 1980; Ross and Gilman, 1980). It is now evident that the hormone-sensitive cyclase consists of at least three separate proteins (Table 3.2): a catalytic

Table 3.2   Properties of Components of the Adenylate Cyclase Complex[a]

Component	Properties
Hormone receptor (R)	Binding site on extracellular face; high affinity for agonist; one or more different receptor type per cell; interacts with G/F component so that GTP binding causes decrease in hormone affinity
Catalytic subunit (C)	When isolated, Mn ATP much better substrate than Mg ATP; not stimulated directly by F^-, GTP, or hormones; sensitive to heat, SH reagents
Regulatory subunit (N or G/F)	Guanine nucleotide-binding protein; fluoride-binding protein; confers upon C ability to employ Mg ATPase substrate; GTPase; mediates regulation of activity of C by nucleotides, fluoride, and hormone; contains cholera toxin substrate; stable to heat and SH reagents; hormones stimulate exchange of GDP for GTP at nucleotide binding (N) site

[a]From Ross and Gilman (1980) and Rodbell (1980). Abbreviations: GTP = guanosine triphosphate; GDP = guanosine diphosphate; SH = sulfhydryl; F^- = fluoride; ATP = adenosine triphosphate; ATPase = ATP hydrolysing enzyme; GTPase = GTP hydrolysing enzyme.

subunit (C) which is relatively inactive in the free state; a guanine nucleotide-binding protein (G/F or N) which also possesses GTPase activity and mediates the action of various regulatory ligands; and the hormone receptor (R) which appears to interact mainly with the regulatory guanosine triphosphate-(GTP) binding protein and not with the catalytic subunit.

On the basis of extensive studies in their own laboratories as well as evidence from studies of others, Ross and Gilman (1980) have proposed a model to describe the mechanism by which hormone–receptor interaction leads to the activation of the cyclase. This is a modified version of previous models discussed by Cassel and Selinger (1977) and by Levinson and Blume (1977). This model is depicted in Figure 3.6. The essential feature of the model is that when GTP occupies the guanine nucleotide binding site, the regulatory subunit G/F (in later discussions, N is employed to designate this same protein) can interact with the catalytic subunit. The complex so formed (C ~ G/F·GTP) is the active catalytic moiety which converts ATP to cAMP.

The assumptions underlying this model are: (1) G/F is the only site of GTP binding and is also the site of GTP hydrolysis; (2) C ~ G/F–GTP is the active catalytic species; (3) hydrolysis of GTP by G/F (k_1) results in an activation of the cyclase; (4) in the absence of hormone, k_{-2} is the rate-limiting step in the regeneration of G/F–GTP; (5) dissociation of GDP is the step regulated

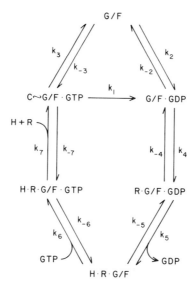

Figure 3.6 Reaction sequence of the components of the adenylate cyclase. G/F symbolizes the guanine nucleotide and fluoride binding regulatory subunit of the enzyme; C, the catalytic subunit; R, the hormone receptor; and H, the hormone. The only active species of the cyclase in the membrane is $C \sim G/F \cdot GTP$. See text for discussion. Redrawn from Ross and Gilman (1980)

by hormone-receptor interaction, a model compatible with the concept of "collision coupling" proposed by Tolkovsky and Levitzki (1978); and (6) hormone binding is a negative heterotrophic process in relation to guanine nucleotide binding. Thus, in this model, binding of hormone to receptor (R + H $\rightleftharpoons$ RH) leads to the association of RH with G/F·GDP, leading to formation of a complex (G/F·GDP·R·H). This association leads to the dissociation of GDP from its binding site, resulting in the formation of G/F·R·H. This complex now binds GTP, resulting in the formation of G/F·GTP·R·H, which promptly dissociates into R·H and G/F·GTP. The latter associates with C, which leads to the formation of the active cyclase complex $C \sim G/F \cdot GTP$ and simultaneously activates the GTPase of the G/F subunit. This leads to GTP hydrolysis, the dissociation of C from G/F leading to G/F·GDP and an inactive cyclase molecule.

In the absence of hormone, k_{-2} is the rate-limiting step in the regeneration of G/F·GTP and $k_2 > k_{-2}$. Hence, very little G/F is formed. In some situations, however, k_{-2} is finite so that addition of a nonhydrolyzable analog of GTP will result in activation of the cyclase in the absence of hormone. In other cases, k_{-2} is close to zero so that such analogs will only sustain activity after hormone activation of the system.

This model accounts satisfactorily for much of the biochemical evidence presently known but does not account for the recent finding of Schlegel et al. (1979). They estimated the dimensions of the various components of the glucagon-sensitive adenylate cyclase in rat liver plasma membrane by em-

Table 3.3 Functional Size of Adenylate Cyclase Components Determined By Target Size Analysis[a]

Enzyme Source		Component (M.W. $\times$ 10^5)				
		RN	C	NC	RNC	R_iN_i
Rat liver:	R = glucagon	6–13	1.5	2.3	3.5	—
Fat cell:	R = catecholamine; ACTH	13	—	2.3	—	>13
	R_1 = adenosine					
Turkey: RBC	R = catecholamine	—	0.9	1.8	2.5	—

[a]From Rodbell (1980). RN = Hormone receptor–nucleotide binding protein in nonactivated cell; C = catalytic subunit in nonactivated cell; NaC = catalytic subunit–regulatory subunit in activated cell; RNC = complex of all three proteins in activated cell; R_iN_i = hormone receptor–nucleotide binding protein in noninhibited cell where agonist acts as an inhibitor of the enzyme.

ploying target size analysis (Kempner and Schlegel, 1979). Their results as well as more recent results (Rodbell, 1980) on other cyclases are summarized in Table 3.3. As predicted from the reaction sequence outlined in Figure 3.6, there was an increase in molecular weight when C shifted from an uncoupled state to one in which C was coupled to N_s (the G/F subunit in Figure 3.6), and a further increase when R and NC were complexed together. However, estimation of the size of RN_s, the receptor–nucleotide regulatory protein complex existing in the unstimulated membrane, gave a value considerably higher than predicted from their dissociated forms. The results have been interpreted (Rodbell, 1980) in terms of a disaggregation coupling model (Figure 3.7) in which, in the absence of hormone, RN_s components associate to form oligomers. These undergo disaggregation into monomers capable of binding GTP when hormone is added. The monomers are capable of associating

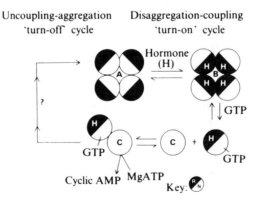

Figure 3.7 Model of how hormone (H) binding induces a disaggregation of RN subunits (A → B) which then allows these subunits to bind GTP, dissociate, and the dissociated subunits bind the catalytic subunit (C) and produce an active cyclase enzyme. From Rodbell (1980), with permission.

with the catalytic subunit of the enzyme to bring about its activation. This type of organization could account for the fact that at low hormone concentrations it is possible to activate more than one cyclase molecule by a single hormone receptor binding event. This would be possible if not all hormone binding sites on the oligomer needed to be occupied in order for disaggregation to occur.

As noted in Table 3.3, Rodbell (1980) has extended this type of analysis to situations in which agents inhibit adenylate cyclase (adenosine in fat cells). In this case as well, the RN_i (Ni nucleotide-binding inhibitory protein) is also considerably larger than the activated enzyme. He has proposed that both types of receptors, those that cause stimulation and those that cause inhibition, are coupled to the cyclase by a nucleotide (GTP) binding unit, N_s and N_i, respectively. The presence of N_i-type units have been described for several muscarinic receptors (Watanabe et al., 1978; Berrie et al., 1978; Blume et al., 1979). From these findings, Rodbell has proposed two generalizations. The first, illustrated schematically in Figure 3.8, is that both stimulating and inhibiting agents that control adenylate cyclase activity do so by interacting with specific RN oligomers (RN_s or RN_i) which possess specific GTP-binding proteins that when activated bind to the catalytic subunit C of adenylate cyclase and either stimulate or inhibit the activity of this enzyme. The second is that other hormones which initiate cell response by acting via surface receptor and bring about other transducing events in the membrane are also coupled to these transducers (e.g., an ion channel) by means of nucleotide binding (regulatory) proteins. In support of this possibility are the findings that GTP affects agonist–receptor binding in several systems including angiotensin binding in the adrenal medulla (Glossman et al., 1974) and α-adrenergic agent binding in the liver (Blackmore et al., 1978). Also, it has been found (Walaas et al., 1979) that insulin activates a cAMP-independent protein kinase in the sacrolemma of muscle cell by a process that is regulated by GTP. The fact that GTP alters hormone binding makes these systems of interest because it has been shown (see Figure 3.6) that when GTP binds to the N subunit of the RN complex, the dissociation

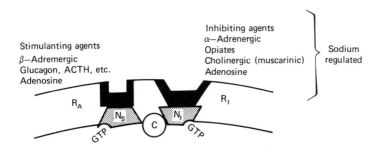

Figure 3.8 Schematic representation of dual regulation of the adenylate cyclase system by stimulatory and inhibitory hormones or neurotransmitters. The hypothesis is that the coupling of both types of receptors (R_A and R_I) to the cyclase (C) is mediated by a nucleotide binding protein (N) that binds GTP. From Rodbell (1980), with permission.

constant for hormone–receptor interaction (R⇌RH) is changed. Hormone is bound less avidly under these conditions (Ross and Gilman, 1980; Rodbell, 1980).

Transduction in the Calcium System

The intramembranous events in the calcium messenger system are not known. The two serious hypotheses as to the molecular basis of generating calcium messages at the plasma membrane are those developed by Michell (1975) based upon earlier observations made by Hokin and Hokin (1955) and by Hirata and Axelrod (1980). The first hypothesis states that changes in phosphoinositol turnover is the basis of calcium gating. The second states that phospholipid methylation plays this role.

In order to understand the first hypothesis and the data relating to it, it is first necessary to review the pathways of phosphoinositide synthesis and degradation (Figure 3.9). The immediate precursor of phosphotidylinositol is CDP-diacylglycerol, which is formed by the reaction of phosphatidic acid (PA) with CTP (reaction 3). Reaction of inositol with CDP-diacylglycerol (reaction 4) leads to PI synthesis. Further phosphorylation of PI (reactions 5 and 6) leads to di- and then triphosphoinositide (DPI and TPI). Dephosphorylation of these compounds regenerates PI (reactions 7 and 8). PI can also undergo hydrolysis to 1-phosphoinositol (and/or 1,2-cyclic phosphoinositol) and 1,2-diacylglycerol (reaction 9).

A peculiar feature of phosphoinositides is that the major fatty acid in their 1-position is stearate and the one in their 2-position is arachidonate. The functional significance of this composition is not known.

Complicating any simple analysis of their transducing role in the plasma membrane are the facts that (1) PI is present in both plasma and subcellular membrane and (2) the enzymes involved in PI turnover are not confined to the plasma membrane but exist, in part, in the endoplasmic reticulum and cytosol.

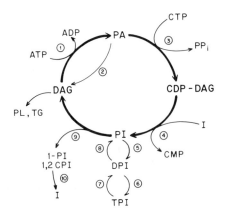

Figure 3.9 The pathways of phosphatidylinositol (PI) metabolism. See text for discussion.

Two different functions, resulting from two different processes, have been attributed to this pathway. The first, proposed by Hawthorne and White (1975), involves the interconversions of DPI and TPI to PI as a means of altering cation (specifically divalent cation) binding to the inner surface of the plasma membrane of cells in the nervous system. It is proposed that these changes in binding are involved in the gating processes in these membranes. This hypothesis will not be discussed further. The interested reader is referred to the review of Hawthorne and White (1975).

The other mechanism is depicted in Figure 3.10, in which coupling of receptors involved in the calcium signaling system alters calcium permeability (gating) in the plasma membrane by altering the turnover of PI. The specific site of action of the hormone–receptor complex is considered to be a stimulation of the hydrolysis of PI to diacylglycerol, 1-phosphoinositol, and 1,2-cyclic phosphoinositol (Figure 3.9).

This proposal is based upon the following facts (see Michell, 1975): (1) Activation of many of the receptors, for example, α-adrenergic and muscarinic cholinergic, which are known to increase the entry of calcium into the target cells, also increases the turnover of PI. (2) Receptors thought to act via adenylate cyclase activation do not increase PI turnover. (3) The increased PI turnover does not depend upon the presence of extracellular calcium. (4) Application of other agents, for example, the divalent cation ionophore A23187, which increase the intracellular calcium by a receptor-independent mechanism, do not enhance PI turnover. (5) The dose-response curves for the activation of PI turnover are similar to the curves of agonist binding to receptor. (6) The change in PI turnover is related to the type of receptor and coupling mechanism and not the to type of cellular response.

Much of the work in studying this system has involved measuring ^{32}P incorporation into PA and PI, reactions which are now believed to constitute late events, namely, the resynthesis of PI and not the primary receptor-mediated events. In some studies, cells have been prelabeled with ^{32}P and the release of [^{32}P]phosphate following stimulation has been measured. The problem with this approach is that of determining the cellular source of the [^{32}P]phosphate.

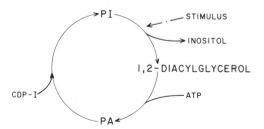

Figure 3.10 Model of calcium gating and PI metabolism in which hormone (neuro-transmitter)–receptor interaction (designed stimulus) leads to an hydrolysis of PI, and this hydrolysis leads to a change in the permeability properties of a calcium channel.

In a recent series of experiments, Fain and Berridge (Fain and Berridge, 1978; Berridge and Fain, 1978) have prelabeled the fly salivary gland with [^{3}H]inositol and then followed the fate of the incorporated label after stimulation of the gland with 5-hydroxytryptamine (5HT). After labeling, 94% of the label was found in the PI fraction. Upon stimulation, there was a breakdown of PI to intracellular 1-phosphoinositol and 1,2-cyclic diphosphoinositol and a considerable release of [^{3}H]inositol to the medium (see Chapter 5). This breakdown correlated in time with an increase in calcium flux across the cell. The release of inositol was seen in the absence of extracellular calcium and was not reproduced by addition of either exogenous cAMP or A23187 agents capable of stimulating secretion. The release occurred as rapidly as the increase in rate of salivary secretion. In this tissue, PI breakdown occurred without an immediate increase in PI resynthesis. As the tissue became depleted of PI, there was a loss of responsiveness to 5HT. Incubation of such glands for 1 hour in the absence of hormone but in the presence of inositol led to a recovery of responsiveness. These results are some of the strongest evidence in favor of the hypothesis that PI breakdown is an integral aspect of the process within the membrane that leads to the change in calcium permeability after the interaction of specific hormones or neurotransmitters with their surface receptors.

The complexities and therefore the regulatory potential of this PI system has become even more evident because of two recent developments. Although originally the arachidonate liberated from phospholipids was considered to arise principally from the action of phospholipase A$_2$ on phosphatidylcholine, recent studies (Rittenhouse-Simmons and Deykin, 1978; Bell et al., 1979; Kennerly et al., 1979; Rittenhouse, 1979) have shown that the diacylglycerol derived from PI breakdown is rich in arachidonic acid and that an enzyme capable of hydrolyzing the acyl bond in this compound is widely distributed. Because arachidonate is the precursor for prostaglandins and hydroxy fatty acids, each of which may influence cell function, it is possible that the release of this fatty acid from diacylglycerol plays some type of messenger function in many cellular responses. Similarly, recent studies of Takai et al. (1979) have shown that the calcium-dependent protein kinase requires 1,2-diacylglycerol for its activation, suggesting that 1,2-diacylglycerol may also play some type of messenger function.

The other recent development relates to the messenger functions of DPI and TPI. As noted previously, Hawthorne and White (1975) discussed the evidence suggesting that the state of phosphorylation of these compounds in the membrane may regulate ionic channels in that membrane. Recent studies by Farese and his associates (Farese et al., 1979; Farese et al., 1980) raise the possibility that *release* of these phosphorylated inositides from the membrane may play a messenger function analogous or complementary to those played by Ca^{2+} and cAMP. They found that the content of both DPI and TPI increased in adrenal cells after adding ACTH to these cells (see Chapter 6) and that the rise in their content correlated with the steroidogenic response of the tissue to this hormone. They also found that addition of DPI to either isolated adrenal tissue or to isolated adrenal mitochondria stimulated the rate-limiting reaction in steroid biosynthesis. From these findings, they suggest that DPI and/or TPI are the final messengers controlling the key intramitochondrial reaction in steroid biosynthesis. However, it is not yet clear from whence the DPI and TPI arise. It is possible that they come from an intracellular source other than the plasma membrane. In keeping with this possibility are the observations of Farese and coworkers that adrenal mitochondria as well as plasma membrane are capable of synthesizing DPI and TPI. It is possible that the DPI and TPI in this tissue arise within the mitochondria and serve a local messenger function. As such, they would function as third messengers, in which case it might well be that they have a specific role in controlling mitochondrial hydroxylase reactions.

Finally, Jolles et al. (1980) have recently described the fact that the phosphoprotein product of a Ca^{2+}-dependent protein kinase is a DPI kinase capable of phosphorylating DPI to TPI. This finding suggests that changes in DPI and TPI metabolism may be a consequence of cAMP- and/or Ca^{2+}-mediated changes in the state of phosphorylation of key enzymes in PI metabolism. Clearly, more work is necessary to define the roles of DPI and TPI, but these recent studies open entirely new prospects as to their regulatory functions.

The other possible mechanism of membrane transduction in receptor–hormone message transfer involving membrane lipids was discovered recently by Hirata and Axelrod (1980). They described a metabolic pathway within the plasma membrane of cells that involves the conversion of phosphatidylethanolamine (PE) and S-adenosyl-L-methionine (SAM) to phosphatidyl-N-monomethylethanolamine (PME) by the enzyme phospholipid methyltransferase I (PMI-I), and then the conversion of PME to PC by two successive methylations of PME to phosphatidylcholine by the enzyme phospholipid methyltransferase II (PMT II) (Figure 3.11). These enzymes are arranged within the membrane bilayer in such a way that the first enzyme employs cytosolic SAM and PE within the inner leaf of the bilayer. The PME so generated then serves as substrate for PMT-II. The PC generated appears in the outer leaflet of the membrane. This shift of PE to PC and the associated translocation of the phospholipid headgroup leads to an increase in membrane fluidity. Activation of this membrane pathway occurs after receptor occupancy in the case of β-adrenergic receptors on the rat red blood cell (Hirata and Axelrod, 1978) in the case of Con A-stimulated lymphocyte mitogenesis (Hirata et al., 1980).

In the case of the β-receptor, Hirata et al. (1979) propose that the phospholipid methylation by increasing membrane fluidity allows for a greater activation of cyclase by hormone. In addition, phospholipid methylation leads to an increase in β-adrenergic receptor number in the red cell (Strittmatter et al., 1979). From these results, it is evident that some receptors are cryptic in membranes but become available when membrane PC

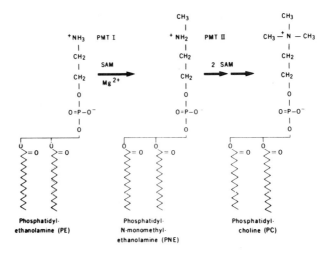

Figure 3.11 The pathway of phospholipid methylation involving the conversion of PE to PME by phospholipid methyltransferase I (PMT-I) and the two-step conversion of PME to PC by phospholipid methyl transferase II (PMT-II). SAM = S-adenosyl-L-methionine. From Hirata and Axelrod (1980), with permission.

content increases. Of equally great interest is the finding (Hirata and Axelrod, 1980) that the phenomenon of down-regulation of receptor number (see above) may involve another feature of this pathway (Mallorga et al., 1980), namely, that of the activation of phospholipase A_2. The methylation of PE to PC is closely coupled to the activation of phospholipase A_2 which catalyzes the conversion of PC to lysophosphatidylcholine (LPC). When C_6 astrocytoma cells are treated with an inhibitor of phospholipase A_2, for example, mepacrine, down-regulation of the cyclase system does not occur as it does in control cells after repeated exposure to β-adrenergic agonists. Conversely, when cells are treated with activators of this enzyme, for example, phorbol esters, the cells become rapidly refractory to cyclase activation by β-adrenergic agonists.

In the case of the mast cell, exposure of these cells to Con A triggers the metabolic pathway PE $\rightarrow$ PME $\rightarrow$ PC $\rightarrow$ LPC (Hirata et al., 1979). There is a considerable literature (see Chapter 8) showing that an influx of calcium into the mast cell triggers the subsequent release of histamine.

The question explored by Ishizaka et al. (1980) is the relationship between activation of the phospholipid methylation pathway and calcium uptake. They found that the treatment of mast cells with the divalent $F(ab')_2$ fragments of antibodies raised against rat basophil leukemia cells (a circulating mast cell) leads to a rapid activation of methylation (Figure 3.12) which precedes in time both calcium uptake and histamine release. These results indicate that phospholipid methylation precedes the changes in calcium flux across the membrane and hence might play some role in regulating the influx of calcium into the cell. To evaluate this possibility, Ishizaka et al. (1980) examined the effect of the methyltransferase inhibitor 5'-deoxyiso-

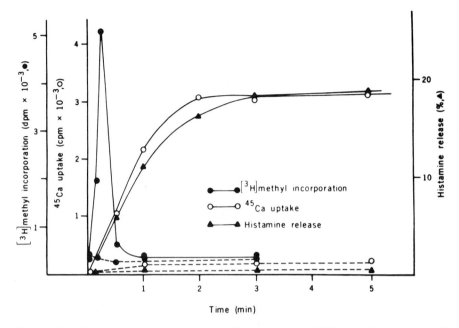

Figure 3.12 Time course of change in phospholipid methylation ([³H]methyl incorporation, ●) calcium uptake (○), and histamine release (▲) in mast cells activated by divalent F(ab')₂ fragments. Cells treated with monovalent fragments (—) showed no response in any of these ways. From Hirata and Axelrod (1980), with permission.

butylthio-3-deazaadenosine (3-deaza-SIBA) on phospholipid methylation, calcium uptake, and histamine release. The inhibitor reduces all three responses more or less proportionally and in a dose-dependent manner. These authors suggest that activation of the methylation pathway by altering membrane fluidity may open calcium ion channels in membrane. The resulting influx of calcium could simultaneously trigger histamine release and, by activating phospholipase A₂, serve as a means of terminating the calcium influx (Figure 3.13).

Since arachidonic acid is one of the major products (along with LPC) of phospholipase A₂ actions and is the precursor of prostaglandins and hydroxyperoxylipids, the methylation pathway and the closely associated arachidonate release may serve as a means of generating messengers, other than Ca^{2+} and cAMP, that serve to couple stimulus to response when surface receptors are activated. In a number of the systems to be discussed in later sections of this monograph, one consequence of cell activation is an increase in phospholipase A₂ activity. It is quite likely that the phospholipid methylation pathway is coupled to and precedes the activation of this enzyme in many of these cellular systems. Yet to be resolved is the relationship of this the phospholipid methylation–phospholipase A₂ pathway, changes in transmembrane calcium influx, and the phosphatidylinositol pathway discussed immediately above. In any case, it is already apparent that the phospholipid

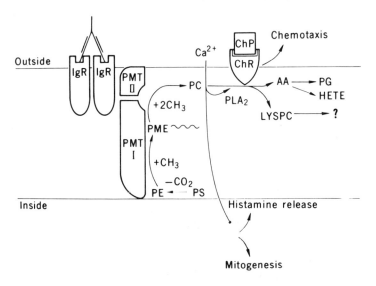

Figure 3.13 Schematic representation of the membrane events taking place in the plasma membrane of a mast cell when its IgE (IgR) is activated. Both PE methylation and activation of phospholipidase A_2 (PLA_2) occur, as well as an increase in calcium influx. See text for discussion. From Hirata and Axelrod (1980), with permission.

methylation pathway plays a role in the membrane events involved in signal generation in both the cAMP and calcium pathways of intracellular communication.

A question which this conclusion raises, particularly in the light of current views of membrane structure (Singer and Nicolson, 1972), is how specific receptors are coupled to messenger generation in a given cell. If the fluid mosaic model structure is accepted as a valid description of plasma membrane structure, then activation of the phospholipid methylation pathway would be expected to have a generalized rather than restricted effect on membrane function. In the case of a cell in which the PE-to-PC conversion and translocation mediated or modulated both cyclase activity and calcium influx, both calcium flux and cAMP production should change upon addition of hormone or neurotransmitter. However, there are many examples, to be discussed subsequently, in which a hormone interacting with its receptor causes a change in only one of these two processes.

The only studies that address this question are those reported by Strittmatter et al. (1979). They found that cultured C_6 astrocytoma cells have both β-adrenergic and benzodiazepine receptors coupled to adenylate cyclase. Both β-adrenergic agonists and benzodiazepine stimulate [^{3}H]methyl group incorporation into the phospholipids of these cells. When added together at maximally effective doses, benzodiazepine and β-agonists increase methylation of phospholipids in an additive manner. These results show that different receptors are located in separate domains of the membrane and are associated with a different group of methyltransferase enzymes. This means that activation of each receptor leads to a localized change in phospholipid methylation. The resulting change in fluidity is restricted to a small domain of membrane lipids. These findings support more recent models of membrane structure (Cullis and DeKruijff, 1979; Jaim and White, 1977; Klausner et al., 1980; Sandermann, 1978) in which there are a variety of separate lipid domains in a biological membrane rather than a single homogeneous one as envisioned in the fluid mosaic model.

As discussed above, although many α-adrenergic receptors appear to have as one of their primary effects a change in the calcium permeability of the plasma membrane, not all of them bring about this change. Another common effect of α-adrenergic receptor occupation is an inhibition of adenylate cyclase activity. Based on the fact that the coupling of β-receptors, and receptors for other peptide hormones, to the adenylate cyclase is influenced by the lipid composition of the membrane, Michell (1975) has proposed that the breakdown of PI might also account for the α-receptor-mediated inhibition of adenylate cyclase. However, this is difficult to reconcile with the membrane events in cases such as the activation of insulin secretion in the pancreatic beta cell (see Chapter 6). In this cell, a metabolite of glucose activates calcium entry, and this change in calcium entry is associated with a change in PI turnover. On the other hand, α-adrenergic agents do not enhance calcium entry but inhibit adenylate cyclase activity. It appears more likely that the α-receptor mediates inhibition of cyclase by the mechanism proposed by Rodbell (Figure 3.8).

Another point raised previously is the fact that in some tissues calcium enters as a consequence of hormone–receptor interaction via a so-called receptor-operated channel, which does not cause a depolarization of the membrane, while in others calcium entry is an indirect consequence of receptor occupancy being caused by a receptor-mediated depolarization of the membrane. It is possible that both types of channels exist in the same cell type. For example, Study et al. (1978) showed that either depolarization (by high K^+) or carbachol interacting with muscarinic receptors caused a calcium-dependent increase in cellular cGMP content. Their results suggest that K^+ increases cGMP by activating voltage-dependent calcium channels and carbachol by activating a nonvoltage-dependent, receptor-operated channel. Both K^+ and carbachol effects were inhibited by D600, so it remains possible that the same calcium channel was being opened by two separate means. A critical question not yet addressed is whether both types of calcium channels are regulated by the PI turnover system. The type of calcium channel seen in the tissues such as parotid, liver, and salivary gland appears to differ from that in nerve endings and heart and chromaffin cells in that Verapamil and its derivatives block the latter in a more or less specific manner but do not have the same effect upon calcium entry into liver or salivary gland. This has been taken as evidence for a fundamental difference between calcium channels in the two types of tissues.

Electrotonic Coupling in Nonmuscle Cells

A further complexity introduced into any discussion of the transducing function in the calcium messenger system is that, in tissues such as skeletal muscle, a message at the cell surface is transduced into a second message generated in a different membrane, the sarcoplasmic reticulum (SR). As discussed above, it is not yet known exactly how the excitatory event—the action potential—on the cell surface triggers the release of calcium bound to the sarcoplasmic reticulum. However, the weight of recent evidence favors the view that some type of electronic coupling between the two membrane systems is responsible. Even if this is the correct explanation of how the intracellular calcium message is generated in the skeletal muscle cell, there is no agreement that it is true for other types of muscle cells. For example, there is considerable evidence in support for a calcium-induced release from SR in the heart. The calcium entering the cell across the plasma membrane is thought to serve as a trigger for the release of calcium bound to the SR (Fabiato and Fabiato, 1978).

The situation in smooth muscles is less well understood (Bolton, 1979). There are smooth muscles in which low concentrations of appropriate agonists cause contraction by inducing the mobilization of calcium from an internal pool, but high agonist concentrations alter the entry of calcium into the cell. If one considers only the circumstances of low agonist concentration, the available data suggests that the internal pool affected by stimulation is that in the sarcoplasmic reticulum. Direct membrane-to-membrane coupling between the surface and SR membrane may mediate this release. A major problem in defining this coupling is that calcium appears to be essential for the maintenance of membrane–membrane interaction.

It is possible that the endoplasmic reticulum (ER) in other cells serves as a primary source of calcium in stimulus–response coupling and in the motility of nonmuscle cells (Hitchcock, 1977). Sites of apposition between endoplasmic reticulum and surface membranes, so-called subsurface cisterns (SSC), have been described in nerve terminals (Henkart et al., 1976), cultured L cells (Henkart and Nelson, 1979; Nelson and Henkart, 1979), and macrophages (Reave and Axline, 1973). Furthermore, the endoplasmic reticulum in a variety of nonmuscle cells, including fibroblasts (Moore and Pastan, 1977), carries out ATP-dependent calcium uptake.

The possible role of the ER in nonmuscle cells has been studied by Henkart and Nelson (1979). They examined the source of the calcium in fibroblasts (L cells) responsible for the plasma membrane hyperpolarization seen either spontaneously or after mechanical or chemical stimulation (Nelson and Peacock, 1972). Previous work by Lamb and Lindsay (1971) had shown a rapid exchange of extracellular with intracellular calcium in L cells. Henkart and Nelson found that microinjection of calcium elicited a plasma membrane hyperpolarization and interpreted their data to mean that the hyperpolarizing activation (HA) of these cells was due to a specific, calcium-dependent increase in membrane K^+ permeability. They showed that HA occurred in cells incubated in the absence of extracellular calcium or in the presence of cobalt or D-600. Longer exposure to either cobalt or zero calcium environment led eventually to a decline in HA, which was interpreted as being due to a decrease in intracellular calcium pools. Furthermore, in a zero calcium environment, any given cell was capable of only a single HA, but multiple HAs were seen if calcium was reintroduced into the medium. The authors concluded that the source of calcium mediating these responses was an intracellular calcium pool. They further showed that these cells possessed specialized appositions of the endoplasmic reticulum with their plasma membranes, which they called subsurface cisterns (SSC). They proposed that these membrane–membrane junctions mediated the coupling between mechanical, chemical, or electrical stimulation of the plasma membrane and the release of calcium from the endoplasmic reticulum.

These studies raise the possibility that surface membrane–endoplasmic reticulum coupling is a widespread cell property, not confined specifically to muscle cells, and that it may function in nonmuscle cells much as it does in muscle to couple plasma membrane excitation to the generation of the intracellular calcium signal by initiating calcium release from the endoplasmic reticulum. This mechanism may operate in secretory cells, at synapses, and even in hepatic cells. As such, it may represent a major transducing mechanism in the calcium messenger system.

It must be noted that there are other systems in which the mechanism by which the coupling of the plasma membrane stimulus to the release of calcium from an internal pool is not known. An example of this situation is the exocrine pancreas, in which acetylcholine (and other secretagogues) interacts with a muscarinic receptor on the cell surface leading to a marked mobilization of calcium from an intracellular pool (see Chapter 6). In this case, neither external Ca^{2+} nor external Na^+ is required for the Ach-induced response. It is possible, therefore, that in some cells in which the calcium signaling system operates there is an additional messenger which couples events at the plasma membrane to events in one or more intracellular membranes to induce the generation of the intracellular calcium signal.

TRANSMISSION

The third step in information transfer (Table 3.1) in membrane transducing systems is that of the transmission of the second messenger from the plasma membrane to the intracellular receptor sites for the particular messenger. Little is known about this process, but significant features of it bear discussion. These relate specifically to how the particular information transfer system is organized both spacially and temporally.

Transmission in the Calcium System

Two simple experiments reported respectively by Baker (1976) and Loewenstein and Rose (1978) point up the complexities of the problem relating to the transmission of the calcium signal. The experiment of Baker was to inject either Ca^{2+} or Mg^{2+} into a restricted segment of an intact squid axon and observe its lateral displacement along the axis with time. The result, shown in Figure 3.14, was that the injected calcium had undergone very little lateral "diffusion" during the same period of time that the Mg^{2+} had. Baker concluded from this result that the calcium but not the magnesium was bound to stationary intracellular buffer systems and was therefore not freely diffusible away from the site of injection. Using a quite different approach, Loewenstein and Rose (1978) came to a similar conclusion. In their experiments, Aequorin, a calcium-sensitive fluorescent protein, was injected into one of the cells of the salivary gland of *Chironamus*. Under resting conditions, there was very little light output. However, if calcium was injected into the cell, there was a marked increase in light output, but only in the immediate vicinity of the site of injection even though sufficient calcium was injected so that, if freely diffusible, it would have been sufficient to raise the calcium ion content sufficiently to activate Aequorin through the entire cell. If, prior to the calcium injection, the cell was treated with an inhibitor of mitochondrial calcium accumulation, then calcium injection elicited an increase in light output from the entire cell.

Loewenstein and Rose (1978) also used a different approach to the same problem. In previous work, they had shown that a rise in the cytosolic calcium ion concentration in one of a pair of electrically coupled cells (through gap junctions) led to an uncoupling of these cells, that is, the gap junctions are normally regions of low resistance to the flow of ionic currents, but develop high resistance if the calcium ion content of the cytosol is raised. Employing the large salivary gland cell, they showed that if microelectrodes were placed in the cells to either side of the central cell and then calcium ion

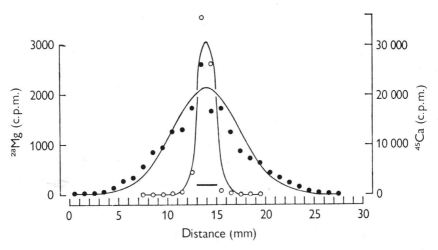

Figure 3.14   Self-diffusion of ^{38}Mg (●) and ^{45}Ca (○) following their injection into the axoplasm of the intact squid axon incubated at 21°C. Measurements were made 510 minutes after injection of the labeled ions. The bar represents the original site of injection. From Baker (1976), with permission.

was injected to one side of the central cell, this cell became uncoupled from its neighbor nearest to the side of injection but remained coupled to its far neighbor. From these results, they concluded that even after a significant rise in the cytosolic calcium ion content in a given region of the cell, there was not a general rise in the calcium ion concentration throughout the cell cytosol or, in other words, that the domain of calcium within the cytosol was restricted by the activities of the intracellular calcium-sequestering systems, most notably the mitochondria and microsomes.

One can calculate that the amount of calcium injected by Loewenstein was greater than that which is likely to enter any given region of the cell across the plasma membrane when the cell goes from a resting to an activated state. This being the case, his results argue that if the only effect of an extracellular messenger upon cellular calcium metabolism is to alter its rate of entry across the plasma membrane, the cytosolic domain in which a rise in the calcium ion concentration will occur will be restricted by (1) the magnitude of the calcium influx, (2) the activity of the plasma membrane calcium pump, (3) the cytosolic buffering systems, and (4) the geometric distribution of calcium-sequestering organelles. However, for calcium to serve its messenger function, there is no need to assume that a uniform rise in the Ca^{2+} concentration throughout the cell cytosol must occur in order for the calcium message to be received and to evoke a response. The critical determinant will obviously be the geometric distribution of the calcium response elements in relation to the geometric distribution of calcium-sequestering systems. The problem is likely to be quite different in polar as compared to nonpolar cells.

The Nonpolar Cells

The induction of histamine release from the mast cell and of insulin from the beta cell of the Islets of Langerhans are two well-studied systems in which stimulus–secretion coupling occurs in a nonpolar cell (Figure 3.15). Each is discussed in later sections (see Chapters 6 and 8). However, at this juncture they serve as useful examples for illustrating the point under discussion. In both, the major signal for the initiation of secretion appears to be an influx of calcium into the cell across the plasma membrane. In both, this signal acts in the immediate region of the cell where it was generated to initiate the exocytosis of secretory granules containing, respectively, histamine and insulin. The intracellular calcium-sequestering organelles are not located in the immediate vicinity of the plasma membrane; hence, upon the alteration of calcium influx there is a significant rise in the calcium ion concentration of the cytosolic domain just beneath the plasma membrane and restricted to that region of the membrane at which the first messenger has acted.

Direct support for this model has come from studies by Lawson and Raff (1979), in which a population of mast cells were exposed to a secretagogue immobilized on large beads. Because of this arrangement, only a small portion of the surface of a given cell could come in contact with first

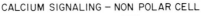

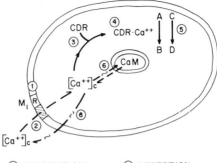

① RECOGNITION   ④ RECEPTION
② TRANSDUCTION   ⑤ RESPONSE
③ TRANSMISSION   ⑥ TERMINATION

Figure 3.15 Calcium signaling in a nonpolar cell. $[Ca^{2+}]_c$ represents cytosolic calcium ion concentration; $[Ca^{2+}]_e$, extracellular calcium; CDR, calmodulin; CaM, intramitochondrial calcium; and A → B and C → D, metabolic pathways within the cell. M_1 represents the first or extracellular messenger, and R its membrane receptor.

messenger if the beads containing first messenger were far enough apart. Under these conditions, it was possible to directly demonstrate that exocytosis occurred only from that part of the cell which was in direct contact with the bead (see Chapter 8). This result fulfills the prediction of the Baker and Loewenstein observations and indicates that in a naturally stimulated cell, the domain of the calcium signal is restricted, In such a circumstance, it is likely that the major function of the calcium-sequestering systems is to restrict the domain of calcium, that is, to terminate the message. However, even in one of the two examples under discussion, insulin release, a more active role of this system is apparent in the sense that mechanisms exist to alter the sequestering function of the intracellular organelles and hence expand the spatial domain of the calcium signal.

Before closing this discussion of signal transmission in nonpolar cells, another example with quite different properties is worth describing. This is the case of the fertilization of oocyte by sperm. Considerable evidence has accumulated showing that calcium ion played some signaling role in the fertilization of the egg. Recently, this has been put on a firm basis by the studies of Ridgeway et al. (1978). Because of the large size of the oocyte, they were able to inject the calcium-sensitive fluorescent protein Aequorin into the oocyte. The light output from the resting cell was low, indicating that in the unfertilized egg, the cytosolic calcium ion concentration is low as in other quiescent cells.

When such an egg was fertilized by a small sperm acting at a very restricted locus on the cell surface, a dramatic event occurred. A wave of light passed across the oocyte from one end to the other. It began at a site just beneath the site of fertilization and spread to the opposite end of the oocyte. By the time it had reached the far end of this large cell, the output of light from the initiating end was already back nearly to baseline values. This propagated wave of light was taken as an indication that a sudden increase in calcium ion concentration took place at the site of fertilization and that this rise in local calcium ion concentration itself or some accompanying ionic event initiated a propagated disturbance longitudinally across the cell which led to calcium release and a rise in cytosolic calcium ion concentration in every region of the cytosol. The basis for this particular mode of signal transmission is not known.

The importance of these observations, aside from their obvious relevance to signaling in the fertilization response, is that intracellular organelles (membranes) other than the sarcoplasmic reticulum in the skeletal and cardiac muscle can serve as a means to propagate a signal from one region of the cell to another. The possibility that this mode of intracellular signal transmission is involved in nonmuscle cells has not been explored in any systematic or meaningful fashion.

The Polar Cells

In contrast to the situation in nonpolar cells, in polar cells the site of signal generation is usually confined to one portion of the cell, the basolateral membrane, and the site of cellular response is confined to another, the luminal membrane (Figure 3.16). In such a situation, particularly in a cell rich in mitochondria and microsomes, it is unlikely that a calcium signal generated at the cell surface can penetrate deep within the cell and diffuse to the luminal membrane to exert its effect there. Five obvious possibilities exist: (1) The calcium-binding characteristics of microsome and mitochondria are modified in these cells so that transcellular propagation of the calcium signal is possible. (2) The calcium signal upon entering the subsur-

CALCIUM SIGNALING – POLAR CELL

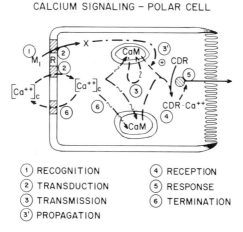

(1) RECOGNITION   (4) RECEPTION
(2) TRANSDUCTION   (5) RESPONSE
(3) TRANSMISSION   (6) TERMINATION
(3') PROPAGATION

Figure 3.16 Calcium signaling in a polar cell. $[Ca^{2+}]$ represents free cytosolic calcium; CaM, intramitochondrial calcium; CDR, calmodulin; and $[Ca^{2+}]_e$, extracellular calcium.

face domain provokes another signal, a third messenger, which is transmitted across the cell; propagation of the signal is via a membrane system such as the endoplasmic reticulum. (4) Calcium binds to its receptor element just beneath the basolateral membrane surface, and this calcium–receptor complex carries the message. (5) When first messenger interacts with the basolateral membrane, an additional signal is generated that acts to modify the intracellular sequestration of calcium so that the calcium signal is propagated across the cell.

There are little data to support several of these alternatives. In the case of the first possibility, there is no evidence that the calcium transport properties of mitochondria and microsomes obtained from polar cells differ, in any fundamental way, from those obtained from nonpolar cells.

It is possible that a calmodulin–calcium-mediated phosphorylation of protein components of the response element could take place in one region of the cell and then diffuse to a different region of the cell where they would interact with cellular constituents to determine cell response. This mechanism would require that dephosphorylation of phosphorylated proteins would be slow compared to their rate of phosphorylation. It would also require diffusion of cellular proteins across considerable distances. As mentioned above, some type of intracellular propagation occurs in the egg, but it is not possible to determine by present means whether this is unique to the egg and specialized tissues such as muscle or whether it is a widespread phenomenon.

The two possibilities that have been considered and for which some experimental evidence exists to support them are the generation of a third messenger and the generation of an additional second messenger that acts to alter intracellular calcium transport. A repeated observation waiting in a sense for an interpretation is the finding that, in many different tissues in which there is clear evidence that the initial membrane transduction event leads to an influx of calcium into the cell, a rise in the cGMP content of the cell is seen (see Rasmussen and Goodman, 1977). In many of these cases, this rise in cGMP concentration depends directly upon the calcium entry and will be seen regardless of the mechanism by which an increase in calcium entry is produced, such as natural agonists, KCl-induced depolarization, or divalent ionophore addition. The significance and function of this third messenger are not known. A rise in cGMP content is not confined to polar cells but is seen in nonpolar cells as well. This observation alone does not eliminate the possibility that cGMP functions to extend calcium signal propagation in polar cells. Several cGMP protein kinases have been discovered, but the function of their phosphoprotein products has not been identified. Likewise, changes in cGMP content are correlated with changes in calcium fluxes in some tissues, but no definable general relationship has been discerned. At the moment, then, the role of this third messenger in signal propagation is not clear.

The situation with cAMP is somewhat clearer. There are systems in which it seems to function as a third messenger and part of its function is to enhance signal propagation. There are other systems in which it is a separate second messenger in which capacity it serves, among other functions, to extend the spatial domain of the calcium message. The latter appears to be the case in the action of a variety of agents upon the beta cell of the pancreas (see Chapter 6). Another example is the case of fly salivary, in which there is evidence that the calcium message is responsible for a specific change in the Cl^- permeability of the luminal membrane even though it is initially generated at the basolateral membrane (see Chapter 5). In this case, cAMP has been shown to induce the mobilization of calcium from an intracellular pool thought to be the mitochondrial pool. By this action, cAMP is responsible for the propagation of the calcium message by altering the calcium-sequestering properties of the intracellular (mitochondrial) sink.

Transmission in the Cyclic AMP System

Scant attention has been paid to the problem of signal transmission in the cAMP system, but many of the same problems exist in this system as in those discussed. The geometric distribution of the various phosphodiesterases and their respective catalytic properties must determine the domain of the cAMP message, much as the distribution of microsomes and mitochondria determines the calcium domain. There is some evidence that compartmentation of cAMP occurs in certain cells, but this evidence is too scant to be of value in defining transmission of the cAMP message. In a polar cell, the cAMP generator adenylate cyclase is located on the basolateral membrane, yet the cAMP response element is thought to be located on the luminal membrane. The tissue possesses active phosphodiesterases, hence it is difficult to envision how the message is transmitted across the cell. This problem has been considered by Swillens et al. (1976) in the case of thyroid-stimulating hormone (TSH) action on the thyroid acinar cell. They base their analysis on the measurement of the known activities of the three components involved: (1) adenylate cyclase, with a basal activity of 2.8×10^{-6} mol/min and a stimulated activity of 11.2×10^{-6} mol/min; (2) soluble phosphodiesterase (PDEI), $K_m = 4 \times 10^{-5}$ M and $V_{max} = 3.7 \times 10^{-5}$ mol/min; and (3) membrane-bound PDE II, with a $K_m = 10^{-6}$ M and $V_{max} = 3.7 \times 10^{-6}$ mol/min. In this situation, the cAMP concentration estimated to exist in the domain of the basal membrane is 10.8×10^{-6} M, and that in the domain of the apical membrane, 10×10^{-6} M. However, these figures must be considered minimal because they ignore important regulatory factors. For example, PDE I in many cells is regulated by the calcium–calmodulin complex. The effect of this regulation is to lower the K_m of the effect for cAMP by a factor of 30. For example, in the case of PTH action on the renal tubule, after an initial 2.5 to 4-fold increase in total cAMP content in the tissue, the cAMP levels fall to values 1.25 to 1.35 times the basal levels. Thus, in these cells the PDE activities dominate the cAMP–messenger system. It is likely that the cAMP gradient from basal to apical membranes is significantly steeper than that calculated by Swillens et al. (1975).

One possible mode of cAMP signal transmission is via the transmission of the catalytic subunit of the cAMP-dependent protein kinase. When cAMP interacts with the protein kinase (RC + cAMP $\rightleftharpoons$ R·cAMP + C) the catalytic subunit (C) dissociates from regulatory subunit (R). The free subunit (C) is the catalytically active form of the enzyme. Hence, it is possible that this free subunit is generated in one part of the cell and translocated to another. Jungmann et al. (1974) have shown the translocation of protein kinase activity from cytosol to nucleus in ovarian cells when activated by LH, and Keely et al. (1975) have described the movement of PK activity from cytosol to particulate fraction. Similarly, Koremman et al. (1974) found a translocation of enzyme from cytosol to microsomal fraction in uterus following a rise in cAMP content, and Palmer et al. (1974) have shown a glucagon-induced increase in nuclear PK activity in liver. All of these findings are consistent with this mode of signal transmission being cooperative under some conditions.

In their studies of the role of cAMP in the action of parathyroid hormone (PTH) on renal tubular phosphate transport and of arginine vasopressin (AVP) action on H_2O flow in different parts of the nephron, Kinne and associates (see Chapter 4) proposed that PTH or AVP act upon an adenyl cyclase confined to the basolateral membrane and that the subsequent rise in cAMP leads to the activation of a protein kinase in the luminal membrane of these polar cells. Activation of this luminal PK leads to the phosphorylation of one or more proteins which are coupled to and responsible for the change in the permeability properties of this membrane. Because cells of the proximal and collecting tubules of the kidney possess considerable phosphodiesterase activity, it is not at all clear how the signal is transmitted from one surface to the other in these cells.

Reception

Once the signal is transmitted within the cell cytosol, the next step in the information transfer process is its intracellular reception (Table 3.1). Specific receptor proteins for both cAMP and calcium have been identified. To date, only two cAMP receptor proteins have been found, but at least nine intracellular calcium receptor proteins are known. These are tropinin C, leiotonin, parvalbumin, calmodulin, regulatory and essential myosin light chains, synexin, and the intestinal calcium-binding protein. Only two of these will be discussed in detail: troponin C and calmodulin.

Cyclic AMP-Binding Proteins

To date, the only cAMP-binding proteins identified in the intact cell are components of a single class of enzyme—protein kinases (Krebs, 1972; Beavo et al., 1975; Hofman et al., 1975). The cAMP binds to a specific regulatory subunit of these enzymes. Two different protein kinases (I and II) can be identified according to their chromatographic behavior. PK I predominants in skeletal muscle, PK II in heart. Multiple forms of the enzyme are seen in other tissues. Also, Severin et al. (1978) have described a protein kinase from brain that differs in properties from either of the muscle enzymes, and many represent therefore a third type. All three enzymes appear to exist as tetramers (R_2C_2) and all bind 4 moles of cAMP per mole of holoenzyme. The catalytic subunit appears identical in all (M.W. 38,000). The difference in the holoenzymes reside in differences in their regulatory subunits (Hofman et al., 1975; Dills et al., 1979; Rosen and Erlichman, 1975; Severin et al., 1978). The contrasting properties of the binding protein from skeletal (PK I) and cardiac (PK II) enzymes are given in Table 3.4. The brain enzyme is not included because it has not been well characterized. Its molecular weight is 50,000, and it can be converted by borohydride reduction into two fragments of 27,000 and 23,000, only the latter of which binds cAMP.

The major difference in the cAMP-binding proteins from muscle is a difference in molecular weight, a difference in suspectibility to phosphorylation, with the R from PK II highly susceptible and that from PK I not, and the differences in their effects upon the activity of the catalytic subunit (Corbin and Lincoln, 1978).

The functional significance of these different types of cAMP receptor proteins is not currently known. Most interesting is the fact that under circumstances where the cyclase system is not activated, all or nearly all the cAMP-binding proteins are associated with PK. This is in marked contrast to the situation with calmodulin, in which case in the resting cell the bulk of it is free in the cytosol. Once the cell is activated and R·cAMP is formed, it is possible that this complex, R·cAMP, serves a messenger function distinct from the released and now active C. The only clue that this might be the case is the report by Jungmann et al. (1974) that in ovarian cells a rise in cAMP content leads to the formation of R·cAMP and C, each of which is then translocated separately to the nucleus.

Table 3.4 Comparison of the Properties of the Regulatory Subunits (cAMP-Binding Proteins) of PK I and PK II

Property	R I	R II
Association	R_2C_2	R_2C_2
cAMP Binding	2 per each R	2 per each R
Molecular Weight	48,000	55,000
Phosphorylation	—	—
cAMP Affinity K_b	0.1 μM	2.8 μM
Mg ATP Binding to holoenzyme	High-affinity site	No high-affinity site

Calcium Receptor Proteins

The subject of calcium-binding proteins has been reviewed recently by Kretsinger (1976, 1979a,b). A summary of their major characteristics is given in Table 3.5. Of particular interest are calmodulin, troponin C, and leiotonin. These are three closely related proteins that appear to have arisen by gene duplication from a common ancestor. The only known function of troponin C is that of coupling stimulus to response in skeletal and cardiac muscle, and the function of leiotonin is that of coupling stimulus to response in smooth muscle. On the other hand, calmodulin couples stimulus to response in a variety of cellular functions.

Evolutionary Interrelationships

The amino acid sequence of the carp cytosolic Ca^{2+}-binding protein parvalbumin has been examined by Kretsinger and Nockolds (1973). They reported that the sequence is unusual in that it contains three regions of homologous sequence repeats, each about 33 residues long. X-Ray crystallographic analysis of the conformation of parvalbumin (Moews and Kretsinger, 1975) suggests that the internal sequence repeats are the sites of a Ca^{2+}-binding pocket of β-antiparallel conformation by two regions of a helix. They have termed this Ca^{2+}-binding repeat sequence the "EF hand" in which helix E, Ca^{2+}-binding loop EF, and helix F represent the basic structural domain (Figure 3.17). Each EF region contains about 33 residues, 12 of which comprise the EF hand of the Ca^{2+}-binding loop.

Determination of the amino acid sequence of troponin C (Collins et al., 1973), essential myosin light chains of rabbit skeletal muscle (Weeds and McLachlan, 1974; Tufty and Kretsinger, 1975), regulatory myosin light chains of rabbit skeleton muscle (Mutsuda et al., 1977), intestinal calcium-binding protein (Hofman et al., 1977) and calmodulin (Vaneman et al., 1977) has shown that these proteins also contain homologous internal sequence repeats. These repeat sequences are similar to those of parvalbumin. This means that parvalbumin, troponin C, calmodulin, essential and regulatory myosin light chains, and the intestinal Ca^{2+}-binding proteins comprise a family of homologous, "EF"-containing proteins.

The general characteristics of the members of this family are summarized in Table 3.5. Although leiotonin is probably a member, it has not yet been characterized and hence has not been included. These proteins are low-molecular-weight proteins containing two, three, or four EF regions. In some cases (e.g., essential and regulatory myosin light chains and cardiac troponin C), the number of "EF" domains does not correlate with the number of Ca^{2+}-binding sites. This could represent a legitimate loss of Ca^{2+} binding by certain "EF" regions, or it is possible that Ca^{2+} binding by these regions occurs under different experimental conditions. Of interest is the specificity of the Ca^{2+}-binding sites. These sites have been classified as either (Ca^{2+}) binding sites (Ca binding unaffected by millimolar concentrations of Mg^{2+}) or $(Ca^{2+}-Mg^{2+})$ binding sites (Ca^{2+} binding is competitive with Mg^{2+}). The

Table 3.5 Ca^{2+} Receptor Proteins

Protein	Molecular Weight	Number of EF Domains	Number of Ca^{2+} Binding Sites	Type of Ca^{2+} Binding Site	Apparent Ca^{2+} Binding K_{diss} (μM)[a]	Physiological Function	Reference
Parvalbumin	12,000	2	2	(Ca^{2+}–Mg^{2+}) site	8.0	Unknown	Potter et al. (1977)
Troponin C							
Skeletal	18,000	4	4	(2) Ca^{2+} sites (2) (Ca^{2+}–Mg^{2+})	20 2	Regulation of actomyosin ATPase	Potter et al. (1977)
Cardiac	18,000	4	3	(1) Ca^{2+} site (2) (Ca^{2+}–Mg^{2+})	200 3.6		
Calmodulin	16,700	4	4	Ca^{2+} sites	(2) 2–6 (2) 10–18	General Ca^{2+} receptor	Wang and Waisman (1979)
Myosin light chains							
Regulatory light chain	19,000	4	1	(Ca^{2+}–Mg^{2+})	2 mM[b]	Regulation of actomyosin ATPase	Weeds et al. (1977) Kuwayama and Yagi (1979)
Essential light chain	17,000–21,000	4	0	—	—		
Intestinal Ca^{2+}-binding protein							
Small form	12,500	2	2	(Ca^{2+}–Mg^{2+})	0.1–1.0	Intestinal Ca^{2+} transport and storage (?)	Wasserman and Feher (1977)
Large form	27,000	4	4	(Ca^{2+}–Mg^{2+})			

[a] K_{diss} of (Ca^{2+}–Mg^{2+}) sites is reported in the presence of millimolar Mg^{2+}.
[b] When the RLC is associated with myosin, the affinity of Ca^{2+} binding increases 100-fold.

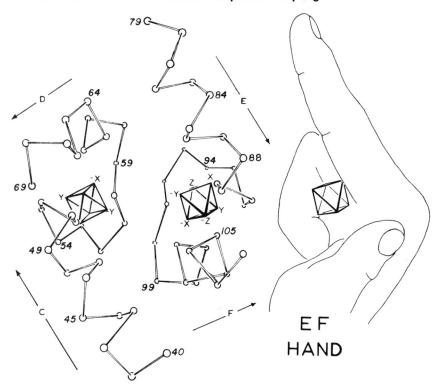

Figure 3.17 Schematic representation of the EF hand or protein structure of each calcium binding site. From Kretsinger (1979), with permission.

affinity of binding of Mg^{2+} by the $(Ca^{2+}$-$Mg^{2+})$ sites is generally three orders of magnitude lower than the affinity of Ca^{2+} binding to these sites. The physiological significance of $(Ca^{2+}$–$Mg^{2+})$ vs (Ca^{2+}) sites is not known.

Kretsinger (1972) first suggested that parvalbumin evolved by gene triplication of a primitive ancestral protein which contained only one EF domain. Later, Collins (1976b) suggested that parvalbumin and troponin C were derived from a common ancestral protein containing one EF region which underwent two successive gene duplications and fusions to produce an ancestral protein containing four Ca^{2+} binding sites. The deletion of one of these sites from the four EF-containing precursor produced parvalbumin. However, an examination of the individual domains of troponin C and calmodulin has revealed that regions 2 and 4 are more closely related to one another than they are to regions 1 and 3 (Vanaman et al., 1977). This result is inconsistent with previous theories of Kretsinger (1972, 1975) or Collins (1976). In view of this observation, Vanaman et al. (1977) and Kretsinger (1979b) have suggested that the existence of an ancestral pair of calcium binding proteins, their subsequent duplication would produce a pair of pairs. Gene fusion would complete the procedure and produce the four EF-domain-containing ancestor.

Kretsinger (1979, 1980) has examined the extent of internal homology of the EF-containing proteins and concludes that the level of internal homology is greatest within calmodulin. This suggests that calmodulin is more closely related to the ancestral protein than to the other proteins. Of the other EF-containing proteins, troponin C has been shown to be the most closely related to calmodulin (Vanaman et al., 1977). Since alignment of the amino acid sequence of troponin C and calmodulin to show maximum homology introduces a three-residue gap in the sequence of calmodulin, Vanaman et al. (1977) suggested that calmodulin arose by duplication of a smaller two EF-domain-containing precursor than troponin C. It would appear that troponin C did not evolve from a calmodulin precursor, but that calmodulin and troponin represent separate evolutionary lines. Barker et al. (1977) have constructed an evolutionary tree of the EF-domain-containing superfamily. The authors suggest that the evolutionary tree can be divided into two main branches and that the myosin light chains have evolved from the calmodulin branch of the tree, while parvalbumin and the intestinal Ca^{2+}-binding protein have evolved from the troponin branch of the tree. The trunk of the tree before this branching is thought to consist of the four EF-containing ancestral protein.

Troponin C
The only calcium-binding protein associated with the contractile elements in skeletal and cardiac muscle is troponin C. This protein has a molecular weight of 12,000, contains four EF domains, and has four calcium-binding sites, two classified as two pure calcium sites and two $Ca^{2+}-Mg^{2+}$ sites (Table 3.5). Potter et al. (1977) have shown that the protein undergoes a conformational change, as measured by circular dichroism, when calcium is bound. This calcium-dependent conformational change is biphasic, with a K_{Ca}^{2+} of 0.27 and 33 μM for the two separate phases representing respectively the binding to the ($Ca^{2+}-Mg^{2+}$) and Ca^{2+} sites.

Leiotonin
This is a recently isolated and incompletely characterized protein in smooth muscle which Ebashi (1979) believes confers Ca^{2+} sensitivity upon smooth muscle actin–myosin systems. Hence, it is thought to play a role in smooth muscle contraction similar to that played by TNC in skeletal muscle. Just as the troponin complex in skeletal muscle consists of several subunits only one of which is the calcium receptor protein, TNC, so in the leiotonin system Ebashi (1979) has described a small (M.W. 17,000) acidic protein that is likely to be a new member of the family of EF hand, calcium-binding proteins listed in Table 3.5.

Calmodulin
Of all the Ca^{2+} receptor proteins, calmodulin has been most intensively studied (for recent reviews see Wang, 1977; Wang and Waisman, 1979;

Wolff and Brostrom, 1979; and Cheung, 1980). Calmodulin (Table 3.5) exists in a variety of tissues (Smoake et al., 1974) and in many different organisms including many plants and probably all animals (Waisman et al., 1975; Charbonneau and Cormier, 1979; Waisman et al., 1978). Calmodulins from a variety of tissues are similar (Table 3.6). They all are asymmetric (f/f_0 1.3) low-molecular-weight proteins (M.W. 15,000 to 19,000) which are highly acidic with an isoelectric point (PI) (pH) of 4.1. They contain about 30% acidic residues ($gl\chi$ + $as\chi$), 45% nonpolar residues, and 55% polar residues (Liu and Cheung, 1976; Walsh and Stevens, 1977). An absence of trp and a high phe/tyr ratio is responsible for the low ultraviolet absorption and the unusual absorption spectrum of the protein. One mole of the unusual amino acid ξ-N-trimethyllysine (Watterson et al., 1976; Vanaman et al., 1977; Miyake and Kakiuchi, 1978; Jackson et al., 1977) has been found per mole of protein, and calmodulin also contains an acetylated N-terminus residue (Ac-Ala) (Vanaman et al., 1977).

A comparison of the amino acid sequence of the bovine brain and rat testes calmodulins suggest that these proteins are virtually identical (Vanaman et al., 1977; Dedman et al., 1978). Also, the calmodulins of bovine heart, bovine brain, and human erythrocyte are indistinguishable by tryptic peptide mapping (Stevens et al., 1976; Jarrett and Kyet, 1979). Despite these findings, discrepancies exist regarding the number and classes of Ca^{2+}-binding sites reported for calmodulin. These discrepancies probably represent variation in the conditions under which the calcium-binding properties have been studied. Most reports indicate that calmodulin binds four mol Ca^{2+} per mol protein with dissociation constants for calcium in the micromolar range when assayed at high ionic strength (> 40 mm). Concentrations of Mg^{2+} as high as 3 mM have no effect on Ca^{2+} binding. At low ionic strength, cation-binding properties become more complicated, and competition between Ca^{2+} and Mg^{2+} for the binding sites may occur (Wolff et al., 1977).

The secondary structure of calmodulin has been examined by several techniques including CD and ORD. The molecule consists of approximately 40% α-helix, 18% β-pleated sheet, and 42% random coil in the presence of Ca^{2+} (Klee, 1977). The changes in calmodulin secondary structure due to Ca^{2+} binding leads to an increase in the content of α-helix, an enhanced resistance to proteolytic inactivation (Ho et al., 1975; Liu and Cheung, 1976), and a decrease in Stokes radius (Kuo and Coffee, 1976a,b).

Because calmodulin contains multiple Ca^{2+}-binding sites, the question has been raised as to whether all four Ca^{2+}-binding sites need to be occupied before a Ca^{2+}-dependent conformational change occurs. Klee (1977) demonstrated that the binding of two moles Ca^{2+} to the high-affinity sites (K_{diss} = 4 μM, Table 3.6) is sufficient for the bulk of the conformation change in the molecule. This result suggests that the binding of only two moles Ca^{2+} is required for enzyme activation. Dedman et al. (1977a,b) have examined the dependence on Ca^{2+} concentration of Ca^{2+} binding, conformation change, and enzyme activation. They reported that 95% of the α-helical change

Table 3.6 Physical and Chemical Ca^{2+} Binding Properties of Various Calmodulins

Parameter	Source					
	Bovine Heart	Rat Testes	Bovine Brain	Porcine Brain	Bovine Adrenal Medulla	Earthworm
Molecular weight	19,000	18,000	15,000	16,500	16,000	18,000
Sedimentation constant $S^0 20$, w	2.0	1.9	1.85	—	1.9	1.95
f/f_0	1.3	1.34	1.2	—	—	1.3
pI (pH)	4.1	3.9	4.3	—	4.3	4.0
E275–278, 1% 1 cm	1.9	2.1	1.0	1.5	—	3.2
Acidic residues (glx + asx) (%)	34	33	33	36	33	34
Number of Ca^{2+}-binding sites						
High affinity	1	4	3 (2)*	2	—	2
Low affinity	2–3	0	1 (2)	2	2	—
Dissociation constants of Ca^{2+} binding (μM)						
High affinity	2.9	2.4	3.5 (1.1)	4	—	6
Low affinity	11.9	—	18 (8.6)	12	20	—
α-Helical content						
+ Ca^{2+}	—	54	57	50	40	—
− Ca^{2+}	—	45	39	30–35	20	—
References	Teo et al. (1973)	Dedman et al. (1977b)	Lin et al. (1974); Liu et al., (1976)	Klee (1977)	Kuo and Coffee (1976)	Weisman et al. (1977, 1978)

^{a}Values according to Watterson et al. (1976).

occurred before threshold enzyme activation and that the maximum enzyme activation by calmodulin corresponded to the binding of about two mole Ca^{2+} per mole calmodulin.

Parvalbumin

Parvalbumins are small (M.W. 12,000), highly acidic (pI 4.0) Ca^{2+}-binding proteins (Table 3.5) found in all vertebrates including fish, birds, amphibians, reptiles, and mammals (Benzonana et al., 1972; Heizmann et al., 1977) and in the white leg muscle of the invertebrate limulus (Anderson et al., 1978). They are present in especially large amounts in the skeletal muscles of vertebrates (Baron et al., 1975). The physiological function of parvalbumin is at present unknown. Pechère et al. (1975) and Gillis and Gerday (1977) have suggested that parvalbumin may play a role in the relaxation cycle of white muscle. In particular, it has been suggested that parvalbumins may serve to shuttle Ca^{2+} between myofibrils and the SR. In support of this suggestion is the observation that Ca^{2+} accumulation by SR is not fast enough to account for the rate of relaxation of a living muscle (Ebashi, 1976).

MODULATION

Once the second messenger has bound to its receptor protein, the question then becomes how the message modulates cellular response.

General Features

The mechanisms of modulation of the cAMP message and the calcium message, via calmodulin, troponin C, and leiotonin, are different. In all cases, the receptor proteins do not possess any intrinsic enzymatic activities but undergo conformational changes when interacting with their respective messenger. As a consequence, they must exist in some multiprotein complex to influence cellular activity. The nature of these complexes is restricted in the case of the cAMP-receptor proteins, troponin C and leiotonin C but not in the case of calmodulin, which interacts with a variety of response elements.

There are at least four mechanisms by which these regulatory proteins could alter the structure and/or function of other proteins. In the first two, the regulatory subunit would be bound to the catalytic subunit in the absence of the messenger. This complex could be either active or inactive. Binding of the messenger to the regulatory site would lead to either activation or inactivation of the system. Conversely, in the second two cases, the regulatory subunit and the catalytic subunits would be dissociated in the absence of messenger. Binding of messenger to regulatory site would lead to an association of regulatory with catalytic subunit and the complex would either be active or inactive.

In the case of the cAMP system, the receptor protein (R) is bound to the catalytic subunit (C) of the protein kinase. In this state, the kinase is inactive

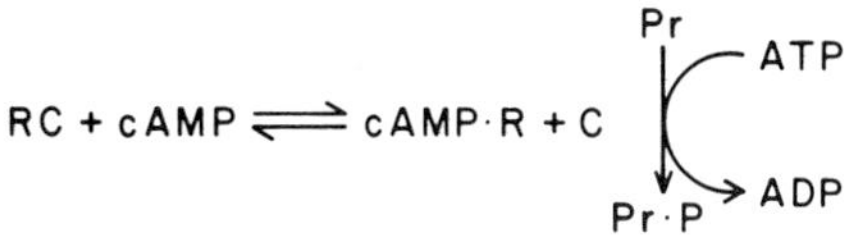

$$RC + cAMP \rightleftharpoons cAMP \cdot R + C$$

$$\begin{array}{c} Pr \\ \diagup ATP \\ \diagup \\ Pr \cdot P \diagdown ADP \end{array}$$

Figure 3.18 Mechanism by which cAMP regulates the protein kinase reaction. RC = Inhibited complex; C = free catalytic subunit; Pr = protein substrate; and R = regulatory subunit or cAMP binding protein.

(Figure 3.18). When the cAMP content of the cell cytosol rises, cAMP binds to R, alters its conformation, and causes its dissociation from C. Free C is now an active protein kinase which catalyzes the phosphorylation of a variety of proteins.

At present, this is the only known modulating mechanism in the cAMP system. However, there are membrane-bound as well as soluble cAMP-dependent protein kinases. It is not yet known how the former are activated by cAMP, but it is possible that they do not involve a dissociation of R from C.

At least two mechanisms are known by which the calmodulin–calcium complex is involved in intracellular modulation (Figure 3.19). The first of these is exemplified by the calmodulin-dependent activation of phosphodiesterase. In this case, in the absence of calcium, calmodulin and phosphodiesterase are separate. A rise in calcium ion content leads to the formation of a calcium–calmodulin complex. The binding of calcium to calmodulin leads to a conformation change in the molecule which in turn leads to its association with phosphodiesterase. This complex, calcium–calmodulin–phosphodies-

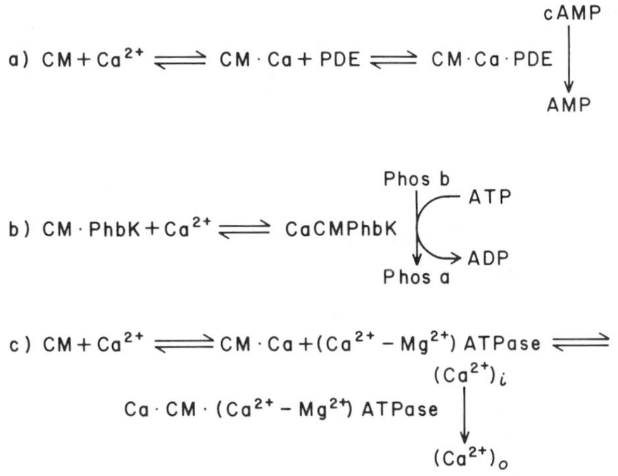

a) $CM + Ca^{2+} \rightleftharpoons CM \cdot Ca + PDE \rightleftharpoons CM \cdot Ca \cdot PDE$ $\begin{array}{c} cAMP \\ \downarrow \\ AMP \end{array}$

b) $CM \cdot PhbK + Ca^{2+} \rightleftharpoons CaCMPhbK$ $\begin{array}{c} Phos\ b \\ \diagup ATP \\ \diagup \\ \diagdown ADP \\ Phos\ a \end{array}$

c) $CM + Ca^{2+} \rightleftharpoons CM \cdot Ca + (Ca^{2+} - Mg^{2+})\ ATPase \rightleftharpoons$

$$Ca \cdot CM \cdot (Ca^{2+} - Mg^{2+})\ ATPase \begin{array}{c} (Ca^{2+})_i \\ \downarrow \\ (Ca^{2+})_o \end{array}$$

Figure 3.19 Mechanism by which Ca^{2+} regulates (a) phosphodiesterase (PDE), (b) phosphorylase *b* kinase (PhbK) activity, and (c) the plasma membrane calcium pump. CM = Calmodulin; Phos b and a represent the nonphosphorylated and phosphorylated forms of phosphorylase. Note that in cases (a) and (b), Ca·CM activates a protein kinase, in case (c), a $(Ca^{2+}-Mg^{2+})$-dependent ATPase.

terase, is the active form of the enzyme. In another system, for example, phosphorylase kinase, calmodulin is a subunit of this oligomeric protein. Allosteric modification of the bound subunit, calmodulin, leads to a calcium-dependent activation of the enzyme. It is possible that in still other systems calmodulin will be found to be a bound inhibitor in the absence of calcium and its calcium-dependent dissociation would lead to an activation of a particular enzyme (see Chapter 10).

Sensitivity Modulation

In describing cellular control systems in terms of information flow, it is generally believed that messenger-mediated cellular response is a consequence of an increase in strength (amplitude) of the message, that is, an increase in the concentration of either calcium and/or cAMP in the cell cytosol. However, this is not the only means of inducing response.

In the calcium control system, examples of both positive and negative sensitivity modulation have been recognized (Figure 3.20). Both result from the cAMP-dependent phosphorylation of a calcium-dependent protein kinase. Positive modulation is seen in the case of phosphorylase kinase (see Chapter 4). When phosphorylated by cAMP-dependent protein kinase, the K_a for activation by Ca^{2+} is 0.5 μM, and when nonphosphorylated it is 3 μM. Conversely, in the case of myosin light chain kinase, cAMP-dependent phosphorylation of this enzyme leads to a decrease in its sensitivity to activation by Ca^{2+} (see Chapter 8). In both cases, the cAMP-dependent protein kinase catalyzes the phosphorylation of a subunit of the calcium-dependent kinase other than its calcium-binding subunit, calmodulin. It thus appears that phosphorylating of this other subunit leads to a change in the affinity of calmodulin for calcium (see Chapter 10).

This conclusion has important implications. It indicates that the affinity of calmodulin for calcium is not a fixed value but varies by a factor of at least 10 or possibly more, depending upon the protein (response element) with which it is associated (Figure 3.20). This means that in a cell containing several calcium–calmodulin-activated enzymes, not each is necessarily activated to the same degree by a given increase in the cytosolic calcium concentration; that is, a graded or sequential type of response can be seen.

Negative sensitivity modulation is also seen in the cAMP messenger system. Administration of insulin modifies the subsequent hepatic response to glucagon without altering the glucagon-dependent rise in cAMP concentration. Even though the [cAMP] rises to the same extent, the activation of both glycogenolysis and gluconeogenesis by glucagon is inhibited. Insulin shifts the apparent dose–response curve to the right; that is, there is less activation of the process at any glucagon or cAMP concentration. Walkenbach et al. (1978, 1980) have recently shown that the effect of insulin is to reduce the sensitivity of the cAMP-dependent protein kinase to cAMP (Figure 3.21). A higher concentration of cAMP is required to induce the dissociation of RC to C and R·cAMP in the enzyme isolated from the insulin-treated cell.

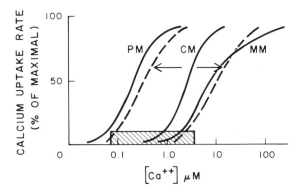

Figure 3.20   Effect of change in the affinity of calcium binding to calmodulin in relation to the control range of cytosolic calcium ion (shaded area). The activities of the two main calcium pumps in the plasma membrane (PM) and mitochondrial membrane (MM) as a function of free calcium content of the cell cytosol define the control range for Ca^{2+} concentration in the cell cytosol. The line labeled CM depicts the calcium binding curve of free calmodulin. The dotted line to the left defines approximately the calcium binding curve for CM when it is a component of the phosphorylated form of phosphorylase kinase. The dotted curve on the right defines the approximate calcium binding curve for CM when it is a subunit of phosphorylated myosin light chain kinase. Note that by controlling the sensitivity of these calmodulin-regulating systems to Ca^{2+}, cAMP-dependent phosphorylation can shift the apparent affinity of CM for calcium from one extreme of the calcium control range to the other.

These two examples demonstrate that control of cellular response by either the calcium or the cAMP messenger system can be achieved directly by *amplitude modulation* (by changing the concentration of calcium ion or

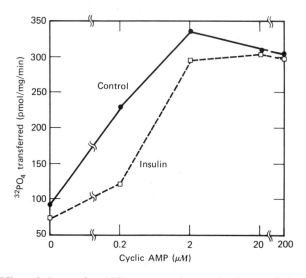

Figure 3.21   Effect of changes in cAMP concentration on the degree of phosphorylation of crude glycogen synthase isolated from control and insulin-treated liver. From Walkenbach et al. (1978), with permission.

cAMP) or indirectly by *sensitivity modulation* (by changing the affinity of the response element for the messenger) (Table 3.7).

An additional important determinant of cellular response is that of hormone receptor number. Levitzki (1978) has pointed out that the circulating concentration of catecholamines, for example, are far below the dissociation constant for the β-receptor. Hence, under physiological conditions only a small percentage of the receptors are ever occupied. Levitzki also pointed out that in a specific cellular response system, the turkey erythrocyte, the hormone concentration necessary to induce a half-maximal effect on Na^+ efflux ($1 \times 10^{-8} M$) is over two orders of magnitude lower than that needed to produce a half-maximal effect on adenylate cyclase ($6 \times 10^{-6} M$). Occupation of 0.016% of the receptors is sufficient to cause an initial tenfold rise in cAMP concentration from 2×10^{-8} to $2 \times 10^{-7} M$, a concentration sufficient to fully activate the cAMP-dependent protein kinase in this cell. Nonetheless, the receptor number is important because if response is a function of the number of occupied receptors (HR), then a reduction in either H or R will reduce the response (H + R $\rightleftharpoons$ HR $\rightarrow$ physiological effect). For example, Nickersen (1956) has shown that irreversibly 99% of the histamine receptors on the cell surface can be blocked and one can still obtain a maximal hormonal response; the decrease in receptor number causes a shift of the dose–response curve to the right.

Thus, an increase or a decrease in receptor number can lead to a type of sensitivity modulation just as a change in receptor affinity can. It is possible therefore to have differentially responsive cell types responsive to different concentrations of circulating hormone merely by having different densities of receptors for the hormone on the cell surfaces. Similarly, a difference in the responsiveness of different intracellular response elements to the same intracellular messenger can be achieved by having a greater or smaller concentration of the response element in relation to other response elements within the same cell. This means that, both at the cell surface receptors and in the interaction of cellular response elements with the intracellular mes-

Table 3.7 Sensitivity Modulation of Cellular Response

Primary Messenger	Effect	System
cAMP	Increased sensitivity to calcium	Glycogenolysis
	Decreased sensitivity to calcium	Smooth muscle contraction
Calcium	Increased sensitivity to cAMP	Calcium uptake by cardiac SR
	Decreased sensitivity to cAMP	?
	Increased sensitivity to cGMP	Glucose transport

senger, *sensitivity modulation* can be achieved either by a change in the affinity of specific receptor for extra- and intracellular messenger, respectively, or by a change in receptor or response element number.

RESPONSE

The ultimate consequence of information transfer is cellular response. Response depends upon the interaction of the intracellular receptor proteins with response elements within the cell.

Cyclic AMP Response Elements

In the case of the cAMP messenger system, the only presently identified type of response element is the catalytic subunit of protein kinase (Robison et al., 1971). The immediate molecular effect of its activities is to change the state of phosphorylation of a variety of proteins leading to a change in their activity which is eventually expressed as a change in cell function. These cAMP-dependent protein kinases are widely distributed in animal cells. A challenge remains, however. This is the challenge of defining the specific substrates for these kinases in particular target tissues and identifying the mechanisms by which the phosphorylated proteins regulate cell function.

Calmodulin Response Elements

In the case of the calcium–calmodulin system, a variety of response elements have been identified. These include general and specific protein kinase, calcium transport systems, and microtubule assembly. The properties of the various response elements which interact with the calcium receptor protein, calmodulin or CDR, are summarized in Table 3.8.

Cyclic Nucleotide Phosphodiesterase

Cyclic nucleotide phosphodiesterases catalyze the hydrolysis of cAMP and cGMP to AMP and GMP, respectively. The presence of multiple forms of cyclic nucleotide phosphodiesterase was first reported by Thompson and Appleman (1971). By chromatography on DEAE cellulose columns of extracts from a variety of tissues including liver (Russell et al., 1973), heart, kidney, mammary gland, lung, and brain (Appleman and Terasake, 1975), three discrete active fractions of phosphodiesterase activity have been resolved. These are referred to as D-I, D-II, and D-III according to their elution from the column by a salt gradient. The D-III form has a low K_m (cAMP) and is particulate; D-II is a soluble enzyme possessing equal activity toward cAMP and cGMP; and D-I is a low-K_m (cGMP) high-K_m (cAMP) enzyme. Because of the Ca^{2+} dependence of this latter enzyme, its properties are further discussed.

The separation of soluble phosphodiesterase into Ca^{2+}-sensitive and Ca^{2+}-insensitive forms was initially reported in rat brain by Kakiuchi et al. (1971). Later it was shown that the activation of this enzyme by Ca^{2+} was

Table 3.8 Properties of Calmodulin-Regulated Response Elements

Enzyme	Tissue	Molecular Weight	Apparent K_m (Ca²⁺)	References
Myosin light chain kinase	Gizzard	105,000	3 μM	Dabrowska et al. (1978)
	Skeletal muscle	90,000	—	Wang and Waisman (1979)
	Platelet	105,000	—	Hathaway and Adelstein (1979)
Phosphorylase b kinase	Skeletal muscle	1.26×10^6	3 M, 0.5 M (activation)	Brostrom et al. (1971)
Protein kinase	Liver	1.3×10^6	0.3 μM	Sakai et al. (1979)
	Synaptosomes	—	0.3 μM	Schulman and Greengard (1978)
Guanylate cyclase	*Tetrahymena pyriformis*	—	8 μM	Nagao et al. (1979)
Tubulin	Brain	110,000	1 μM	Nishida et al. (1979)
NAD kinase	Plant	—	0.25 μM	Anderson and Cormier (1978)
Modular binding protein I	Brain	85,000	—	Sharma et al. (1979)
Modulator binding protein II	Brain	70,000	—	Sharma et al. (1978)
Plasmalemma Ca²⁺ pump	Red blood cell	125,000	0.8 μM	Niggli et al. (1979); Waisman et al. (1981)
Adenylate cyclase	Brain	—	2.5 μM (activation) 200 μM (inhibition)	Brostrom et al. (1978)
Phosphodiesterase	Heart	155,000	2.3 μM	Ho et al. (1977)

mediated by calmodulin (Kakiuchi et al., 1973). The kinetic properties of the calmodulin-dependent, partially purified phosphodiesterase of brain and heart have been characterized in many laboratories (see Figure 1.20) (Teo and Wang, 1973; Ho et al., 1977; Wallace et al., 1978; Klee et al., 1978). The enzyme catalyzes the hydrolysis of both cAMP and cGMP. Ho et al. (1976) have suggested that the activation of bovine heart phosphodiesterase by calmodulin results in a fivefold increase in V_{max} and a decrease of about 30-fold in the K_m (from 1.5 mM to 0.2 mM) when cAMP is used as substrate. Similar results have been reported by Klee et al. (1978). When cGMP is used as substrate, a decrease in K_m of about fiftyfold (from 0.26 mM to 9 μM) and no change in V_{max} (remains at about 30% of the V_{max} for cAMP) are seen (Ho et al., 1976).

The calcium–calmodulin-regulated brain phosphodiesterase is of considerable interest because it has opened an additional avenue of research. In 1974, Weiss and coworkers (Weiss et al., 1974) reported that the drug Trifluoperazine acted as a specific inhibitor of the calcium-activated enzyme (Figure 3.22). Subsequent work has shown that this drug and other drugs of the phenathiazine type act by binding specifically to the calmodulin moiety of the calmodulin–enzyme complex (Weiss and Levin, 1978). More spe-

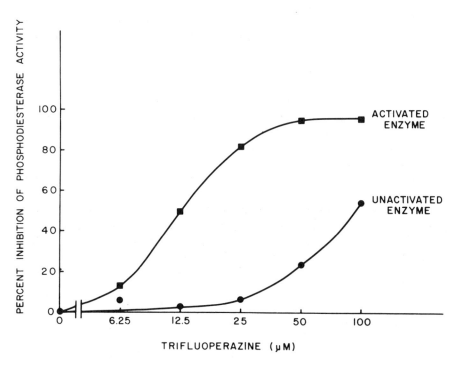

Figure 3.22 Inhibition of calmodulin-activated PDE by increasing concentrations of trifluoperazine. Note that the Ca·CM-activated enzyme is considerably more sensitive to inhibition by the drug than is the unactivated enzyme. From Weiss et al. (1974), with permission.

cifically, these drugs bind to calcium–calmodulin much better than to a calcium-free calmodulin. When the calcium–calmodulin complex is bound to PDE, addition of the drug does not cause a dissociation of the two proteins but inhibits the activity of the enzyme presumably by inducing a conformational change in calmodulin which is transmitted to the PDE. This result means that the complex of calcium–calmodulin–PDE can exist either in an active or inactive state.

These findings have considerable medical significance as a means of developing a better understanding of the mode of action of this class of drugs. They also offer a new investigative tool with which to probe calcium–calmodulin-mediated events in many different systems. A few examples of their use in this way are cited in other sections of this monograph.

Adenylate Cyclase

The direct stimulation of the adenylate cyclase of the plasmalemma by hormone–receptor complex is believed to be the usual mechanism responsible for activation of the cAMP second messenger system. That Ca^{2+} might be involved in adenyl cyclase regulation was suggested by Birnbaumer (1973), who demonstrated that the enzyme derived from a variety of tissues was strongly inhibited by low concentrations of Ca^{2+}. Brain tissue, on the other hand, was found to possess adenylate cyclase activity which exhibits a biphasic response to Ca^{2+}. Low Ca^{2+} concentrations activated and higher concentration inhibited the enzyme. An examination of brain tissue by Brostrom et al. (1975) and Cheung et al. (1975) has revealed that calmodulin mediates this calcium-dependent stimulation of adenylate cyclase. Brostrom et al. (1978) have demonstrated the existence of calmodulin-dependent adenylate cyclase activity in all areas of rat brain, in human neuroblastoma, and in glioma cell lines. An examination of porcine kidney medulla, frog erythrocyte, and rat and rabbit hearts failed to reveal calmodulin-stimulated adenylate cyclase. On the other hand, Valverde et al. (1979a,b) have reported the presence of calmodulin-stimulated adenylate cyclase in pancreatic islets.

The biphasic response of brain adenylate cyclase to Ca^{2+} has been examined by Brostrom et al. (1977) and Wescott et al. (1979). Their results suggest that brain contains separate calmodulin-sensitive and -insensitive forms of adenylate cyclase. The calmodulin-insensitive form has been shown to be inhibited by Ca^{2+}. The calmodulin-sensitive adenylate cyclase displays a biphasic response to Ca^{2+} stimulation (Figure 3.23) at low Ca^{2+} [$K_m(Ca^{2+})$ $2.5 \mu M$] and inhibition at higher Ca^{2+} [$K_m(Ca^{2+})$ 200 μM] (Brostrom, 1978. Gnegy et al. (1976) have reported that calmodulin regulates the stimulation of adenylate cyclase activity by the putative neurotransmitter dopamine. Brostrom et al. (1979) have analyzed the possible role of calmodulin in the regulation of cAMP production in response to norepinephrine in intact glial tumor cells. Their results suggest that in these cells, calmodulin mediates the increase in cAMP production induced by norepinephrine because Trifluoperazine inhibited this response.

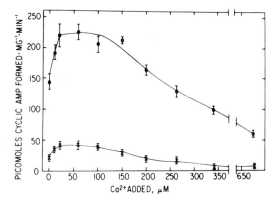

Figure 3.23 Adenylate cyclase activity in glial tumor cell homogenates as function of Ca^{2+} concentration in the presence (●) and absence (×) of 100 μM norepinephrine. From Brostrom et al. (1976), with permission.

In conclusion, it appears that in many tissues (other than neural tissue agents), influencing Ca^{2+} concentration could regulate cAMP synthesis in a reciprocal fashion; that is, agents that increase Ca^{2+} would be expected to inhibit cAMP synthesis. Presumably, this mechanism does not require calmodulin. In other tissues such as brain, Ca^{2+} (mediated by calmodulin) appears to be essential for the activation of neurotransmitter-stimulated adenylate cyclase. In the absence of Ca^{2+} and calmodulin, transmitter activation of adenylate cyclase is greatly reduced.

Phospholipase A₂

Specific phospholipases that hydrolize the acyl bond of the fatty acid in the Sn2-position of phospholipids are widely distributed in nature (Van den Bosch, 1980). Those bound to the plasma membrane of many different cells show an absolute requirement for Ca^{2+}. In many cases, one of the consequences of hormonal stimulation of a particular cell by a specific hormone or extracellular messenger is a calcium-dependent activation of the enzyme. This process has been particularly well studied in human platelets (see Chapter 8). Of interest in the present context are the observations of Wong and Cheung (1980). These investigators showed that calmodulin mediated the effects of Ca^{2+} on platelet phospholipase A_2. The mechanism by which calcium–calmodulin regulates this enzyme is not known. It seems likely that the general mechanism by which Ca^{2+} regulates the activity of this plasma membrane-bound enzyme will prove to be via calmodulin. Regulation of this membrane-bound enzyme by calcium–calmodulin represents a relatively unexplored area, but one which is likely to prove of great significance in our eventual understanding of how the calcium messenger system regulates the function of the plasma membrane. The relationship of phospholipase A_2 activity to PI turnover has been discussed above.

Calcium Pumps

The maintenance of low cytosolic Ca^{2+} concentrations is the function of membrane Ca^{2+} pumps in the plasmalemma, the mitochondria, and the microsomes. The two well-characterized pumps, the plasmalemma Ca^{2+} pump of the human red blood cell and the canine heart microsomal pump, are regulated by calcium ion.

The red blood cell plasmalemma Ca^{2+} pump catalyzes the energy-dependent uphill transport of Ca^{2+} from the cytosol (Ca^{2+} concentration 0.1 μM) to the extracellular fluid (Ca^{2+} concentration 1 mM) (Schatzmann and Vincenzi, 1969). The isolation of highly purified inside-out vesicles composed of plasma membrane has allowed characterization of the red blood cell Ca^{2+} pump. An apparent K_m for Ca^{2+} of 0.8 μM has been reported by Waisman et al., 1981a,b,c,), a value in accordance with the physiological concentration of Ca^{2+} in these cells. The stimulation of Ca^{2+} pumping by calmodulin in inside-out red blood cell membrane vesicles (see Figure 2.3) has been reported by several groups (MacIntyre and Green, 1978; Hinds and Vincenzi, 1978; Larson and Vincenzi, 1979; Waisman et al., 1981a,b,c). Presently available data support the view that calmodulin stimulates the activity of this ATPase by simple ligand (CDR)–enzyme association and not by a covalent modification, as is thought to be the case with calmodulin control of calcium ATPase activity in the sarcoplasmic reticulum (Jarrett and Kyte, 1979).

Recently Kuo et al. (1979) have demonstrated the regulation of the synaptic plasmalemma Ca^{2+} pump by calmodulin, so it is likely that this action of calmodulin is widespread. Hormonal regulation of the red blood cell or synaptic Ca^{2+} pump has not been reported. However, Pershadsingh and McDonald (1979) have reported that the adipocyte plasmalemma Ca^{2+} pump is inhibited by physiological concentrations of insulin. Also, Ziegelhoffer et al. (1979) have observed the phosphorylation and activation of the heart sarcolemmal Ca^{2+} pump by the cAMP-dependent protein kinase. Together these results suggest that the plasmalemmal Ca^{2+} pump may represent a target for both cAMP- and calcium-dependent protein kinase.

LePeuch et al. (1980) have reported that both calcium and cAMP regulate Ca^{2+} transport in cardiac SR. They have shown that the regulatory protein of the Ca^{2+} pump, phospholamban, is phosphorylated at different sites by a calmodulin-stimulated protein kinase and by the cAMP-dependent protein kinase. Calmodulin-dependent phosphorylation is capable of activating sarcoplasmic Ca^{2+} uptake. The cAMP-dependent phosphorylation does not activate Ca^{2+} uptake in the absence of calmodulin but amplifies the activation brought about by calmodulin-dependent phosphorylation. The microsomal Ca^{2+} pump in other tissues may also be regulated by hormones. Waltenbaugh and Friedmann (1978) have reported that glucagon increased the Ca^{2+} uptake of liver microsomes.

The Ca^{2+}-stimulated Mg ATPase of membranous preparations has been generally interpreted to be a reflection of the Ca^{2+} transport system

(Schatzmann and Vincenzi, 1969). This ATPase has been demonstrated in a variety of tissues including the microsomes of brain (Saermark and Vilhardt, 1979), liver (Waltenbaugh and Friedmann, 1978), adipose tissue (Bruns et al., 1977), and kidney (Moore and Landon, 1979), as well as in the plasma membrane of red blood cells (Schatzmann and Bürgin, 1978), heart cells (Ziegelhoffer et al., 1979), kidney cells (Moore et al., 1974), pancreatic islet cells (Lambert and Christophe, 1978), adipocytes (Pershadsingh and McDonald, 1979), and synaptosomes (Ohashi et al., 1970). If these pumps are regulated by similar mechanisms as the red blood cell plasmalemma and the cardiac microsomal pump, then it is reasonable to suggest that (a) calmodulin acts as a cytosolic Ca^{2+} sensor which activates the Ca^{2+} pumps and terminates the Ca^{2+} second message, and (b) hormones which act to stimulate or inhibit the Ca^{2+} pumps (e.g., via cAMP) could alter the temporal and/or spatial domains of the Ca^{2+} message.

Protein Kinases and Membrane Function

Calcium-mediated phosphorylations mediating membrane function have been studied by Schulman and Greengard (1978a,b). They found a Ca^{2+}- and calmodulin-stimulated protein kinase in the particulate fraction ($105,000 \times g$ pellet) of a number of tissues including spleen, skeletal muscle, heart, vas deferens, adrenals, and lung. Interestingly, a comparison of the phosphoproteins found in these membranes by SDS gel electrophoresis reveals a dissimilar pattern of phosphoprotein bands for each tissue. This suggests that tissue-specific regulatory effects of a calmodulin-stimulated protein kinase may be achieved by the varied tissue distribution of the substrates for this kinase. Carstens and Weller (1978) have reported a similar multifunctional protein kinase that is activated by cAMP rather than calcium in the membranes of a variety of tissues. So it is quite likely that in many cells membrane functions are controlled by actions of both types of kinases acting in either a coordinate or redundant fashion.

An example of the role of the calmodulin-stimulated protein kinase in the regulation of membrane function has been revealed from the studies of brain synaptosomes (functionally intact, pinched-off nerve endings). DeLorenzo and Friedmann (1977a,b) first suggested that the molecular mechanisms mediating the effects of Ca^{2+} on neurotransmitter release could involve the action of Ca^{2+}-dependent protein phosphorylation. DeLorenzo and Friedmann (1978) have demonstrated a direct correlation between Ca^{2+}-specific synaptosomal phosphorylation and Ca^{2+}-specific transmitter release. The regulation of these events was subsequently shown to be mediated by calmodulin (DeLorenzo et al., 1979). Besides the calmodulin-dependent regulation of synaptosomal membrane phosphorylation and norepinephrine release, these investigators have also implicated calmodulin in the release of acetylcholine and dopamine. It is interesting to note that calmodulin-stimulated phosphorylation of synaptosomal membranes produces only two phosphoproteins of molecular weight 80,000 and 86,000 (Krueger et al.,

1977), which are found only in nerve tissues (Sieghart et al., 1979). Sieghart et al. (1979) also report that these phosphoproteins can be phosphorylated at different sites by cAMP- and Ca^{2+}-dependent protein kinase, suggesting that both cAMP and Ca^{2+} are involved in the control of neurotransmitter release.

Soluble Protein Kinase

Garrison et al. (1979) reported that angiotensin II and vasopressin stimulate the phosphorylation of 10 to 12 soluble hepatic proteins by a mechanism that requires Ca^{2+} and is independent of changes in cAMP or the activity of the cAMP-dependent protein kinase (Chapter 7). The proteins whose phosphorylation is stimulated by this mechanism have molecular weights identical with those whose phosphorylation is increased by glucagon through an activation of the cAMP-dependent protein kinase (a mechanism which is not dependent on the presence of extracellular Ca^{2+}). These findings imply that the activity of many soluble proteins may be regulated by a redundant biochemical mechanism involving phosphorylation by either a Ca^{2+}- or a cAMP-dependent protein kinase.

The major cAMP-dependent protein kinase first isolated was that responsible for catalyzing the phosphorylation of phosphorylase b kinase, converting it from its "inactive" to its "active" form. Later, it was shown that this same kinase catalyzed the phosphorylation of glycogen synthase, converting it from its "active" to its "inactive" form. Roach et al. (1978) demonstrated that the calcium-dependent protein kinase phosphorylase b kinase is also capable of catalyzing the phosphorylation of glycogen synthase. Recently, DePaoli-Roach et al. (1980) have shown that three additional fractions of protein kinase from rabbit skeletal muscle could catalyze the phosphorylation of glycogen synthase. Hence, at least five mechanisms exist for the phosphorylation of this enzyme. The cAMP-dependent protein kinase and the Ca^{2+}-dependent protein kinase (phosphorylase kinase) bring about the phosphorylation of different sites on the glycogen synthase molecule (DePaoli et al., 1980). The cAMP-dependent kinase catalyzes the preferential phosphorylation of a M.W. 12,000 CNBr fragment of the enzyme, whereas phosphorylase kinase catalyzes the phosphorylation of a M.W. 21,000 CNBr fragment. At higher phoshorylation levels, cAMP-dependent protein kinase also catalyzes the phosphorylation of this latter fragment. Either phosphorylation alone is sufficient to reduce the activity of glycogen synthase, although phosphorylation of the M.W. 12,000 site has a greater effect than phosphorylation of the M.W. 21,000 site. In addition, one of the other kinases catalyzes the phosphorylation of the enzyme at a third site also associated with a decrease in activity.

These findings are of great importance from the point of view of understanding the mechanisms by which the two messenger systems regulate the same cell function. The fact that Ca^{2+}-dependent and cAMP-dependent protein kinases may use the same protein substrate but catalyze the phosphorylation of different sites on the substrate molecule means that the function of the same regulated protein may be modified by phosphorylation of one of several sites on the molecule. Given this possibility and the findings of DePaoli et al. (1980) that these sites are not equivalent in terms of their influence on protein function, it is likely that when a complex system such as hepatic gluconeogenesis is activated by the calcium messenger system rather than the cAMP system, a slightly different pattern of control would result. This appears to be the case. The inhibition of pyruvate kinase is more marked when glucagon (cAMP) rather than norepinephrine (Ca^{2+}) stimulates hepatic gluconeogenesis (Garrison and Borland, 1979).

Microtubule Assembly

Tubulin, the subunit protein of microtubules, is a heterodimer composed of two polypeptide chain (α and β) of molecular weight 55,000 each. It exists in the cytosol as well as being associated with membranous structures such as presynaptic membranes (Kornguth and Sunderland, 1975). Cytoplasmic microtubules may play a role in the intracellular transport of the secretory granules toward the cell apex during protein secretion (Rossignol et al., 1977). Together with the microfilaments framed from actin, microtubules comprise the cytoskeleton and are thought to be essential for cell motility and mitosis (Dedman et al., 1979).

A role for Ca^{2+} in the regulation of microtubule assembly was first suggested by Olmsted and Borisy (1973). They demonstrated the in vitro inhibition of microtubule polymerization by Ca^{2+}. Later, Salmon and Jenkins (1977) reported the stimulation of *in vitro* depolymerization of microtubules by Ca^{2+}. Nishida and Sakai (1977) showed that porcine brain extracts contain a factor capable of conferring Ca^{2+} sensitivity to the microtubule assembly process. In the presence of this factor, micromolar levels of Ca^{2+} inhibited microtubule assembly or promoted microtubule disassembly. Marcum et al. (1978) identified calmodulin as the factor which conferred Ca^{2+} sensitivity to this system. They found that 10 μM Ca^{2+} and an eightfold molar excess of calmodulin over tubulin was required to completely inhibit microtubule assembly. At physiological ionic strength, a calcium concentration of 1 μM is necessary to completely inhibit microtubule assembly (Nishida et al., 1979; Kumogai and Nishida, 1979). Under these conditions, a calmodulin/tubulin ratio of 1.5/1.0 was reported, and a Ca^{2+}-dependent binding of calmodulin to tubulin dimer was observed.

The physiological significance of calmodulin-regulated microtubule assembly–disassembly has been investigated by comparing the cellular distribution of fluorescent antibodies to calmodulin and tubulin during mitosis (Welsh et al., 1978; Welsh et al., 1979). Parallel studies with tubulin and calmodulin antibodies show that calmodulin does not accompany all microtubular profiles during mitosis but appears to be localized in specific areas of the mitotic apparatus. For instance, at metaphase, tubulin antibodies decorate the complete spindle and show bundles passing from spindle poles to chromosomes and also transversing the metaphase plate, whereas calmodulin is concentrated near the spindle poles with strands projecting to the chromosomes. Since the spindle poles are thought to act as nucleating sites for microtubule assembly–disassembly, it is possible that calmodulin is restricted to these areas because these are the regulatory sites of microtubule assembly–disassembly.

Troponin C, Leiotonin, and Calmodulin in the Regulation of Contraction

The control of contractile responses in various muscles appears to involve in some way these three calcium receptor proteins (Szent-Gyorgyi, 1976; Ebashi et al., 1978). The most thoroughly studied is troponin C, which functions in skeletal and cardiac muscle to couple the calcium signal to the contractile apparatus. As noted previously, this apparatus, which consists of thin actin filaments arrayed between thick myosin filaments, is in a repressed state in the absence of calcium but can become activated in the absence of calcium if the regulatory complex of proteins consisting of troponin and tropomyosin is removed from the muscle. This complex, thus, acts normally to prevent the interaction of skeletal muscle myosin with actin. Tropomyosin is a long, filamentous molecule. These molecules are arranged end to end and form two continuous strands wound around the groove of the double helix made up of actin molecules. The troponin molecules are globular and sit at regular sites upon the tropomyosin. Troponin consists of three subunits—TN-C, TN-I, and TN-T. The I subunit is an inhibitory subunit which, if present without a C subunit, keeps the contractile system relaxed but which is unresponsive to calcium. Addition of TNC confers calcium sensitivity to the system. When the entire complex is present, addition of calcium by changing the conformation of TN–C leads to a shift in the conformation of the tropomyosin molecules along the actin filament away from the groove, thereby allowing the interaction of myosin with actin to form so-called active complexes (Figure 1.8). The key point is that these proteins are informational molecules, and the information flow is from troponin via tropomyosin to actin. No enzymatic steps are involved, only changes in protein conformation that lead to the intermolecular transmission of information.

Too little is known about leiotonin to discuss its mode of action. Ebashi (1979) has proposed that it acts in operationally analogous fashion to troponin C, it regulates the conformation and therefore the functional properties of the thin filament. There is, however, considerable evidence that the regulation of smooth muscle contraction involves events in the heavy (myosin) chains (Szent-Gyorgyi, 1976; Lehman and Szent-Gyorgyi, 1975), and specifically that this regulation involves the phosphorylation and dephosphorylation of myosin light chains by a protein kinase–protein phosphatase system (see Chapter 8).

The myosin of a variety of muscle and nonmuscle cells has been shown to contain a kinase which phosphorylates a single site on the regulatory light chain (RLC). In nonmuscle cells such as platelets, alveolar macrophages (Hathaway and Adelstein, 1979), brain cells (Dabrowska and Hartshorne, 1978), and hamster kidney cells (Verna et al., 1979), it is believed that the myosin light chain kinase-catalyzed phosphorylation of the RLC is the event responsible for activation of the contractile apparatus of these cells. Similarly, in smooth muscle, the phosphorylation of the RLC by myosin light chain kinase is believed to be responsible for the regulation of contraction (Sobieszek, 1977). In skeletal and cardiac muscle, myosin light chain kinase-catalyzed phosphorylation of the RLC occurs physiologically (Bárány et al., 1979), but the physiological significance of this phosphorylation is not known.

The calcium-sensitive component of the myosin light chain kinase in smooth muscle is calmodulin (Dabrowska et al., 1978). The same holds true in the skeletal muscle (Yagi et al., 1978; Waisman et al., 1978) and in platelets (Hathaway and Adelstein, 1979). Approximately 150 ng/ml calmodulin is needed to activate the smooth muscle enzyme to half its maximal activity (Dabrowska et al., 1978). The role of this system in regulating smooth muscle contraction is discussed in Chapter 7.

TERMINATION

The final step in cellular information transfer is the termination of the message. Little investigative attention has been paid to this aspect of cell activation. However, inadvertently several key discoveries have been made. The most interesting is the finding that calcium–calmodulin activates the plasma membrane calcium pump so that from the moment the calcium message increases in intensity, it initiates the events responsible for the subsequent decrease in its intensity.

Another aspect of the termination process is that in many tissues, for example, in mast cells, the calcium channel in the plasma membrane remains open only for a brief time even in the continued presence of the extracellular stimulus. The other features of the mitochondrial and microsomal membrane calcium pumps which indicate that they participate in calcium message termination are discussed in Chapter 2.

Even less attention has been paid to message termination in the cAMP system other than to identify the various phosphodiesterases in the cell (Table 3.8). There are at least three enzymes (D-I, D-II, and D-III) that can be separated chromatographically. D-III is a particulate low-K_m (cAMP) enzyme; D-II is a soluble enzyme possessing equal activity toward cAMP and cGMP; and D-I is a soluble low-K_m (cGMP), high-K_m (cAMP) enzyme regulated by calmodulin–calcium. Few studies have addressed the question of the relative importance of these various enzymes in the control of the cAMP messenger system function in particular cell responses. However, by analogy with the properties of the calcium messenger system, it can be suggested that the different phosphodiesterases play different roles. The soluble nonregulated enzyme must function to set upper limits on the in-crease in cAMP concentration and so functions in this system the way mitochondrial calcium uptake does in the calcium messenger system. The membrane-bound enzyme in liver is regulated by the redox state of the cell cytoplasm (see Chapter 7), that of the red cell is regulated by calcium–calmodulin (see Chapter 4), and that in some nerve cells is regulated by the state of phosphorylation of the membrane (Wolff and Brostrom, 1979). Likewise, one of the soluble enzymes (D-I) is regulated by calmodulin–calcium.

The regulation of these enzymes must determine the fine control of cAMP concentrations in intact cells. It is a generally recognized phenomenon that upon activation of the adenylate cyclase system in a particular cell by a specific extracellular messenger, there is an initial three- to fourfold rise in the cAMP content of the cell, which usually falls within minutes to values 1.25- to 1.5-fold greater than the basal values. This phasic type of response depends upon the presence of calcium, indicating that this ion exerts some type of control in the intact cell, probably that of regulation by PDE and adenylate cyclase activity.

In this regard, it is of particular interest that Wang and coworkers (1975) have shown that the calcium–calmodulin-mediated change in soluble PDE activity is also enhanced by cAMP, but only in the presence of Ca^{2+}. The cAMP by binding with the catalytic site on the PDE enzyme increases its rate of association with calcium–calmodulin. This means that cAMP regu-lates its own hydrolysis (messenger termination) by a calcium-dependent process. Thus, there is evidence in both messenger systems that each mes-senger regulates some key component of signal termination. In the calcium system, calcium–calmodulin controls the activity of the calcium pump in the plasma membrane; and in the cAMP system, cAMP regulates the activity of the soluble phosphodiesterase which is a major factor in messenger hy-drolysis in most cells.

The key point in terms of understanding the simple elegance of modulation in both systems is that the steady state concentration of the messenger in the activated cell is only slightly greater than that in the resting cell. Neverthe-less, this small change is sufficient to shift the cell from inaction to action. One can show quite readily that this small rise in cAMP is seen within the context of a system in which both cAMP synthesis and hydrolysis are high, because if one adds a phosphodiesterase inhibitor, the cAMP concentration increases 15- to 20-fold. Thus, control of information flow is determined by a rapid generation and a rapid termination of message flow. This is also true in the case of the calcium messenger system. For example, in the fly salivary gland (see Chapter 5), the transcellular flux of calcium in the gland cell is 20-fold greater in the hormonally activated cell than in the resting cell, but the steady state increase in cytosolic calcium ion concentration is barely detectable.

Is it worth emphasizing these control characteristics in both messenger systems (Table 3.9). From the point of view of our discussion of the mechanisms of message termination, both systems exemplify the dynamic balance between message generation and message termination. The latter is equally as important as the former in determining the nature of the ultimate cell responses.

INTEGRATIVE ACTION OF HORMONES AND NEUROTRANSMITTERS

Years ago, Sherington (1947) wrote a monograph entitled, *The Integrative Action of the Nervous System,* in which he developed the concept that even the smallest motor event in a limb required the interplay of a variety of different neurons innervating a number of different muscles for even a simple movement to be executed properly. Similarly, one recognizes the integrative function of the endocrine system in the organism as exemplified by the interplay of insulin, epinephrine, glucagon, thyroxine, cortisol, and growth hormone, in coordinating the functions of liver, muscle, heart, and brain in terms of their fuel metabolism.

However, the integrative functions of hormones and neurotransmitters upon cell function have not been stressed. It is, nonetheless, the hallmark of their actions. If, for example, we consider the action of ACTH upon the adrenal cortex, at the most superficial level of analysis, we conclude that the primary consequence of ACTH action is an increase in the rate of adrenal steroid biosynthesis and secretion. However, if we analyze the consequences of ACTH action more fully, we discover that this hormone has a variety of short- and long-term effects on cell function all important to the fulfillment of its primary task. These include an increased uptake of cholesterol, an increased uptake of acetate leading to an increase in rate of cholesterol synthesis, and an increased rate of cholesterol ester hydrolysis. All of these increase the supply of the prime substrate, cholesterol, for steroid biosynthesis. The hormone also increases the rate of transport of cholesterol from cytosol to mitochondrial matrix space and therein increases the rate of conversion of cholesterol to pregnenelone. The process of steroid synthesis requires increased supplies of reducing equivalents which in turn require an

Table 3.9 Common Control Characteristics of the Two Messenger Systems

1. The messenger operates within very restricted concentration ranges
2. Upon cell activation, there is a transient marked increase in messenger concentration
3. Sustained cellular response is maintained with messenger concentrations barely higher than those found in the resting cell
4. Under conditions of sustained response, there are high rates of messenger generation and messenger termination
5. There are multiple mechanisms for regulating message termination
6. Both messenger generation and messenger termination are highly regulated

increased rate of utilization of energy yielding substrates. To meet and even anticipate this demand, ACTH stimulates glucose uptake, glycogenolysis, and hexose monophosphate shunt activity. If hormonal exposure of the adrenal cells is prolonged, two other changes occur. The individual cells undergo hypertrophy, and the cell number increases, that is hyperplasia supervenes. Both responses increase the total capacity of the adrenal glands to produce steroid hormones.

The information just summarized indicates that ACTH has an integrative action on the adrenal cell. It is possible to consider a situation in which the hormone acting on the cell generates a cAMP and/or a calcium message which alters the function of the single enzyme complex involved in the conversion of cholesterol to pregnenelone. In such a situation, all the other changes in cell function would ensue because of alterations in various feedback control loop. For example, the stimulation of the activity of the enzyme would lead to a fall in cholesterol concentration which, in turn, could act as a feedback inhibitor of cholesterol uptake and synthesis. With a fall in cholesterol concentration, both uptake and synthesis would be released from feedback inhibition and would increase in rate. However, the available evidence does not support this view. Rather, the available data strongly support an alternative view in which the cAMP and/or calcium messengers act at a number of independent sites within the cell to integrate the activities of the various enzymes and transport systems involved in the total response of the cell to this hormone. This is not to deny that feedback regulation is an important aspect of metabolic control, but to emphasize that superimposed on this type of more basic type of regulation is the integrative type of controls characteristic of hormonally regulated cellular processes.

This integrative type of cellular control is also a characteristic of neurotransmitter-induced cellular responses. Two examples can serve to validate this statement. The first is the action of acetylcholine at the neuromuscular (N–M) junction; the second is the action of acetylcholine in the adrenal medulla.

In the cases of skeletal muscle, the release of acetylcholine at the N–M junction causes a rise in the cytosolic calcium ion concentration, which has two major and simultaneous actions. It induces the muscle to contract, and it causes a net breakdown of glycogen and an increase in glucose uptake, both of which increase the supply of energy-yielding substrate and therefore eventually increase the availability of ATP to counterbalance the increased utilization of ATP during the contractile process.

In the case of the adrenal medulla, acetylcholine also causes a rise in the cytosolic calcium ion content. This in turn, both directly and indirectly, causes both a release of stored catecholamines and an activation of the enzymes involved in the biosynthesis of catecholamines. If the stimulation is sustained, then an increase in the capacity to synthesize catecholamines also increases.

These examples are but a few of the many known instances in which it has been clearly established that the action of hormone or neurotransmitter mediated by the synarchic messengers cAMP and calcium is an integrative one in that these messengers act at multiple control points within the cell to integrate the metabolic activities of that cell and thereby determine the eventual response of the cell to the extracellular messenger.

CONCLUSION

An analysis of the properties of cellular control systems in terms of their serving as a means of transferring information from cell surface to cell interior is a convenient way in which to compare the properties of the cAMP and calcium messenger systems. Such a comparison reveals that these two systems are operationally similar, but differ mainly in the molecular details by which the respective messengers, cAMP and calcium, are generated, and by which they (the messengers) modulate the activity of cellular response elements.

Synarchic Regulation

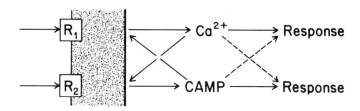

INTRODUCTION

Logically, one might consider two possible modes of biochemical evolution underlying the development of biological systems involved in intercellular communication. On the one hand, primitive cells might have developed rather primitive control devices that were discarded as better ones evolved. Hence, the mechanisms underlying the response of a group of amebae during aggregation might bear little or no relationship to those underlying the response of the human liver to changes in the concentration of the specific pancreatic hormone glucagon. Likewise, one might anticipate that mechanisms that underlie synaptic transmission in the nervous system would be quite different from those that function in the stimulatory action of the peptide hormone angiotensin upon aldosterone secretion from the zona glomerulosa of the mammalian adrenal cortex. On the other hand, primitive solutions of stimulus–response coupling might have been of such simple elegance and evolutionary adaptability that they survived through the millennia by being modified, embossed, and adapted to new functions to meet new evolutionary demands but retaining throughout their basic properties. If so, then the biochemical events involved in the response of a swimming paramecium to an external impediment might have a basic similarity to the response of the uterine muscle cell to the peptide hormone oxytocin.

The most compelling argument that there is a universal system of stimulus–response coupling with ancient evolutionary roots is the existence of the major components of both the cAMP and Ca^{2+} messenger systems in all animal cells. Neither the calcium channel which exists in the paramecium nor the adenylate cyclase found in the cellular slime mold *Dictyostelium discoideum* differ appreciably from their counterparts in a variety of mammalian cells. However, this universal occurrence of the components of these two cellular information transfer systems by itself does not constitute sufficient evidence to warrant the conclusion that these two intracellular agents, calcium and cAMP, act as synarchic messengers in stimulus–response coupling in nearly all animal cells. It is possible that the two systems convey a different type of information from cell surface to cell interior, and function rather independently of one another. Against this possibility is the considerable data showing that, in nearly every cell type examined, the calcium and cAMP messenger systems are intimately interrelated, and do not provide distinctly different types of information, but instead interact to integrate cellular response to a specific class of extracellular stimuli. Before presenting a model of this universal system of synarchic regularion, it is worth reviewing the various known interrelationships between the effect of cAMP and of calcium.

INTERRELATIONSHIP BETWEEN CALCIUM ION AND CYCLIC AMP

Summary of General Interrelationships

The various interrelationships between these two messengers are summarized in Table 4.1. Three general themes are apparent in these relation-

Table 4.1   Interrelationships Between Calcium and Cyclic AMP in Cellular Control Systems

1. Control of cAMP metabolism or action by calcium ion
    a. Increase soluble phosphodiesterase activity
    b. Increase membrane-bound phosphodiesterase activity
    c. Increase adenylate cyclase activity
    d. Decrease adenylate cyclase activity
    e. Alter sensitivity of cAMP-dependent activation of phosphodiesterase
    f. Alter sensitivity of cAMP-dependent activation of microsomal calcium pump
2. Control of calcium metabolism or action by cAMP
    a. Increase calcium uptake of ER
    b. Increased activity of plasma membrane calcium pump
    c. Increased permeability of plasma membrane to calcium
    d. Decreased permeability of plasma membrane to calcium
    e. Increased efflux of calcium from cells by control of Na^+–Ca^{2+} exchange
    f. Increased mitochondrial calcium exchange
    g. Increased sensitivity of calcium receptor protein to calcium signal
    h. Decreased sensitivity of calcium receptor protein to calcium signal
3. Control relationships between the two messenger systems
    a. Sequential control
    b. Coordinate control
    c. Independent control
    d. Redundant control
    e. Hierarchical control
    f. Antagonistic control

ships: (1) calcium regulates cAMP metabolism, thereby extending or limiting the cytosolic domain of cAMP; (2) cAMP regulates calcium metabolism, extending or restricting the calcium domain; and (3) the two messengers act either coordinately, sequentially, antagonistically, hierarchically, or redundantly to control eventual cellular response.

The specific types of controls of calcium metabolism by cAMP and of cAMP metabolism by calcium in any particular cell type define the relationship between these two messengers within a given cell. In some cells, a rise in Ca^{2+} concentration leads to a rise in cAMP concentration and in others, to a fall in cAMP; and in still others, to a biphasic response depending on the magnitude of the change in $[Ca^{2+}]$. The converse is also true.

A number of specific examples of one or the other of these $cAMP–Ca^{2+}$ interactions in particular cells or tissues are listed in Table 4.2. Although not exclusive, this list is not totally inclusive. Many of these are discussed in considerable detail in the ensuing chapters. Data concerning the control characteristics of many other tissues are less complete than those cited, but the available data strongly suggest that in many $cAMP–Ca^{2+}$ interactions similar to those listed will be found to serve the function of coupling stimulus to response. Finally, the $cAMP–Ca^{2+}$ relationship in one particular cell type, the nonnucleated red cell, is worth reviewing briefly as a confirmation of the university of this relationship.

Table 4.2   Calcium–Cyclic AMP Interactions In Stimulus–Response Coupling

1. Effects of calcium on cAMP messenger systems
   a. Stimulates cAMP production—brain, adrenal cortex, pancreatic islets, adrenal medulla, slime mold
   b. Stimulates cAMP hyrolysis—brain, heart, liver, kidney, fly salivary gland, many other tissues
   c. Activates phosphoprotein product of cAMP-dependent protein kinase, glycogenolysis in many tissues
2. Effects of cAMP on calcium messenger system
   a. Increases calcium entry across plasma membrane—heart, synapse
   b. Increases calcium release from mitochondria—kidney, liver, fly salivary gland, others
   c. Increases calcium uptake by microsomes—heart, uterus, liver, smooth muscles
   d. Increases calcium efflux across plasma membrane—smooth muscle, heart
   e. Decreases sensitivity of response elements to calcium—smooth muscle, heart
   f. Increases sensitivity of response element to calcium—phosphorylase *b* kinase, liver, muscle
3. Interrelated activities
   a. cAMP-dependent and calcium-dependent protein kinases act upon same protein substrate—liver, brain, adrenal cortex
   b. Regulate sequential steps in metabolic or transport process—secretion in fly salivary gland, glycogenolysis

Cyclic AMP Metabolism in the Erythrocyte

The simplest cell in the mammal is the erythrocyte. It possesses neither nucleus, mitochondria, nor endoplasmic reticulum. Hence, there is a single membrane system enclosing a cell cytosol. Nevertheless, the erythrocyte of rodents contains a catecholamine-sensitive adenylate cyclase and phosphodiesterase activity (Sheppard and Burghardt, 1969). A similar catecholamine-sensitive cyclase has been studied in avian and anuran erythrocytes (Helmreich et al., 1977; Lefkowitz et al., 1976; Kahn, 1976). It is noteworthy that in addition to activating the cyclase, catecholamines induce the release of calcium from the membranes of turkey erythrocytes (Steer et al., 1975) and from the intact human erythrocytes (Rasmussen et al., 1975; Nelson and Heustis, 1980).

The physiological function of this hormonal system in the red cells is not known, but Nelson and Heustis suggest that a calcium-dependent protein kinase may regulate the degree of phosphorylation of band 2 protein in the membrane. This protein interacts with spectrin in the cell and may thus play a role in controlling the shape of the red cell. In any case, it represents the very simplest of systems in which to explore the nature of the interaction between the cAMP messenger and calcium messenger systems and to explore whether such an interaction is a universal attribute of cellular control systems.

The response of isolated rat erythrocytes to isoproterenol addition is shown in Figure 4.1. After hormone addition, there is an initial three- to

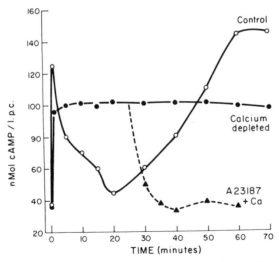

Figure 4.1 Time course of change in cAMP content of rat red cells after exposure to isoproterenol (added at time zero). In normal cells, the response is triphasic (○). In calcium-depleted cells (●), there was a single phase of response, and the cAMP content fell promptly if the calcium ionophore A23187 was added (▲) to the calcium-depleted cells in a calcium-containing medium.

fourfold rise in cAMP content (phase I) followed shortly by a fall to values near basal values (phase II) and then a subsequent sustained four- to fivefold increase in cAMP content (Rasmussen et al., 1979; Clayberger et al., 1981). Thus, even in this simple system there is evidence for a complex flow of information in the cAMP messenger system.

The system has the following features: (1) The triphasic response does not occur in calcium-depleted cells; rather, a monophasic response is seen (Figure 4.1). (2) The activity of the adenylate cyclase is the same in cells from all three phases as judged by the change in cAMP concentration upon addition of the phosphodiesterase inhibitor Ro 20/1724 (Figure 4.2). (3) There is a shift of calmodulin (CDR) from cytosol to membrane after iso-proterenol addition. (4) This shift in CDR from cytosol to membrane is associated with a calcium-dependent activation of membrane-bound phos-phodiesterase (MPDE). (5) The activity of MPDE is higher in phase II than in phase III or in control cells (Figure 4.3). (6) The activity of Ca^{2+}/Mg^{2+} ATPase in the membrane is higher in phase III than in phase II or in control cells (Figure 4.3). And (7) cAMP-dependent phosphorylation of the mem-brane causes an increase in calmodulin binding and an activation of membrane-bound PDE.

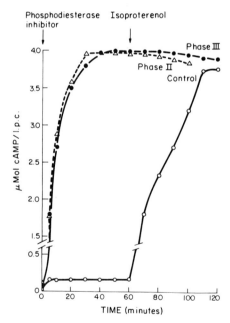

Figure 4.2 Cyclic AMP content of rat renal cells as function of time after addition of a PDE inhibitor and isoproterenol. The control cells (○) were exposed to the inhibitor at time zero and then at 60 minutes treated with isoproterenol (IP). Phase II cells (△) were obtained by exposure of rat cells to IP for 15 minutes, washed, and exposed to the PDE inhibitor at time zero. The Phase III cells (●) were preincubated with IP for 1 hour before the PDE inhibitor was added at time zero.

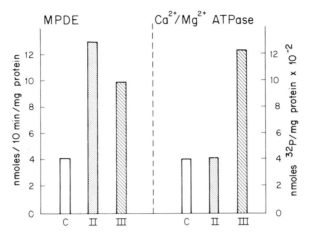

Figure 4.3 Amount of membrane-bound phosphodiesterase activity (MPDE) and Ca^{2+}/Mg^{2+} ATPase activity of red cell membranes isolated from control (C), phase II, and phase III cells.

These data suggest the following sequential model. The association of isoproterenol with its receptor leads to the activation of adenylate cyclase and possibly a release of membrane-bound calcium. This latter possibility is likely in view of the report of Nelson and Huestis (1980) showing that addition of catecholamines to human cells induces a calcium-dependent phosphorylation of a membrane protein. The initial rise in cAMP content is a result of the cyclase activation (phase I). The subsequent fall is due to the association of calcium–calmodulin to the MPDE either because of a cAMP-dependent phosphorylation of the membrane and/or a rise in cytosolic calcium concentration. The increased activity of MPDE leads to a fall in cAMP concentration (phase II). The final rise in cAMP content (phase III) appears to occur as a consequence of the activation of Ca^{2+}/Mg^{2+} ATPase, a decrease in cytosolic calcium, and a dissociation of calmodulin from the MPDE. A decrease in activity of the MPDE leads to a rise in cAMP concentration. This model leads to the important conclusion that components of the calcium messenger and cAMP messenger systems interact even in a simple cell, the nonnucleated erythrocyte.

A UNIVERSAL MODEL OF STIMULUS
RESPONSE COUPLING

From the foregoing summary and the data to be presented in succeeding chapters, one can conclude that nearly all cells employ the same system for coupling stimulus to response. As noted previously, the term stimulus–response coupling as used in the present context covers not only the stimulation of so-called excitable tissues by neurotransmitters but also so-called nonexcitable tissues by either hormones, neurotransmitters, or other extracellular messengers. Thus, stimulus can be either a neurotransmitter, a hormone, or a metabolite. However, not all such stimuli act via this universal system. Only those stimuli that alter cell function by interacting with a surface membrane receptor are included. Even this classification is too broad. Only those extracellular messengers that interact with surface receptors and evoke the specialized response (or work function) of the particular cell appear to employ the synarchic messengers cAMP and calcium. The response of a given cell type may be contraction, secretion, heat production, or a change in the activity of a particular metabolic or transport pathway. The term synarchic messengers implies that these two intracellular substances, calcium and cAMP, act in concert to regulate the particular response observed and rarely if ever act in isolation to control cell function.

The essential features of this universal system can be most simply represented by a schematic model (Figure 4.4). In this model, one or more

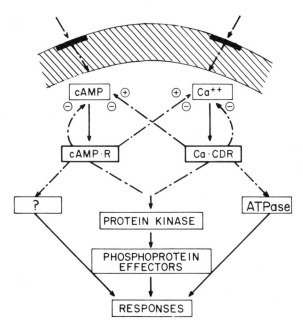

Figure 4.4 Schematic representation of the components involved in synarchic regulation of cell function. The hatched area at the top represents the plasma membrane, and the dark patches are receptors for hormones or neurotransmitters. When these interact with the appropriate agonist, either an increase in cAMP or Ca^{2+} occurs within the cell. These two intracellular messengers interact with their respective intracellular receptor proteins (cAMP·R and Ca·CDR). These interactions lead to activation of one or more protein kinases which in turn utilize a variety of proteins as substrates. The products, phosphoproteins, determine the cellular response. In addition, Ca·CDR is known to activate some response elements by allosteric modification rather than covalent modification rather than covalent modification. An example is the Ca^{2+}/Mg^{2+} ATPase of the red cell membrane. At present, mechanisms other than protein kinase activation have not been identified in the case of cAMP·R, but a prediction of the model is that they will be found. Finally, a critically important component is that the two intracellular messengers regulate each other's concentration and their own concentrations by various feedback effects. CDR = Calmodulin; R = the cAMP receptor component of protein kinases.

extracellular messengers acting on surface receptors coupled respectively to the calcium- and cAMP-mediated limbs of the information flow sequence initiate cell response by causing an increase in the intracellular concentrations of the two messengers. These, in turn, act, and interact, in four important ways. The first is that they regulate the metabolism of each other, that is, there is a dialogue between the two limbs. The two systems are nearly always coupled by this type of messenger interaction. The second is that they modify the sensitivity of the response elements of their partner so that the system has features of both amplitude and sensitivity modulation, that is, they are coupled in this fashion as well. The third is that they regulate the activity of cellular response elements by a common biochemical mechanisms—the controlled phosphorylation of enzymes, of transport and structural proteins, and possibly even of complex lipids, that is, they are coupled in this way, too. Finally, the control of response elements is not stereotyped because at least the Ca^{2+}–CDR complex and probably the cAMP–R complex can control the activity of response elements by means other than regulating protein phosphorylations. This individual, noncoupled feature of their relationship is of critical importance in determining the plastic, as opposed to the stereotyped, nature of these systems in specific settings.

It is instructive to compare this schematic representation of synarchic regulation (Figure 4.4) to those depicted in Figure 1.5, representing, as they do, the more historical and traditional view of the functions of calcium in excitable tissues and of cAMP in hormonally controlled systems. The validation of the more complex model depicted in Figure 4.4 is presented in the succeeding chapters. However, before doing so, it is worth discussing the particular variations on this universal theme that will form the organizational basis of the ensuing discussion.

Given the complexity of the system depicted, and the number of different relationships between Ca^{2+} and cAMP listed in Tables 4.1 and 4.2, there is every reason to expect that the various components of the system will exhibit different relationships and assume different roles in coupling different stimuli to the response of different cells. In fact, it is the very high potential for variation which probably underlies the great evolutionary success and survival of this control system. Its hallmark is clearly its plasticity.

Nonetheless, if one surveys our current knowledge of Ca^{2+}–cAMP interrelationships, one discovers that there are not an infinite but a very finite number of variations on the universal theme. These are depicted schematically in Figure 4.5. The first and most obvious relationship (Figure 4.5a), *coordinate control,* is one in which the intracellular messengers are both generated in response to a single extracellular stimulus, and both participate in a coordinate fashion to regulate cellular response. The second relationship (Figure 4.5b), *hierarchical control,* is one in which separate extracellular stimuli (or different concentrations of the same stimulus) cause the separate activation of the Ca^{2+} and cAMP systems, and these two intracellular messengers interact in some type of hierarchical fashion to produce a complementary enhancement of cellular response. The third relationship (Figure 4.5*c*), *sequential control,* is one in which primary activation of one of the two limbs of the system is followed by the activation of the second as a consequence of an increase in the strength of the first intracellular message. This type of control also has the feature that the secondary messenger augments or extends the domain of response of the primary message. The fourth relationship (Figure 4.5*d*), *redundant control,* is one in which separate extracellular stimuli acting on the separate limbs of the system initiate the same cellular response. The last relationship (Figure 4.5*e*), *antagonistic control,* is one in which the two limbs of the system are activated by separate extracellular stimuli but in which a rise in the intracellular concentration of one messenger blunts or antagonizes the effect of the other.

Although, as will be discussed, there are cellular systems that represent

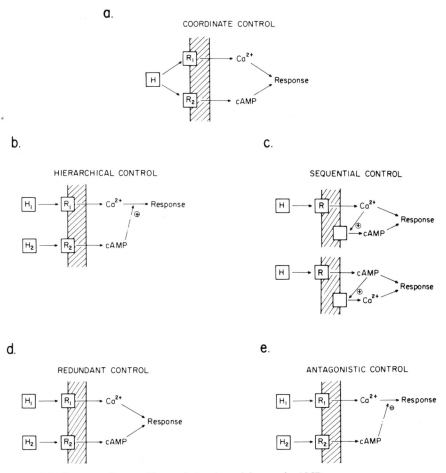

Figure 4.5 Patterns of synarchic regulation by calcium and cAMP.

rather pure examples of each of these variations, in many other cases a particular cellular response system exhibits some type of mixed pattern, with one particular variant being the major and another the minor chord of the universal theme. Nonetheless, this classification, by focusing attention on the major relationship in a given tissue, is of considerable value in drawing attention to the organizational grandeur of this control system and in providing a focus for the discussion of both its universality and particularity.

An additional modality of control not illustrated in the model (Figure 4.4) is that of a suppression of cAMP production or a decrease in calcium entry into the cytosol as a consequence of first messenger action. Such controls do not invalidate the basic model but extend to an additional domain. Primary controls of this negative or inhibitory type appear less common than the more usual positive or stimulatory controls. However, a less systematic search has been made for such elements. They may be considerably more common than presently realized.

To emphasize the universal interrelationship between these two messenger systems in stimulus–response coupling, one need only review the list of interactions seen and the tissues in which they are found (Table 4.1). The data summarized in this table are incomplete because specific relationships are not known or have not been looked for in many tissues. An appraisal of the list shown in Table 4.2 leads to the conclusion that there is no distinction between excitable and nonexcitable tissues in the nature of these interrelationships. Liver and heart share a common cAMP-dependent regulation of ATP-dependent calcium accumulation by microsomes. Brain and kidney share a calcium-dependent control of cAMP hydrolysis. Fluid secretion in the fly salivary gland and glycogenolysis in the rat liver are controlled by operationally similar mechanisms.

EVALUATION OF MODEL

General Features

Before proceeding, it is worthwhile offering a critique of the model. The point that is likely to be questioned immediately is the fact that, as depicted, the calcium message arises from a transduction event (an increase in the permeability of a calcium channel) in the plasma membrane. Yet, as has been made clear in the previous discussion (see Chapter 3), the calcium signal may arise either from the extracellular pool as depicted in Figure 4.4, or from one or more intracellular pools, for example, from the sarcoplasmic reticulum in the case of skeletal muscle. However, if one views the situation in the model (FIgure 4.4) in a less literal sense, then the model represents the essential truth, which is as follows: there is an operational similarity between all cell systems in which calcium is used as messenger, in that an event, electrical or chemical, on the cell surface leads to a rise in cytosolic calcium ion concentration. This rise is a direct consequence of the excitatory event at the cell surface membrane, which may cause a release of calcium from and/or a change in calcium permeability in this membrane or give rise to some signal, chemical or electrical, that causes a release from and/or a change in calcium permeability in an intracellular membrane. This model emphasizes this operational similarity, but it is obvious that in terms of a particular system under study, it is necessary to define the precise details of this transduction event.

The second general point concerns the respective modes by which the cAMP receptor protein and the calcium receptor protein, calmodulin, regulate cell function. Both are capable of regulating the activity of an important class of regulatory proteins namely, protein kinases. Calmodulin regulates a number of other calcium-dependent processes that do not involve this class of enzymes. This would appear to be a significant difference between the modulating function of these two messengers. However, the possibility that the cAMP receptor protein complex may regulate the function of proteins other than protein kinase has not been critically evaluated. It seems likely that when it is, effector elements will be discovered that respond to cAMP·R. In this regard, it is of considerable interest that the regulatory subunit (R) of cAMP-dependent protein kinase can serve as a substrate for cGMP-dependent protein kinase (Geahlen and Krebs, 1980). The true import of the phosphorylation of this regulatory subunit by another protein kinase system has not yet been determined, but it would appear likely that this event is of significance in determining the control properties of the cAMP messenger system. The opposite may also be the case since this protein (R) acts as an inhibitor of cGMP-dependent protein kinase, that is, it appears to be the preferred substrate for this enzyme.

A third point concerns the illustration of a single calcium receptor protein, calmodulin, when in fact there are several—parvalbumin, leiotonin C, and troponin C. Again this is a detail of minor importance. All four proteins are structurally and operationally similar. It is of interest that more than one cAMP receptor protein has also been described (see Chapter 3).

Fourth, as illustrated, a single class of enzymes, the protein kinases, are shown to be activated by either cAMP or calcium. The implication here is not necessarily that the identical enzymes are involved. Clearly, in the case of the phosphorylase system, the cAMP-sensitive protein kinase and the calcium-sensitive protein are different enzymes. However, in a situation such as the hepatic responses to norepinephrine and glucagon, where the same ten proteins are phosphorylated whether calcium or cAMP, respectively, serves as primary messengers, it is not clear if the same or different enzymes are involved. One of at least four possibilities can be considered: (1) the ultimate protein kinase is calcium dependent and cAMP changes the sensitivity of the system to calcium; (2) the ultimate protein kinase is cAMP-dependent and calcium changes the sensitivity of the system to cAMP; (3) each messenger acts on a different protein kinase and each kinase uses the same proteins as substrates; or (4) the two different messengers act on the same protein kinase. Regardless of which of these mechanisms operate, the operational results in terms of information flow are comparable.

The final point concerns the interrelationships between calcium and cAMP in terms of regulating each other's concentration. This is on the surface the least stereotyped aspect of their relationship. Calcium can stimulate either cAMP synthesis or hydrolysis. Cyclic AMP can stimulate either a rise or fall in the intracellular calcium ion concentration by affecting calcium exchange across any or all three calcium transporting membranes—plasma membrane, endoplasmic reticulum, and inner mitochondrial membrane.

The Role of Cyclic GMP

It is necessary to anticipate another objection to the model: its failure to include cyclic GMP (cGMP) guanylate cyclase, and cGMP phosphodiesterase. The problem is that the role of cGMP remains elusive. The more we learn, the less we know. In some ways, it appears to be a variant of the cAMP system, but in others it is quite different. A major problem is that some guanylate cyclases are particulate, others are soluble. In some cases, these cyclases, particularly the soluble ones, appear to be activated by calcium ion. It is not yet clear what role the calcium-mediated rise in cGMP plays in stimulus–response coupling. There are several examples of cGMP-dependent protein kinases but as yet no definition, in physiologically meaningful terms, of the function of the phosphorylated products. A major type of experimental observation that helped define the role of cAMP was the fact that when exogenous cAMP or one of its analogs is added to many hormonally responsive cells, the exogenous nucleotide mimics many of the effects normally produced by the usual first messenger in the same tissue.

This approach has been nowhere near as successful with cGMP. In some tissues, its addition alters cell behavior; but, for example, in the liver the change in behavior is similar to that seen after cAMP addition. Additional confusion is added by the fact that in the case of catecholamine-responsive systems, in which two types of receptors are recognized, the β-receptor is always coupled to adenylate cyclase but the α-receptor interacts with agonists to bring about different primary responses. In the case of the parotid gland, the primary effect appears to be a stimulation of the calcium messenger system. Similarly, in the liver, α-receptor activation leads to turning on of the calcium signaling system.

It would be tempting to generalize from these data and propose that this is as universal as β-receptor–cyclase coupling. Unfortunately, there are examples in which α-adrenergic receptor activation causes primarily a fall in cAMP concentration within the cell. This occurs in the beta cells of the Islets of Langerhans, a tissue in which increased calcium entry, stimulated by the presence of glucose, leads to insulin secretion but in which α-adrenergic stimulation leads to an inhibition of insulin release. It seems most unlikely that calcium entry is increased under these circumstances, but it is well documented that the cAMP content of the cells falls. Still other evidence indicates that the extracellular messenger does not activate the guanylate cyclase directly but does so indirectly by changing the cytosolic calcium ion concentration. The widespread occurrence of this phenomenon surely indicates that the cGMP system is intimately coupled to the calcium messenger system. It is the nature of this coupling that remains elusive.

One of several possibilities exist. One possibility is that in these tissues many of the effects of calcium are not mediated by a direct calcium–calmodulin activation of a response element but indirectly via a cGMP-dependent reaction, for example, by a cGMP-dependent protein kinase reaction. However, in smooth muscle in which the response element is known, namely, myosin light chain kinase, calmodulin is a regulatory sub-unit of this enzyme (see Chapter 8). In this case, therefore, calcium plays a direct messenger role between excitation and contraction. In contrast to smooth muscle, in the adrenal cortex according to Sharma and Sawhney (1970), ACTH induces a rise in cGMP concentration; a cGMP-dependent protein kinase is present and exogenous cGMP stimulates steroidogenesis (see Chapter 6). On the other hand, both the ACTH-induced increase in cGMP concentration and the effect of exogenous cGMP on steroidogenesis require the presence of Ca^{2+}. Hence, in both smooth muscle and adrenal cortex, cGMP appears to play the role of a modulator of the calcium messenger system. The question still is one of defining this role.

If cGMP serves as a positive feed-forward modulator in the calcium messenger system, it may do so by one of two mechanisms: either by altering the *amplitude* of the calcium messenger and/or by altering the *sensitivity* of one or more calcium response elements to the actions of calcium (Figure 4.6). The first possibility has been explored in the case of smooth muscle. Andersson et al. (1975) have shown that cGMP blocks the cAMP-dependent stimulation of calcium uptake by a microsomal fraction from intestinal smooth muscle. In physiological terms, this would represent a means of increasing cytosolic calcium ion concentration. In this case, the

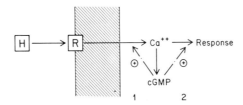

Figure 4.6 Proposed role of cGMP as a positive feed-forward modulator in the calcium messenger system. A hormonally induced rise in cytosolic Ca^{2+} concentration leads to an increase in cGMP content. Thus, this rise in turn, acts by (1) enhancing the amplitude (concentration) of the original calcium message and/or (2) increasing the sensitivity of the calcium response element to calcium.

cGMP/cAMP concentration ratio, by determining the balance between influx and efflux of calcium across the microsomal membrane would determine the steady-state level of cytosolic calcium ion concentration and hence the contractile state or tonus of the muscle. If one could generalize from this observation, it would be to suggest that, in those systems exhibiting an antagonistic pattern of regulation by the synarchic messengers, calcium and cAMP, the calcium-mediated rise in cGMP acts to oppose the cAMP control, and in this sense cGMP and calcium exhibit a sequential messenger pattern.

The possibility that cGMP regulates the sensitivity of the myosin light chain kinase to calcium has not been explored, to my knowledge, but it would be of interest to explore this possibility. On the other hand, sensitivity modulation of a response involving cGMP and Ca^{2+} has been described recently by Baker and Carruthers (1980). The effect of insulin on glucose transport in the barnacle muscle was studied by perfusion of the cell with Ca^{2+}, cAMP, and cGMP, In this case, raising the cAMP concentration caused a decrease in glucose transport which was independent of Ca^{2+} concentration. On the other hand, raising the calcium ion concentration led to an increase in rate of glucose entry into the cell. Similarly, a rise in cGMP concentration led to an increase. Of particular note was the observation that the calcium ion concentration determined both the magnitude of the response to cGMP and the K_a of cGMP activation. When calcium concentration was 0.12 to 0.27 μM, then the response to cGMP was small, but when calcium concentration was 0.91 μM, then the stimulation of sugar transport by cGMP was much greater and was produced by a lower concentration of cGMP ($K_a = 4.1 \times 10^{-7}$). In the case of this response element, calcium and cGMP interact and calcium alters the sensitivity of the system to activation by cGMP, that is, a system in which sensitivity modulation of a cGMP-dependent response is controlled by Ca^{2+}.

A similar situation has been described in the case of a cGMP-dependent protein kinase (Yamaki and Hidaka, 1980). Calmodulin is a regulatory submit of the enzyme. An increase in calcium ion concentration causes an increase in the sensitivity of the enzyme to activation by cGMP. However, of considerable interest is the observation that calmodulin activates the enzyme in the presence of EGTA and 10 nM Mg^{2+}.

These data point the way toward defining the role of cGMP in regulating both cellular calcium metabolism and the sensitivity of cellular response elements to activation by calcium. Considerably more information is needed before one can relate these few examples to a general model of cGMP in synarchic regulation, but the present data are all consistent with the hypothesis that cGMP acts as a modulator in the calcium messenger system. However, the situation is not completely resolved because in cardiac muscle the cGMP content rises after acetylcholine administration, which leads to a negative inotropic effect, a circumstance in which the temporal and/or spacial domain of the calcium message is reduced.

Alternative Modalities of Stimulus— Response Coupling

Before drawing the conclusion that the cAMP–Ca^{2+} duality is the basis for the action of all extracellular messengers which regulate cell function via membrane transducing mechanisms, it is necessary to define the action of insulin, somatomedin, and other nutritive hormones on cell function. These other extracellular messengers also interact with cell surface receptors and thereby alter cell function, but in doing so do not appear to employ either cAMP or Ca^{2+} as messengers. These include hormones such as insulin, somatomedin, and epidermal growth factor. One could argue that these hormones function differently than those extracellular messengers that control the synarchic system. In the case of insulin, for example, the hormone does not induce cells to perform their specific work functions but rather is a major energy storage hormone. If one restricts the class of extracellular messengers (which interact with surface receptors) to those that induce cells to perform their particular work function (secretion, contraction, metabolism), then the evidence supports the hypothesis that these work functions are regulated by the synarchic messenger system. However, a problem still exists, that of how cell growth is regulated and whether one considers this a work function or not.

There is increasing evidence that somatomedins are general growth hormones. They apparently exert their effects through the transfer of information by messengers other than Ca^{2+} and cAMP. Hence, one could, to keep the distinction clear, classify growth as a nonwork function. Unfortunately, there is a difficulty. In many tissues and particularly in cells grown in tissue culture, both cAMP and Ca^{2+} have been postulated to play a modulatory role in the growth and/or differentiation of these cells.

A particular example in an intact tissue is the response of the adrenal cortex to the hormone ACTH. As is discussed subsequently (see Chapter 6), both Ca^{2+} and cAMP have messenger functions in coupling ACTH stimulation (via a surface receptor) to response, that is, the increased secretion of steroid hormones (a work function of this tissue). In addition, prolonged stimulation of the gland by ACTH causes both a hyperplasia and hypertrophy of glandular tissue (a clear growth response). The presumption, yet to be proved, is that Ca^{2+} and cAMP are also the messengers involved in mediating this growth response. Hence, for the present, it is necessary to conclude that although as a generalization these synarchic messengers couple stimulus to response in the case where a specific work function of the tissue is evoked, these two intracellular messengers may have roles in modulating types of intracellular processes other than a highly specialized work function.

Single Messenger Systems

A question of paramount importance is whether there are examples of stimulus–response coupling in particular tissues or cells in which the evidence clearly establishes that either Ca^{2+} or cAMP alone is solely responsible for coupling stimulus to response. The answer to this question is not clear, often because the system is incompletely studied. However, there are at least two systems in which considerable data exist that have been interpreted in terms of a model in which one or the other of these messengers is solely responsible for stimulus–response coupling. These are skeletal muscle contraction in which calcium is considered the sole messenger and the hormonal regulation of fluid transport in the amphibian urinary bladder in which cAMP is considered the sole intracellular messenger. Each of these conclusions will be considered.

Skeletal Muscle Contraction

As discussed in the first chapter, the central role of calcium in stimulus–response coupling was defined first in skeletal muscle. Likewise, the first intracellular calcium receptor protein to be isolated was troponin, the calcium-dependent regulator of actin–tropomyosin–myosin interactions in skeletal muscle. The question of interest to our present thesis is the possible role, if any, of cAMP in the regulation of muscle contraction and muscle cell function.

As reviewed briefly previously (Chapter 1) and in more detail in a subsequent section of this chapter, there is an intimate relationship between Ca^{2+} and cAMP in the control of glycogen turnover in muscle. Hence, in terms of the control of this function of skeletal muscle, there is substantial evidence that the synarchic messengers, calcium and cAMP, act in both a hierarchial and redundant sense. However, there is much less information as to the role of cAMP in regulating the contractile state of skeletal muscle. Nonetheless, there is a basic observation that indicates that cAMP does, in fact, influence the contractile state. The observation is that β-adrenergic agents have an inotropic effect on skeletal muscle from both mammals and amphibia (Bowman and Nott, 1969; Krnjevic and Miledi, 1958). Part of this effect is exerted at the level of the N–M junction where cAMP enhances neurotransmitter (acetylcholine) release (see Chapter 6). Another part of this effect is directly exerted upon muscle cell function. In producing this direct effect, β-adrenergic agonists do not change the degree of membrane depolarization or the size of the action potential, but probably act by altering the behavior of the voltage-dependent calcium channel in the plasma membrane and possibly the T system in the muscle cell (Oota and Nagai, 1977; Varagic and Kentera, 1978; Varagic et al., 1979). These effects lead in some ill-defined fashion to an enhanced release of Ca^{2+} from the sarcoplasmic reticulum, which is the immediate cause of the enhanced contractile response. However, the effect, whatever it is, is independent of the cAMP-mediated changes in glycogen metabolism (Kentera and Varagic, 1975).

Parenthetically, cAMP-dependent protein kinases can employ proteins of the troponin–tropomyosin–actin–myosin complex as substrates *in vitro*. Whether such phosphorylations occur *in vivo* following β-agonist application to intact muscle tissue is not yet clear (Barany et al., 1980; Stull et al., 1980; Entman et al., 1978).

In conclusion, it is clear that skeletal muscle represents a tissue in which the calcium messenger system plays the dominant role in coupling stimulus to response. Nonetheless, there is strong evidence that cAMP serves as a synarchic messenger with calcium in regulating muscle glycogen metabolism and that it also may serve a hierarchical function in the control of the contractile response.

Toad Urinary Bladder

The earliest studies of the second messenger function of cAMP focused on those systems in which the peptide or amine hormone initiated a metabolic response. These systems included the control of glycogen metabolism in the liver and other tissues, of steroid hormone production in the adrenal, and of carbohydrate metabolism in the liver fluke. The discovery that the peptide hormone vasopressin might also mediate its cellular effects by controlling adenylate cyclase activity represented a significant step in broadening the focus of investigative attention because the major effect of this hormone is to alter the transport properties of epithelial membranes.

The first studies of vasopressin action showed that addition of vasopressin to the inside surface of the isolated frog skin enhanced the net flux of Na^+ and H_2O across this tissue (Ussing and Zehran, 1951; Koefoed-Johnsen and Ussing, 1953). Leaf (Leaf, 1965, 1967) then demonstrated that the isolated amphibian urinary bladder also responded to vasopressin with an increase in mucosal to serosal Na^+ flux. In addition, Bentley (1958, 1960, 1966) and Sawyer (1958) showed that the tissue was normally relatively impermeable to H_2O even if an osmotic gradient existed across the tissue. This finding alone demonstrated that this is a "tight" epithelium, and all available evidence supports the view that the flow of both ions and H_2O across this tissue is through an intracellular rather than paracellular route. Treatment with vasopressin or one of its many analogs was found to lead to a marked increase in the bulk flow of H_2O (driven by the osmotic gradient) across the tissue.

Following establishment of these facts plus the fact that vasopressin treatment increased the tissue permeabilities to urea and tritiated H_2O (Leaf, 1965), the toad urinary bladder became a favorite object for the study of the mechanism of action of this hormone. As far as is presently known, this tissue is the structural and functional homolog of the mammalial collecting tubule. In terms of their biochemical responses to vasopressin, they appear to be very similar, although their transport capabilities are somewhat different. However, there is no question that they are both "tight" epithelia which share the same capabilities as regards the control of H_2O permeability and flow by vasopressin.

In order to understand this capability, it is necessary to point out that the plasma membrane of most mammalian cells is freely permeable to H_2O.

Hence, if a difference in the osmotic activity develops in the solutions on the two sides of the membrane, H_2O flows across the membrance to reestablish osmotic equilibrium. The unique feature of the toad bladder is that if a dilute solution ($<$50 mos$M$/l) is placed in contact with the mucosal surface of the cell and a isotonic solution ($>$220 mos$M$/l) on the serosal side, there is very little flow of water across the tissue (Sawyer, 1958). Addition of vasopressin leads to a dramatic increase in the rate of H_2O flow. Investigations by Peachy and Rasmussen (1961) showed that the subcellular membrane with the unusual permeability property was the luminal membrane of the epithelial cells.

As one might anticipate, when vasopressin is added to the mucosal solution of the resting bladder, there is no change in H_2O permeability; but if added to the serosal solution, a prompt change in H_2O flow is seen. The same is true for the vasopressin-mediated increase in Na^+ flux, and there is evidence that a major effect of vasopressin in terms of controlling transcellular Na^+ transport is that of increasing the rate of Na^+ entry into the cell across its luminal face (Leaf, 1967). Although the hormone apparently acts initially on one side of the cell, the processes ultimately regulated are on the opposite side of the cell.

Once it was shown that exogenous cAMP could mimic the effects of vasopressin on both Na^+ flux and bulk water flow (Orloff and Handler, 1962, 1967), rapid progress was made in defining the role of cAMP in this tissue. It was established that all of the following Sutherland criteria were met in terms of identifying cAMP as the second messenger in vasporessin action: (1) vasopressin addition leads to an increase in the tissue content of cAMP (Handler et al., 1965); (2) theophylline and other phosphodiesterase inhibitors enhance the physiological effects of vasopressin (Orloff and Handler, 1962); (3) exogenous cAMP mimics the effects of vasopressin (Orloff and Handler, 1962); (4) there is a hormone-sensitive adenylate cyclase in a particulate (plasma membrane) fraction of the cell homogenate (Bar et al., 1970); and (5) cAMP-dependent protein kinases are present in the tissue (Kirchberger et al., 1972). Furthermore, the cAMP content of the epithelial cells *in situ* increases after vasopressin addition as measured by an immunofluorescent method (Goodman et al., 1975).

From these data, a model of vasopressin action was constructed (Figure 4.7). In this model, the hormone interacts with specific receptors on the basolateral membrane of the cell. This interaction leads to the activation of adenylate cyclase. The subsequent rise in cAMP concentration by activating soluble and/or particulate protein kinases (Kuchenberg et al., 1973; Dousa et al., 1972) leads to the phosphorylation of one or more proteins in, or on the cytoplasmic face of, the luminal membrane. The phosphorylation of this protein(s) is postulated to be the mechanism by which changes in the water, urea, and Na^+ permeabilities of this particular cellular membrane are altered.

Considerable support for this model of hormone action came from the

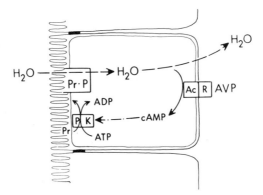

Figure 4.7 Model of the action of vasopressin (AVP) on H_2O flow in the toad bladder or mammalian renal collecting duct. The concept is that AVP binds to a receptor (R) coupled to adenylate cyclase (AC) on the basolateral cell membrane. As a consequence, intracellular cAMP concentration increases and activates an intrinsic protein kinase (PD) in the luminal membrane. The resulting phosphorylation of a protein (Pr·P) is responsible for the change in permeability of this membrane. As shown, the model depicts only the effect of vasopressin on H_2O permeability. As discussed in the text, a separate phosphorylation event is presumed to underlie a hormone-induced change in luminal membrane Na^+ permeability.

work of Schwartz et al. (1974). Because of technical problems, it has not yet been possible to prepare basolateral and luminal membranes from the epithelial cells of the toad bladder. However, these workers developed a method, employing free-flow electrophoresis, for the isolation of luminal and contraluminal (apical and basolateral) membranes of the epithelial cells in the papillae of bovine kidneys. These cells are predominantly cells of the vasopressin-responsive collecting duct, the homolog of the toad bladder. Examination of the properties of these membranes showed that, as predicted by the model, nearly all of the vasopressin-stimulated adenylate cyclase was found in the contraluminal membrane and practically none in the luminal membrane of the cell. Conversely, the luminal membrane, but not the contraluminal membrane, possessed an intrinsic cAMP-responsive protein kinase which in the presence of cAMP led to the phosphorylation of protein substrates in this membrane.

In spite of this impressive evidence, the final validation of this model has not been achieved. In order to do so, it is necessary to show that phosphorylation of a specific membrane protein leads to a specific change in the permeability of the luminal membrane to H_2O, Na^+ and urea. To date, this has not been accomplished. In fact, the situation is clearly more complex than this simple model suggests. It has been found that the different transport pathways for Na^+, H_2O, and urea are affected differently by different treatments of the tissue (Petersen and Edelman, 1961; Levine et al., 1973, 1976; Carvounis et al., 1979; and Stadel and Goodman, 1978). The available results argue that either the effects on H_2O flow and Na^+ transport are mediated by two different receptors in the same cell or by similar receptors in the two major transport cells in this tissue, the granular and mitochondrial-rich cells. If the former, it would be attractive to assume that different intracellular messengers mediated these separate effects. However, from the very onset, it has been clear that exogenous cAMP can change both Na^+ transport and H_2O flow. These results are incompatible with a dual messenger system coupled individually to dual response elements. It has not yet been possible to determine whether Na^+ transport is the property of one cell type, for example, the mitochondrial-rich cell, and H_2O flow a property of the other, namely, the granular cell. It is clear that granular cells are involved in the transepithelial flow of H_2O (Peachey and Rasmussen, 1961), but it is less clear whether the mitochondria-rich cells are involved. The cell types responsible for Na^+ transport is not known. Regardless, if one accepts the fact that the changes in Na^+ and H_2O movements are mediated separately, then in terms of the model (Figure 4.7), more than one protein in the luminal membrane would have to undergo phosphorylation in response to the hormone.

In searching for these presumptive substrates for cAMP-dependent protein kinase, DeLorenzo and coworkers (DeLorenzo and Greengard, 1973; DeLorenzo et al., 1973; Walton et al., 1975) actually discovered that phosphorylation of a specific protein was *decreased* in intact toad bladders following exposure to either antidiuretic hormone or monobutyryl cAMP. Addition of cAMP to bladder homogenates led to a similar decrease in the phosphorylation of this protein. The dephosphorylation of this protein was found to be catalyzed by a membrane-bound phosphprotein phosphatase. Although DeLorenzo et al. (1973) concluded that this protein might function to regulate either the Na^+ and/or H_2O permeability of the luminal membrane, Ferguson and Twite (1974) showed that low doses of AVP which induced a maximal increase in Na^+ transport did not alter the dephosphorylation of this protein, but higher doses which altered H_2O flow also altered its state of phosphorylation. Ferguson and Twite (1974) concluded that the protein was not involved in regulating Na^+ permeability but was involved in the control of H_2O flow.

However, studies by Schwartz et al. (1979) have shown that this is not the case. They found that the protein which undergoes a cAMP-dependent phosphorylation is the regulatory subunit of the cAMP-dependent protein kinase. Association of this subunit with cAMP leads to its dephosphorylation and thus to an increase in the content of free regulatory subunit which associates more readily with the catalytic unit than does the phosphorylated regulatory subunit. Schwartz et al. (1979) suggest that this dephosphorylation is a component of the feedback control of the cAMP response and is involved in the termination rather than the initiation of the physiological response. These results and conclusions mean that at present a major feature of the model (Figure 4.7) remains to be validated. This feature is that phosphorylation of luminal membrane proteins is directly responsible for the hormone-induced changes in Na^+, urea, and/or H_2O fluxes across this cell surface.

The action of vasopressin on the toad bladder has been repeatedly cited as one of the most thoroughly studied systems in which the second messenger model of cAMP action has been validated. It is one of the systems in which the dominant role of cAMP as second messenger has been emphasized. Nevertheless, even in this system, there is evidence that calcium ions play a role in mediating the responses to this hormone. The strongest evidence is that relating changes in calcium ion to Na^+ transport, but the evidence is controversial. On the one hand, Gristein nnd Erlij (1978) and Wiesmann et al. (1977) have presented evidence in support of the concept that a rise in intracellular calcium ion content inhibits the action of vasopressin. On the other, Balaban and Mandel (1979) have studied the effect of the ionophore A23187 upon Na^+ transport in the frog skin and concluded that ionophore induces a calcium-dependent increase in Na^+ transport in this tissue. It is not immediately obvious why the results of Balban and Mandel (1979) in the frog skin differ from those of Wiesmann et al. (1977) in the toad bladder. It is of interest that A23187 in the toad bladder causes a transient increase in Na^+ transport followed by an inhibition, so it is possible that this tissue responds to A23187 with a marked rise in intracellular calcium which rapidly exerts an inhibitory effect on the tissue.

Further indirect support for a messenger role of Ca^{2+} in regulating Na^+ flux has come from studies conducted in MDCK cells. These cells are derived from the canine kidney and grow successfully in tissue culture. Although cultured for many years, the cell line has retained some of its differentiated structure and functions. Most striking, they retain their epithelial morphology, that is, the cells are polar (Leighton et al., 1969) and form into oriented sheets when grown on a surface. They can also be cultured on membrane filters and, when forming as monolayers on these filters, are capable of vectoral Na^+ and H_2O transport (Misfeldt et al., 1976; Cereijido et al., 1978). These transport processes are responsive to dibutyryl cAMP and PDE inhibitors (Valentish et al., 1976) and to vasopressin and prostaglandins (Rindler et al., 1979).

Studies by Rindler et al. (1979a,b) have shown that in the presence of Ouabain (an inhibitor of the Na^+ pump), sodium uptake across the mucosal face of these cells takes place via a saturable neutral carrier machanism. Pretreatment of the cells with A23187 led to a calcium-dependent, tenfold increase in rate of Na^+ entry into the cells. At the very least, these data support the view that changes in the calcium ion content of the cell are capable of increasing the Na^+ permeability of the mucosal cell membrane.

There are only a few studies relating Ca^{2+} to the hydro-osmotic effects of vasopressin Earlier work had shown that vasopressin causes a transient increase in the efflux of calcium from the toad bladder (Cuthbert and Wong, 1974; Schwartz and Walter, 1969). Although the earlier work by Wiesmann et al. (1977) had shown that the addition of ionophore (A23187) inhibited the effect of vasopressin on Na^+ transport, the studies of Hardy (1978) have shown that under appropriate conditions A23187 can cause a marked increase in the bulk flow of H_2O across the tissue. Depending upon conditions,

A23187 can either (1) produce a hydroosmotic response comparable to that produced by submaximal doses of vasopressin, (2) inhibit by 50% the response elicited by a maximal vasopressin dose, or (3) have an additive effect on the action of submaximal doses of hormone. Levine and coworkers (1981) have approached the question of calcium action by employing the drug trifluoperazine. This drug is thought to act by binding to, and inhibiting the action of, calcium–calmodulin. These investigators showed that 10 μM trifluoperazine inhibited by 30 to 50% the hydro-osmotic response to vasopressin, methylisobutyxanthine (an inhibitor of PDE), and exogenous cAMP. They took these results to mean that calcium as well as cAMP plays a messenger role in vasopressin action. A particular feature of their results was that the drug had no effect on the initial change in water flow seen after vasopressin addition but did reduce the maximal response achieved. It did not act simply by altering the cAMP concentration. These results are most consistent with some type of sequential model in which the initial response is mediated by cAMP and with the involvement of a cAMP-mediated rise in Ca^{2+} concentration or a cAMP-mediated increase in the sensitivity of a calmodulin-regulated event to calcium ion (sensitivity modulation) in maintaining the response.

These data do not prove that calcium ion serves a second messenger function in vasopressin action. However, they do show that under appropriate experimental circumstances, a change in intracellular calcium ion concentration can induce either of the major effects of the hormone on Na^+ and H_2O flow. They are, therefore, consistent with the possibility that even in this issue, in which a "pure" cAMP second messenger function has been postulated, the calcium messenger system is also involved in mediating hormone action.

The Universal Versus the Particular

In defining synarchic regulation and in developing the information in support of its universal role in stimulus–response coupling, the particularity of stimulus–response coupling in each cell type will be alluded to repeatedly. However, the very existence of this particularity may raise the concern that there are so many individual variations on this universal theme that the concept of universality loses its meaning, In order to put this question into focus, it is useful to contrast the synarchic system with other universal systems of cell function. Although any number of possible examples come to mind, one could, I suspect, obtain nearly complete agreement that the Krebs cycle is a universal component of the metabolic machinery of all prokaryote cells. The thesis to be considered, then, is whether the synarchic system underlying stimulus–response coupling is as universal a characteristic of cellular function as is the Krebs cycle. Having just reemphasized the number of particular variations on the synarchic theme, the question would appear rather extreme because our concept of the Krebs cycle is that of a stereotyped system of enzymes, located within the mitochondria serving the single, universal function of oxidizing acetyl CoA to CO_2 and in the process, by its coupling to the mitochondrial electron transport chain, generating ATP. If, on the other hand, we consider the activity of the Krebs cycle enzymes in their natural setting and how these enzymes individually and collectively function in different cell types, it becomes apparent that the same duality between the universal and the particular is as much a property of the functioning of these enzymes as it is of the functioning of the synarchic system underlying stimulus–response coupling.

Three particular variations in the functioning of the Krebs cycle enzymes and related systems for transporting Krebs cycle intermediates into and out of the mitochondria will be discussed to illustrate the validity of this conclusion.

The first tissue to be considered is the flight muscle of insects. When active, this tissue has one of the highest known rates of oxidztive energy production and utilization. This capacity is met by a tissue rich in mitochondria that are capable of high rates of oxidative phosphorylation. To most efficiently serve this single functional demand, the mitochondria are organized so that, other than pyruvate, practically none of the Krebs cycle intermediates crosses the mitochondrial membrane. Hence, the intramitochondrial concentrations of these intermediates, are kept at high levels, and these intermediates are essentially isolated within the mitochondrial matrix space. There, they serve only their classic function of rapidly and efficiently converting acetyl CoA, derived from pyruvate, to CO_2 and H_2O with the generation of the ATP necessary to supply energy for the rapidly contracting flight muscle. This particular cell, in terms of its organization of the Krebs cycle, can be considered the prototype of a tissue in which the Krebs cycle enzymes function solely in their classic, cyclic sense.

However, if our discussion of this tissue is broadened to include the machinery of oxidative phosphorylation, a universal associate of the Krebs cycle enzymes, then a particular variation on a universal theme becomes apparent even in this classic system. The universal theme under consideration is that the electrons that flow from substrate to O_2 in mitochondria are derived from the oxidation of acetyl CoA via the Krebs cycle. This is not strictly the case in the flight muscle. This tissue depends heavily on the carbohydrate stored as trehalose an energy-yielding substrate during times of energy demand. The trehalose, once converted to monosaccharide units, is metabolized via the glycolytic sequence to pyruvate. During the operation of this sequence, NAD^+ is converted to NADH at the glyceraldehyde phosphate dehydrogenase step. This shifts the NAD/NADH ratio to a lower value. This shift would, in turn, cause a conversion of pyruvate to lactate and thereby limit pyruvate availability for Krebs cycle activity. In addition, it would result in the accumulation of lactate. However, this does not happen because there is a specific mitochondrial flavoprotein, an α-glycerophosphodehydrogenase, coupled to the electron transport chain which serves to shuttle cytosolic reducing equivalents directly to the electron transport chain in the mitochondrial membrane, thereby keeping the cytosolic NAD/NADH high and pyruvate available for mitochondrial oxidation. In order to have a highly efficient and coupled oxidation of glucose to CO_2 and H_2O, it is essential to have an energetically favorable mechanism to shuttle cytosolic reducing equivalents to the mitochondria, by a component of the mitochondrial electron transport systems other than the classic components, for example, α-ketoglutarate or succinic dehydrogenase, of the mitochondrial system.

The second tissue to be discussed is mammalian adipose tissue. This tissue has as its particular metabolic functions the synthesis of triglycerides in times of energy substrate availability and the hydrolysis of triglyceride and release of the fatty acids derived therefrom in times of energy substrate need. In the case of triglyceride synthesis from glucose, the acetyl CoA derived from glucose catabolism is generated by the intramitochondrial pyruvate dehydrogenase complex. In order to serve as substrate for fatty acid synthesis, this acetyl CoA must be transported out of the mitochondria. In large part, it is not transported directly as acetyl CoA but is first converted into mitochondrial citrate (Figure 4.8). This intermediate is transported to the cytosol and is cleaved there to oxaloacetate (OAA) and acetyl CoA by a reaction requiring ATP. The cytosolic acetyl CoA is then converted to malonyl CoA, the substrate needed for the initiation of fatty acid synthesis, and a step requiring ATP. The cytosolic OAA undergoes reduction to ma-

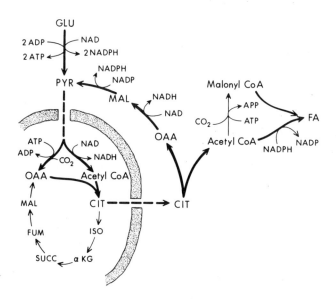

Figure 4.8   Schematic representation of the pathways of carbon in an adipocyte involved in the synthesis of fatty acid from glucose. The shaded area represents the inner mitochondrial membrane.

late, which in turn is oxidized to pyruvate, the two reactions acting as a transhydrogenase to convert a mole of NADH, generated by glycolysis, to NADPH, one of the reducing equivalents needed for fatty acid synthesis. The pyruvate is reconverted to intramitochondrial oxaloacetate by a third reaction requiring ATP. The simplest of bookkeeping shows that sufficient ATP is generated by glycolysis (one molecule per pyruvate molecule) and by the pyruvate dehydrogenase reaction (three molecules per pyruvate) to supply that needed for the reactions of fatty acid synthesis. Hence, the only enzymes of the Krebs cycle active under these circumstances are pyruvate dehydrogenase and citrate synthase. The two carbon units are shuttled out of the mitochondria as a six-carbon unit, regenerated in the cytosol with the production of the four-carbon OAA, which by a series of reactions is recycled to intramitochondrial OAA to initiate another cycle of the two-carbon shuttle. This cycle operates in a fashion similar to that of the classic Krebs cycle, but exists both in the mitochondrial and cytosolic compartments and serves primarily to move two-carbon units from one subcellular compartment to another.

The significance of this cycle in the context of our present discussion is that under this particular metabolic circumstance in this particular tissue, only two of the eight Krebs cycle enzymes are involved. The others are essentially inoperative, although present. If one contrasts this situation with that found in the insect flight muscle, the difference is striking: in this universal biochemical pathway, the Krebs cycle, there is a striking variation in the participation of its component enzymes in the metabolic processes in particular tissues.

The third example to be discussed is the mammalian liver. In this tissue, the mitochondria are the site of numerous crossroads in energy metabolism. They possess the same capability for shuttling two-carbon units, via citrate, to the cytosol for fatty acid synthesis as that just described for the mitochondria of the adipocyte. The shuttling of Krebs cycle intermediates across the mitochondrial membrane and the utilization of only some of the cycle enzymes are also features of both the urea cycle and the process of gluconeogenesis. In each instance, the flux of carbon units through a segment of the pathway is far greater than the flux through the entire cycle. For example, in the case of gluconeogenesis from alanine, only pyruvate carboxylase and malate dehydrogenase are active; the enzyme pyruvate dehydrogenase, which was involved in conversion of glucose to fat, is largely inoperative in the mitochondria of liver cells producing glucose from lactate or alanine. Thus, the Krebs cycle, rather than operating as a stereotyped system of metabolic reactions, operates as a highly plastic metabolic transducer providing not only reducing equivalents for oxidative phosphorylation but, under appropriate circumstances, carbon units for fatty acid, glucose, and/or urea synthesis.

The fantastic plasticity of this system of enzymes as they subserve the metabolic function of the liver stands in sharp contrast to the very stereotyped pattern of their activity in the insect flight muscle. The difference in organizational complexity of this metabolic system in the two types of tissue is as great as the difference in complexity of the synarchic system found in the fly salivary gland on the one hand and the pancreatic beta cell on the other. The former exhibits a rather stereotyped pattern of coupling between stimulus and response in which cAMP and calcium serve as coordinate messengers (see Chapter 5). The latter exhibits aspects of both hierarchical and sequential patterns of stimulus–response coupling (see Chapter 6). Thus, just as in the control system designated synarchy, so in the metabolic sequence known as the Krebs cycle one can recognize a number of particular variations on a universal theme. In neither case does this recognition invalidate the concept that these two components of metabolism are universal attributes of prokaryote cell organization and function.

A second question concerning synarchic regulation is the evolutionary value of a dual rather than a single messenger system. The answer lies in the concept of plasticity of metabolic response, which will be mentioned repeatedly in the ensuing discussion. Plasticity implies, first of all, that a cell's response to a particular extracellular stimulus is modulated by the other extracellular messages being received by the cell. It also implies that a cell's response can vary even though the strength of the intracellular signal does not change. However, the most important feature of this concept of metabolic plasticity is that integration of information in the temporal as well as spatial domain is possible. Plasticity also has a feature of key importance to the process of biological evolution. This feature is that of a capability to have one of the elements in the system undergo change without impairing the functional capabilities of the entire system. The system underlying synarchic regulation is, above all else, highly adaptable. The present-day evidence of different patterns of calcium–cAMP interactions in different cell types is testament to the evolutionary plasticity of the system underlying synarchic regulation.

Relation to the Cell Ionic Net

Another aspect of the model of synarchic regulation worthy of comment is its relationship to the cell ionic net. The major theme to be developed in the succeeding discussion is that in nearly all animal cells there is an intimate relationship between the cAMP and calcium messenger systems in mediating responses to extracellular stimuli acting via transducing elements in the plasma membrane. However, there is another theme that will appear repeatedly but will not be so explicitly developed. This theme is the interrelated changes in ion fluxes across plasma and intracellular membranes. In an effort to draw attention to these ionic relationships, the term ionic net was introduced to denote the fact that changes in the membrane flux (Rasmussen et al., 1976), and therefore the intracellular distribution of one ion, alter those of a number of other ions. Rarely if ever does one observe a change in the flux of a single ion. In the original enunciation of this concept, the relationship between calcium, hydrogen, and phosphate fluxes across the mitochondrial membrane and of calcium-mediated changes in K^+ permeability of the plasma membrane was identified. Since that time, any number of additional ionic interactions have been described. These include Na^+-mediated calcium efflux across both mitochondrial and plasma membranes, calcium-mediated changes in sodium and chloride permeability across luminal membranes of secretory cells, K^+-mediated changes in calcium movements, and calcium-dependent calcium fluxes across microsomal and plasma membranes.

These discoveries add additional evidence in support of the concept that the ionic milieu within the cell serves an integrative function in regulating the metabolism of that cell and that upon cell activation there is a concerted change in this ionic milieu which is an important aspect of the integrated response of the cell to stimulation. Unfortunately, because of the complexity of these ionic interactions and the difficulties in measuring intracellular ionic activities, it is not yet possible to provide a quantitative basis for this concept. Nonetheless, as this information becomes available, it seems certain that the importance of this ionic net in controlling cell function will become increasingly evident.

As originally discussed, the regulatory role of this net was given a biochemical basis because the activities of many enzymes are a function of the cation, hydrogen ion, and anion concentrations in their environment. A change in the relative and/or absolute concentrations of these ions within various cellular compartments would lead to changes in the activities of many different enzymes within these compartments. There is another equally interesting mechanism by which this ionic net may regulate cell function. A corollary of changes in ionic fluxes across membranes is a flow of ionic currents across the cell. Jaffe and Nucciteli (1977) have reviewed data from a variety of systems which support their view that these ionic currents play an important regulatory role in the process of embryonic differentiation. The concept can easily be extended to a consideration of any cellular response in which there is a vectorial component to the response. Thus, information may be imparted to the cell not only by changes in ionic activities within a cell compartment but by the direction and magnitude of ionic currents across the cell.

Calcium and Junctional Communication

The cells in nearly all organized tissues are joined one to another by junctions of several kinds, but the ones of interest to our discussion are low-resistance junctions (so-called gap junctions) that provide a pathway for the direct flow of hydrophilic ions and molecules from the cytosol of one cell to that of its immediate neighbor (Furshpan and Potter, 1968; Loewenstein, 1968; Loewenstein et al., 1978; Loewenstein and Rose, 1978). These junctions display low electrical resistance (high ionic conductivity) and are permeable to small molecules of M.W. 1600 or less, indicating a channel some 14 Å in diameter.

The presence of these channels allows passage of ions and small molecules between cells in an intact tissue, but they are relatively leak-proof to the exterior or extracellular fluids. This means that although we normally treat an analysis of hormone action in the context of single cells, the real tissue response element is a multicellular unit of eight to ten cells coupled via these cell-to-cell channels. To date, relatively little attention has been paid to this structural feature of tissues in considering regulation of metabolic activity. Nonetheless, it may be of considerable significance. For example, in the urinary bladder of the toad there appears to be a functional multicellular unit composed of a single mitochondrial-rich cell surrounded by four to six granular cells (Davis et al., 1974a,b, 1978). If these are coupled electrically as well as anatomically it is quite likely that they function as a single unit rather than as separate entities.

Of importance to our present discussion is the fact that an increase in the calcium ion content of the cell cytosol leads to a decrease in the permeability of these cell-to-cell channels (Rose and Loewenstein, 1975; Loewenstein, 1968; Loewenstein and Rose, 1978; Loewenstein et al., 1978; Rose and Rick, 1978; Rose et al., 1977; Rose and Loewenstein, 1976; Deleze and Loewenstein, 1976). The effect of increasing the free calcium concentration is to produce a graded decrease in the permeability of the membranes in these junctions (Rose et al., 1977; Loewenstein et al., 1978). When the calcium ion content rises above $5 \times 10^{-5} M$, the junctional permeability falls drastically so that the cells become electrically uncoupled and impermeable to ions (including calcium) and all small molecules. When the calcium ion concentration is raised progressively from the resting value to $5 \times 10^{-5} M$, there is a selective decrease first in the permeability of larger molecules and then in the permeability of smaller molecules, and finally an electrical uncoupling reflecting a decrease in ionic permeability.

Within the context of our present discussion, the question of most immediate interest is whether these channels have a role in regulating cell function and particularly responses to extracellular message. A corollary to this question is whether cAMP influences the properties of these channels. First of all, it should be noted that a fall in intracellular pH will decrease junctional permeability by increasing the intracellular calcium ion concentration (Rose and Rick, 1978). Hence, any metabolic activity which leads to a shift in pH will influence intercellular communication. Secondly, Petersen and Iwatsuki (1978) have shown that when cholinergic agonists stimulate exocrine secretion in the acinar cells of the pancreas, there is evidence of electrical uncoupling between the cells consisted with the postulated increase in cytosolic calcium ion concentration in these activated cells. Clearly, physiological stimuli can bring about a sufficient change in cytosolic calcium ion concentration to influence this cell-to-cell channel. However, these observations do not address the question of whether such a change plays any regulatory role. It is possible, as suggested by Loewenstein and Rose (1978), that this calcium-dependent decrease in junctional permeability is a protective device that leads to uncoupling of damaged (calcium-permeable) cells from their neighbors. However, if this were its only significance, one must logically ask why such junctions are formed in the first place.

Loewenstein (1968) has suggested that a major function of this channel is the regulation of tissue growth. He has found a strong correlation between the growth control competence of cells and their ability to form cell-to-cell channels. Conversely, he has shown that cells unable to form such channels are also growth control incompetent. These results suggest that cell-to-cell channels are of great importance in intercellular communication and could play an important role in embryonic growth and development. It has been shown that these junctions remain open throughout the cell cycle (O'Lague et al., 1970) and are thus obvious conduits for the transmission of information for both the initiation and feedback inhibition of growth in multicellular tissues (Furshpan and Potter, 1968; Wolpert, 1971; DeHaan and Sachs, 1972).

One of the more interesting studies designed to test this hypothesis was that carried out by Caveney (1978). The system under study was epidermal growth in the larva of the beetle *Tenebrio*. The cells in this tissue are ionically coupled (Warner and Lawrence, 1973; Caveney, 1974). and gap junctions make up 20 to 30% of their junctional membranes (Caveney and Podgorski, 1975). Caveney showed that cell coupling fluctuated during the process of metamorphosis. He also found that treatment of isolated tissue with the hormone β-ecdysone induced a decrease in intercellular resistivity (an increase in conductance). This hormone stimulates the growth of this tissue, so it is postulated that the fall in resistivity facilitates the transmission of morphogens from one cell to the next thereby coordinating the growth response. Caveney also showed that incubation of the β-ecdysone-treated tissue with 10^{-3} M cAMP inhibited the effect of the hormone. Similarly, treatment with A23187 caused a reversal of the β-ecdysone effect. This author postulates that cAMP is one of the feedback regulators of the growth process.

From the point of view of our thesis, these results extend the possible relationship of the calcium and cAMP messenger systems into the realm of another calcium-regulated process. In this case, based on the analysis of this relationship in the control of the function of other response elements, cAMP might function to increase the cytosolic calcium ion content and/or alter the sensitivity of the calcium response element to the calcium messenger as it does in the case of phosphorylase *b* kinase.

There is a considerable literature on the possible interrelated roles of calcium and cAMP in the regulation of cell division, growth, and proliferation in other types of animal cells (Berridge, 1976; Abell and Monahan, 1973; Boyton et al., 1974; Pastan et al., 1974; Rebhun, 1977; Whitfield, 1973; Rasmussen and Goodman, 1977). This literature will not be reviewed in the present monograph, not because it is not of interest but because it represents at the moment a field with a great number of facts but few unifying themes and represents the possibility of a different regulatory relationship between

Ca^{2+} and cAMP than in the situations presently being discussed. In particular, the present discussion relates to clearly defined extracellular messengers acting through surface receptor to initiate a cellular response to a highly specialized cell type. The situation in terms of differentiation, mitosis, and growth represents an ill-defined one in which it is not yet clear how the information flow is regulated.

RESPONSE ELEMENTS

Definition

In the final analysis, a major determination of the particular variation of the universal theme under discussion is the nature of the interaction of the Ca^{2+}- and cAMP-regulated response elements. In no other response system has this been more completely elucidated than in the case of the regulation of glycogen metabolism. Furthermore, the studies of the regulation of glycogen metabolism have been of great historical significance in the development of concepts in this field. For these reasons it is worth considering the regulatory properties of this system in detail.

Before doing so, however, it is worth considering the meaning of the term response element. As employed throughout this monograph, it is used to denote those enzymes, membranes, or structural elements which are the components responsible for mediating a particular cellular response. Thus, the enzymes involved in the gluconeogenic pathway; the Cl^- channel and K^+ pump of the luminal membrane of the fly salivary gland; the enzymes in the pathway of steroid biosynthesis; the enzymes associated with glycogen particles and regulating glycogen turnover; and the components (secretory vesicles, microfilaments, and/or microtubules, and plasma membrane) that participate in the exocytotic process of insulin, parotid enzymes, and neurotransmitter secretion are each response elements in a particular cell. In some cells, for example, the fly salivary gland, there is only a single such element; but in others, there are several, for example, the enzymes regulating glycogen metabolism and those involved in gluconeogenesis. Although the term is imprecise, it is nevertheless useful in focusing attention on a response unit rather than on a single enzyme or transport step as the important component of the cell being controlled by the synarchic messengers.

A Prototypical Response Element: The Enzymes of Glycogen Metabolism

As noted in the first chapter, the discoveries of the respective roles of cAMP as second messenger and calcium as coupling factor involved studies of hepatic glycogenolysis on the one hand and skeletal muscle contraction on the other. A common response element to the two messengers, the bidirectional system of glycogen synthesis and glycogenolysis (Fischer et al, 1971), is found in skeletal muscle as well as in liver. The behavior of this prototypical response element in skeletal muscle is reviewed here in more detail than in an earlier discussion (see Chapter 1). Particularly, since work in the past decade in several laboratories (Cohen, 1973, 1978; Cohen et al., 1978; Foulke and Cohen, 1979; Walsh et al., 1979; DePaoli-Roach et al., 1979; Jett and Soderling, 1979; Itarte and Huang, 1979; Huang et al., 1979; Brostrom et al., 1971; Wang et al., 1976; Kilimann and Heilmeyer, 1977) has identified a number of new properties of this control system. Rather than review this experimental work in detail, a summary of the main conclusion will be given, a model constructed, and the implications of this model to our central thesis discussed.

Glycogen synthesis and glycogen breakdown occur by separate pathways: synthesis is controlled by the enzyme glycogen synthase; degradation is controlled by the enzyme phosphorylase. The conversions of each enzyme from a less active to a more active state, and vice versa, involve phosphorylation by protein kinase(s) and dephosphorylation by phosphoprotein phosphatase(s). The phosphorylated form of phosphorylase (phosphorylase *a*) is the more active form, and the dephosphorylated form of glycogen synthase is the more active. In the intact muscle cell, there is coordination of these conversions so that in times of increased metabolic demand, phosphorylase is converted to its active form and glycogen synthase to its inactive form. Thus, both are converted from nonphosphorylated to phosphorylated forms by the activity of protein kinase(s). When the need no longer exists and glycogen storage (resynthesis) is required, both enzymes are converted back to their nonphosphorylated forms by protein phosphatase(s).

The situation is complicated by the fact that (1) there is more than one protein kinase; (2) there is more than one site of phosphorylation on several of the protein substrates; (3) some of the substrates are phosphorylated by more than one protein kinase; (4) there is more than one protein phosphatase; (5) one of these protein phosphatases has more than one substrate; (6) there are two different ways in which the system is regulated *in situ:* by β-adrenergic agents activating a membrane adenylate cyclase and by neural stimulation inducing the release of calcium from the SR; (7) there is an inhibitor protein which undergoes phosphorylation and thereby becomes both a substrate for and inhibitor of the protein phosphatase; (8) glycogen synthase phosphorylation may be controlled by protein kinases in addition to the cAMP-dependent and calcium-dependent ones; (9) one of the subunits of phosphorylase *b* kinase is calmodulin, the calcium receptor protein; and (10) the affinity of the calmodulin subunit of this enzyme for calcium is changed when other subunits of the enzyme undergo phosphorylation.

A useful way in which to present these facts in a coherent manner is to trace the flow of information in the case of both hormonal (Figure 4.9) and neural (Figure 4.10) activation of skeletal muscle glycogenolysis.

When epinephrine acts upon the skeletal muscle β-receptor (Firgure 4.9), the cAMP concentration rises, and this leads to an activation of cAMP-

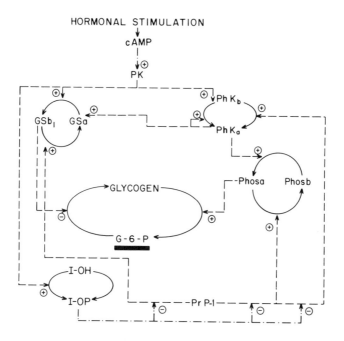

Figure 4.9 Schematic representation of the control of skeletal muscle glycogen metabolism by hormonal stimulation (by catecholamines). Modified from Cohen (1978).

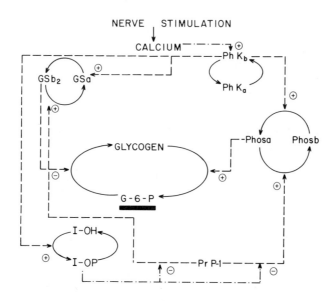

Figure 4.10 Schematic representation of the control of glycogen metabolism in skeletal muscle in response to nerve stimulation. Modified from Cohen (1978).

dependent protein kinase. The active catalytic units of this enzyme catalyze the phosphorylation of three proteins—glycogen synthase (GSa), phosphorylase kinase b (PhK$_b$), and the inhibitor protein (I-OH). As a consequence of glycogen synthase phosphorylation, the inactive phosphorylated enzyme GSb$_1$ is produced and glycogen synthesis inhibited. The phosphorylated form of PhK (PhK$_a$) catalyzes the conversion of phosphorylase b (Phos b) to Phos a. The latter catalyzes the breakdown of glycogen to G-1-P, and this is converted to glucose-6-phosphate (G-6-P). PhK$_a$ also catalyzes the autophosphorylation of PhK$_b$ and the phosphorylation of Gs$_a$, thus augmenting the action of PK. The conversion of I-OH to I-OP by PK leads to the production of phosphoprotein which, by serving as a preferential substrate for phosphoprotein phosphatase-1, PrP-1, inhibits the dephosphorylation of Phos a, PhK$_a$, and GSb$_1$. When stimulation ceases, the pool of I-OP is used up, and then PrP-1 catalyzes the inactivation (dephosphorylation) of Phos a, PhK$_a$, and GSb$_a$. There is an additional positive control of GSa activity by insulin (not shown) that involves both a shift to the right in the affinity of inactive PK for cAMP and an insulin-induced increase in glucose-6-phosphate which acts as a feed-forward activator of GSa.

When the muscle is stimulated neurally to contract repeatedly, the increase in calcium not only activates the contractile system but also the phosphorylase system (Figure 4.10). In this case, calcium activates Phos K$_b$ (the dephospho form of the enzyme). This leads to a Phos b-to-Phos a conversion, a GSa-to-GSb$_2$ conversion, and the I-OH-to-I-OP conversion. GSb$_1$ (Figure 4.9) and GSb$_2$ (Figure 4.10) indicate that the amino acid residues (serine) phosphorylated in GSa by PK differ from those phosphorylated by PhK. As a consequence of the calcium signal, the same physiological responses, inhibition of glycogen synthesis and activation of glycogen breakdown, are seen as after epinephrine action even though the protein kinase reaction responsible for the initiation of the response is different.

Cohen (1978) has shown that PrP-1 and PK are present in significant amounts in many tissues and that their content does not correlate with glycogen content of these tissues. From these observations, he proposes that this system might well have similar properties in other tissues but control the activity of other enzymes in these tissues, for example, pyruvate kinase in liver or acetyl CoA carboxylase in lactating mammary gland. In order to complete this scheme and account for the numerous and increasing number of instances in which calcium-dependent and cAMP-dependent protein kinases catalyze the phosphorylation of the same proteins, a universal calcium-dependent protein kinase must also exist. It is not clear whether or not this is phosphorylase kinase or some other calcium-dependent kinase.

A number of the control characteristics of the glycogen system have been found in other systems and hence represent general mechanisms by which the activity of response elements are controlled. For this reason, it is worth summarizing briefly these characteristics (Table 4.3).

Any discussion of the control properties of this prototypical response

Table 4.3   Control Characteristics of the Glycogen Synthase–Phosphorylase System

1. In a bidirectional controlled metabolic pathway, the key forward and reverse reactions are regulated by separate enzymes
2. There is coordinate control of the forward and reverse reactions
3. There is also a degree of plasticity because there are independent controls that can operate on either the forward or reverse reaction but not on the other
4. Phosphorylation and dephosphorylation are an elegant mechanism by which control of enzyme function is achieved
5. The activity of the response element can be controlled by either a cAMP-dependent or a calcium-dependent protein kinase
6. When the two different kinase catalyze the phosphorylation of a response element protein, they usually phosphorylate it at different sites
7. Phosphorylation of a regulated enzyme at one of several sites can modify its enzymatic function, but different site phosphorylations do not usually produce comparable changes in function
8. By the phosphorylation of a response element, the cAMP-dependent protein kinase can alter the responsiveness of that response element to calcium
9. The sensitivity of a cAMP response element (PK) to cAMP can be altered

element would be incomplete without mention of its mode of operation in other tissues. In the case of the skeletal muscle, as just discussed, the system operates as an example largely of redundant control, but in the running athelete it operates as a sequential or hierarchial system. Likewise, in the liver (see Chapter 7), the system appears to exhibit aspects primarily of redundant and sequential control. In the heart, however, it is likely that under usual circumstances, the system is not switched on and off with each heart beat nor that it serves as a source of gluconeogenic substrate for the organism in times of energy deprivation. Rather, it appears to serve only the local needs of the heart. In that capacity, it is unlikely that it ever exhibits redundant control; sequential control is more likely. There is less information available concerning its regulation in smooth muscle, but there is clear evidence showing that glycogenolysis in smooth muscle is stimulated by the calcium messenger system independent of the cAMP messenger system. It is not yet clear whether in this type of cell, cAMP serves any activating function, nor has the possibility of antagonistic control of this response system in such a tissue been seriously considered. However, such type of control is a distinct possibility in light of other aspects of the calcium–cAMP relationship in smooth muscle (see Chapter 8).

CONCLUSION

The basic theme developed in this chapter is that Ca^{2+} and cAMP function as interrelated intracellular messengers in nearly all animal cells. More specifically, it has been proposed that they function as *synarchic messengers* in stimulus–response coupling when differential animal cells are induced to perform their specialized function by a group of extracellular stimuli (hormones, neurotransmitters, metabolites, ions) which exert their effects by interacting with specific membrane receptors.

The general properties of this system have been discussed. Likewise, the properties of the enzyme complex regulating skeletal muscle glycogen metabolism have been considered. Also, a brief categorization of the major recognized variants of synarchic regulation has been presented. In the succeeding chapters, a detailed consideration of these variations on this universal theme will be undertaken, both to provide support for the general model and to indicate the fact that, by very minor variations in the way different components within the universal system interact, a marked change in the behavior of the overall system can be achieved. Over and over again, what will become evident is the elegant simplicity yet complex beauty inherent in this universal cellular control device.

5

Coordinate Control

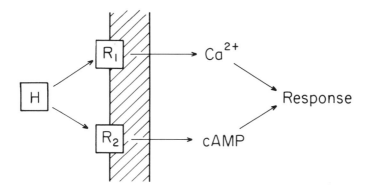

INTRODUCTION

The prototypical examples of synarchic regulation are those in which cAMP and Ca^{2+} act in a coordinate fashion to determine cellular response. The term coordinate as employed in this context has three key aspects: (1) the same hormone induces an increase in the concentration of both Ca^{2+} and cAMP in the cytosol; (2) these two messengers interact to regulate each other's concentration; and (3) they act on different components of the cellular response unit to determine cellular response.

Two examples of this type of control are considered. Both are examples of hormonally regulated processes. The first is the action of the parathyroid hormone (PTH) in regulating gluconeogenesis in the isolated mammalian renal tubule; the second is the action of 5-hydroxytryptamine (5HT) in regulating fluid and electrolyte secretion in the fly salivary gland. At the moment, there is no good example, to my knowledge, of this type of control in the nervous system, but it seems likely that eventually one will become evident.

Although both have been extensively studied, the situation in the fly salivary gland is more clearly delineated because of its greater functional simplicity. Nevertheless, the characteristics of the PTH-mediated response are considered first because historically, it was the studies in this system which led to many of the studies in the fly salivary gland.

RENAL GLUCONEOGENESIS AND
PARATHYROID HORMONE

The kidney is one of two organs in which glucose is produced from noncarbohydrate precursor. The anatomical site of this process is the proximal renal tubule (Guder and Wieland, 1972). Hormones capable of stimulating renal gluconeogenesis include parathyroid hormone (PTH), catecholamines, and angiotensin (Bowman, 1970; Guder and Wieland, 1972; Roobol and Alleyne, 1973; Kurokawa et al., 1973; Nagata and Rasmussen, 1968, 1970a,b; MacDonald and Saggerson, 1977; Guder and Rupprecht, 1975; Guder, 1979; Melson et al., 1970; Kaminsky et al., 1970; Klahr et al., 1973; Kurokawa and Massry, 1973; Friedricks and Schoner, 1973). However, the process is also responsive to changes in extracellular H^+ and calcium and phosphate ion concentrations. Exogenous cAMP and fatty acids also stimulate this process (Krebs et al., 1963; Pagliara and Goodman, 1969; Guder and Wieland, 1972; Roobol and Alleyne, 1973; Kurokawa and Rasmussen, 1973a,b). Of most immediate interest are the facts that either exogenous cAMP or changes in extracellular calcium ion concentration can stimulate renal gluconeogenesis. Because of these findings plus the observation by Chase and Aurbach (1967) that PTH increases urinary cAMP excretion, the hormonally responsive renal tubule was one of the first systems in which the interrelated roles of calcium and cAMP were examined (Nagata and Rasmussen, 1968; Nagata and Rasmussen, 1970a,b; Rasmussen, 1970; Kurokawa and Rasmussen, 1973a,b,c; Kurokawa et al., 1973). As already noted (see Figure 1.11), the effect of the hormone on glucose production required the presence of extracellular calcium even though, in the absence of calcium, it caused a similar rise in the cAMP content of the tissue. Furthermore, the action of exogenous cAMP on glucose formation required calcium. Hence, at the very least, calcium was required for the expression of the cAMP effect. However, as shown in Figure 5.1, PTH caused a calcium-dependent increase in cellular calcium content (Borle, 1970) and a calcium-dependent increase in glucose formation. These findings raised the possibility that PTH caused an increase in calcium entry into the cell as well as an activation of adenylate cyclase.

On the basis of detailed studies of the interrelated roles of calcium and cAMP in regulating gluconeogenesis from a variety of substrates, we (Nagata and Rasmussen, 1970a,b; Kurokawa and Rasmussen, 1973b; Rasmussen, 1970) concluded that both calcium and cAMP served interrelated messenger functions in the action of PTH upon renal gluconeogenesis and developed a model of hormone action in which there was coordinate control of renal tubular metabolism by Ca^{2+} and cAMP (Figure 5.2).

This model was based on the following facts: First, cAMP but not PTH enhanced glucose formation from pyruvate and lactate in the absence of added Ca^{2+} in the medium. Second, the effect of PTH upon glucose formation from all substrates was Ca^{2+} dependent. Third, the effects of PTH upon

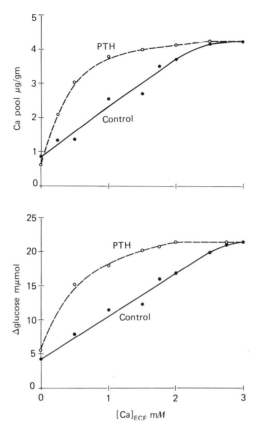

Figure 5.1 Plots of total cell calcium and of change in medium glocuse content as function of the extracellular calcium concentration in the presence ($\bigcirc$) and absence ($\bullet$) of parathyroid hormone (PTH). From Rasmussen et al. (1972), with permission.

cAMP production and glucose formation were not necessarily correlated. For example, when Ca^{2+} was removed from the medium, PTH caused a sustained increase in cAMP content of isolated renal tubules but did not enhance gluconeogenesis even though a decrease in pH stimulated glucose formation under similar conditions (Figure 1.11). When 1.0 mM Ca^{2+} was added to the medium, PTH produced a much smaller rise in cAMP content but a maximal stimulation of glucose production. Fourth, the addition of phosphate to the medium of tubules incubated in the presence of PTH and Ca^{2+} led to a fall in the rate of gluconeogenesis but a rise in the cAMP content. This pattern was explained by the fact that increasing phosphate concentration led to a shift of calcium from cytosol to mitochondria and thereby to a decrease in cytosolic free calcium ion. This, in turn, led to a decrease in calcium-dependent glucose production even though, because of feedback control of cAMP concentration by calcium, the cAMP content of the tissue increased. It was reasoned that if intracellular cAMP were the

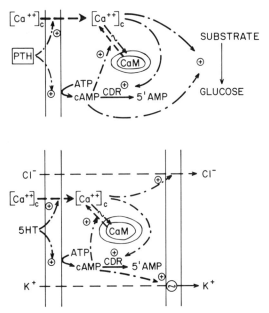

Figure 5.2 Models of the mechanism by which PTH regulates metabolism within the renal tubule (top) and by which 5HT regulates KCl and fluid secretion in the fly salivary gland (bottom). In both cases, the hormone appears to activate calcium entry and adenylate cyclase. As a consequence, both Ca^{2+} and cAMP concentrations increase within the cytosol. Both influence one or more metabolic steps and both regulate each other's concentrations.

primary regulatory of gluconeogenesis, then an increase in extracellular phosphate, by increasing cAMP content, should increase rather than decrease glucose formation. Fifth, Borle (1973), working with isolated tissue culture cells derived from kidney, showed a PTH-mediated increase in calcium uptake by these cells (Figure 5.1). Sixth, PTH and exogenous cAMP show partially additive effects under certain conditions (Guder and Wieland, 1972). Seventh, theophylline and other phosphodiesterase inhibitors do not enhance the effect of PTH on glucose formation (MacDonald and Saggerson, 1977). Eighth, the injection of PTH and of calcium *in vivo* lead to similar changes in metabolite profiles in quick-frozen segments of renal cortex (Nagata and Rasmussen, 1968).

In spite of these facts, more recent discussions have assumed that cAMP is the major and perhaps the only messenger in PTH action (Guder and Rupprecht, 1975; MacDonald and Saggerson, 1977; Guder, 1979). These authors ignore the fact that PTH has a marked effect upon calcium exchange in isolated renal cells (Borle, 1970, 1972; Borle and Uchikawa 1978, 1979; Uchikawa and Borle, 1978). It could be argued that the studies of Borle in isolated cells derived from kidney tissue and grown in tissue culture are no longer representative of intact renal cortical cells, having lost their polarity and specialized functions. This might be a valid argument, except for the fact that Uchikawa and Borle (1978) have recently shown similar effects of PTH upon calcium exchange in isolated renal cortical slices.

The other feature of Borle's data is that although initially he reported (Borle, 1973) that PTH, but not exogenous ¢AMP, stimulated calcium uptake in kidney cells, in later work he has shown that cAMP also increases calcium uptake into renal cells when this is examined in cells chronically exposed to cAMP (Borle and Uchikawa, 1979). From these latter data, it could be argued that PTH acts only on adenylate cyclase and that the resultant rise in cAMP content of the cells leads to all the changes in cellular calcium metabolism. However, a comparison of their data concerning the effect of PTH and exogenous cAMP (Borle and Uchikawa, 1979) shows that the effect of PTH upon total cellular calcium accumulation is twice that of cAMP, even though the relative increase in the cytosolic pool is greater in the presence of cAMP. Also, at comparable concentrations of PTH and cAMP, there are differences in the effects of these agents upon rates of glucose formation (Kurokawa et al., 1973). This concentration of exogenous cAMP has a greater stimulatory effect on glucose formation from lactate than does PTH, even though these two agents have comparable effects upon glucose production from malate, succinate, and α-ketoglutarate. Hence, it seems likely that both calcium and cAMP serve to couple stimulus to response when PTH alters renal gluconeogenesis and that PTH has a direct plasma membrane effect upon cellular calcium uptake (Figure 5.2).

The evidence concerning the messenger roles of calcium and cAMP in the action of other hormones is less complete. Initial studies of Klahr et al. (1973), Kurokawa and Massry (1973), and Friedricks and Schoner (1973) showed that the stimulatory effect of catecholamines was correlated with their ability to enhance the cAMP content of this tissue. The results of more recent studies do not support this view. Guder and Rupprecht (1975) and MacDonald and Saggerson (1977) have shown that there is no correlation between catecholamine-induced glucose formation and changes in cAMP content. They find that the effects of catecholamines are mediated by α-receptor rather than β-receptor activation and probably involve calcium as messenger. A similar conclusion has been reached in the case of the action of angiotensin II. The stimulation of glucose formation by this hormone is not associated with any change in tissue cAMP content, and omission of calcium markedly inhibits its effect (Gruder, 1979).

Thus, in the renal cortical cells, it seems likely that control of gluconeogenesis involves both a coordinate control system regulated by PTH which involves both calcium and cAMP as messengers, and a redundant control system in which other extracellular agents such as angiotension and epinephrine regulate glucose formation employing only the calcium messenger system. The latter circumstances is similar to the situation found in the control of hepatic gluconeogenesis (see Chapter 7).

The precise steps controlled by cAMP or calcium are still an unresolved matter. There is some evidence to suggest that one of the effects of calcium is that of altering the uptake of α-ketoglutarate and possibly other substrates by mitochondria (Roobol and Alleyne, 1973; Mason, 1974). In addition, it seems likely that Ca^{2+} activates phosphoenolpyruvate carboxykinase and inhibits pyruvate kinase (Kurokawa and Rasmussen, 1973a). All of these effects would occur as a consequence of a rise in the calcium ion content of the cytosol and thus can be encompassed in a model in which a rise in cytosolic calcium ion concentration is one of the signals for hormone action.

PTH has an additional metabolic effect, that of increasing the mitochondrial synthesis of 1,25-dihydroxyvitamin D_3 (1,25(OH)$_2$-D_3). It is not immediately apparent how a rise in the cytosolic Ca^{2+} concentration can be employed to regulate the activity of an enzyme which is a component of the inner mitochondrial membrane and whose substrate site faces the mitochondrial matrix space. The fact that such an event does occur raises the interesting question of how the information of hormone–receptor interaction is transmitted to an intramitochondrial hydroxylase. This question will be discussed again in relation to ACTH action on the adrenal cortex (see Chapter 6), but at this point it is worth considering the action of PTH on this renal hydroxylase.

REGULATION OF INTRAMITOCHONDRIAL REACTIONS BY CALCIUM

The major observations concerning the ionic control of 25-hydroxyvitamin D_3 1α-hydroxylase which catalyzes the reaction $25(OH)D_3 \rightarrow 1,25(OH)_2D_3$ were carried out by Bikle, Murphy, and Rasmussen employing isolated renal mitochondria from the D-deficient chick (Bikle et al., 1975; Rasmussen et al., 1972; Bikle and Rasmussen, 1974a,b, 1976; Bikle et al., 1976; Bikle and Rasmussen, 1978a,b). The activity of this enzyme was stimulated by an increase in the extramitochondrial Ca^{2+} concentration between 10^{-8} and 10^{-5} M, and this stimulation was blocked by ruthenium red (Figure 5.3a). However, the enzyme was also stimulated by increasing the extramitochondrial K^+ concentration (Figure 5.3b), and ruthenium red did not block its action. Increasing the Na^+ concentration had no effect on its activity. Of equal interest, the effect of calcium was modified by the Pi concentration of the medium (Figure 5.4a). At an optimal Pi concentration of 1 mM (line C, Figure 5.4a), the enzyme was most sensitive to activation by calcium. Likewise, changes in Pi concentration had a biphasic, calcium-dependent effect on enzyme activity (Figure 5.4b). Increasing the acetate but not the chloride concentration of the medium also enhanced activity, but increasing the HCO_3^- concentration at a fixed pCO_2 caused an inhibition of the calcium- or potassium-mediated stimulation even though this rise in HCO_3^- concentration enhanced calcium uptake. If, however, the pCO_2 was raised at the same time the HCO_3^- concentration was raised, then a marked enhancement of enzyme activity occurred (Figure 5.4b).

The finding that K^+, or K^+ plus valinomycin, stimulated hydroxylase in a manner similar to that seen with calcium means that a rise in Ca^{2+} is probably not increasing the activity of the enzyme by a specific interaction of

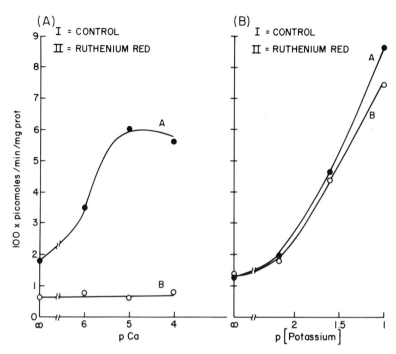

Figure 5.3 Rate of $1,25(OH)_2D_3$ synthesis as function of the Ca^{2+} concentration (A) or K^+ concentration (B) in the presence (●) or absence (○) of ruthenium red. Note that ruthenium red blocks the effect of calcium but not potassium. From Bilke et al. (1976), with permission.

Ca^{2+} with a site on the enzyme but by some mechanism shared in common with K^+ but not with Na^+. The transport of Ca^{2+} and K^+ across the mitochondrial membrane is driven by the membrane potential, but that of Na^+ is not because there are specific carriers within the membrane for the first two but not the third cation. Ca^{2+} and K^+ induce a proton efflux from the mitochondria under conditions in which they stimulate hydroxylase activity. However, simply the uptake of Ca^{2+} by the mitochondria is not sufficient to activate the enzyme because Ca^{2+} uptake occurs when HCO_3^- serves as an anion, but very little stimulation of hydroxylase activity is seen. This inhibitory effect of the HCO_3^- anion can be reversed simply by increasing the pCO_2 in the incubation medium.

In order to interpret these complex data, it is necessary to review the structural organization of this hydroxylase. Although its characteristics have not been completely elucidated, they appear (Henry and Norman, 1974; Ghazarian et al., 1974) to be similar to those found for comparable hydroxylase in adrenal cortical mitochondria. In the latter, the roles of a flavoprotein, nonheme iron, and cytochrome P450 have been defined. A model of such a system is presented in Figure 5.5. The hydroxylase contains a flavoprotein NADPH dehydrogenase which faces the cytosol and, when oxidized, liberates protons into the cytosol and transfers electrons to a nonheme iron

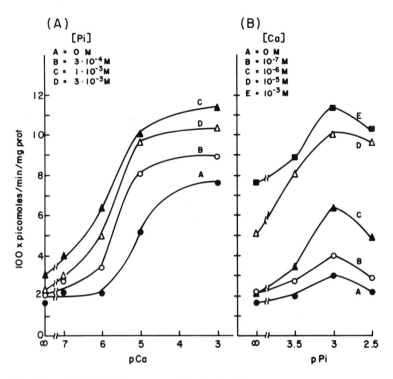

Figure 5.4 Rate of 1,25(OH)$_2$D$_3$ synthesis in isolated chick mitochondria as a function of CA^{2+} concentration (A) or phosphate ion concentration (B). In each case, the data show the effect of the opposite ion on the response curve of the other. From Bilke et al. (1975), with permission.

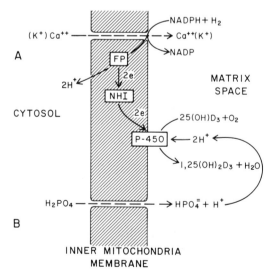

Figure 5.5 Model of the electron transport chain coupled to 1α-hydroxylase in the inner mitochondrial membrane of the kidney. See text for discussion.

and then to a cytochrome P450 which faces the matrix space. The activity of the dehydrogenase can be stimulated by the transport of Ca^{2+} or K^+ (site A) across the membrane; and if protons are available within the matrix, the dehydrogenase is the rate-controlling step. On the other hand, because the membrane is nearly impermeable to protons, the source and sink of protons created by the flow of reducing equivalents through the chain are separated so that protons generated by the dehydrogenase cannot be used in the hydroxylation reaction. The requirement for protons within the matrix is met by the translocation of H_2PO_4, acetate, or any other anion (site B) that can donate a H^+ in the matrix space. Hence, phosphate and acetate stimulate the hydroxylase and enhance the effect of calcium. On the other hand, HCO_3^-, which does not donate a proton, does not stimulate but actually inhibits the reaction by causing a further alkalinization of the matrix space. When one raises the pCO_2, the CO_2 diffuses into the matrix and reacts with H_2O to form H_2CO_3, which then serves as a proton donor thereby explaining the fact that an increase in pCO_2 reverses the inhibitory effect of HCO_3^-.

These data lead to the conclusion that the hydroxylase system is controlled at two sites, A and B. At site A, either Ca^{2+} or K^+ uptake, by collapsing the membrane potential, stimulate the flow of reducing equivalents through Fp to NHI and stimulate respiration and protein efflux. At site B, permeant proton-donating anions enter the mitochondria in response to Ca^{2+} or K^+ uptake and liberate protons within the matrix space. These protons are essential for the actual hydroxylase reaction.

Under physiological conditions, it is known that PTH stimulates this reaction *in situ*. From the data of Borle and Uchikawa (1978, 1979), it is known that when the hormone activates the renal cell, there is a rise in cytosolic calcium ion concentration and a significant increase in the rate of exchange of mitochondrial calcium as well as a net increase in total mitochondrial calcium. Thus, under physiological circumstances, calcium may play a major role in the PTH-mediated control of this hydroxylase. However, this type of control depends not on the specific interaction of calcium ion with a receptor protein but on the increased rate of calcium exchange across the mitochondrial membrane.

In the renal cell, PTH increases the exchange of calcium across both the plasma membrane and the mitochondrial membrane. If these transport processes in the plasma membrane are coupled in any way with the NADH and NADPH dehydroxygenase systems in the plasma membrane, these increased rates of calcium exchange may have a more general function than that of regulating steroid and sterol hydroxylases in the mitochondrial membrane. To distinguish this type of control from that exerted by specific interactions with receptor proteins, it is useful to classify the latter as control by *receptor coupling* and the former as control by *ion–electron transport coupling*.

In spite of the fact that an interaction of Ca^{2+} with a specific receptor protein is apparently not the basis for calcium-mediated changes in the activity of this particular mitochondrial enzyme, there are other such enzymes within the mitochondria whose functions are apparently controlled by Ca^{2+}. These include the interconverting enzyme of the pyruvate dehydrogenase system (Denton et al., 1972) and NAD-isocitric dehydrogenase (Denton et al., 1978). An increase in the intramitochondrial calcium concentration has also been reported to increase the rate of oxidation of β-hydroxybutyrate (Malmström and Carafoli, 1976), succinate (Ezawa and Ogata, 1977), and fatty acids (Otto and Ontko, 1978). How these effects of calcium are mediated is not known.

FLY SALIVARY GLAND

Anatomically, the salivary gland of the blow fly *Calliphora erythrocephala* consists of two portions—the abdominal and thoracic portions. The first is primarily an organ of secretion producing a copious quantity of an isotonic KCl. The thoracic portion is resorptive in nature and reaccumulates part of the KCl so that the final product, the saliva, is a hypotonic KCl secretion. The abdominal portion of the gland secretes digestive enzymes if the flies are fed for several days before the glands are obtained. The studies to be discussed concern only the behavior of the abdominal portion of the gland. Parameters such as fluid secretion, enzyme secretion, and membrane potential have been studied in a single gland, whereas changes in cAMP, calcium, and phosphoinositide metabolism have been studied in 4 to 50 glands. The secretory behavior of the individual gland varies somewhat but is sufficiently consistent that it is possible to relate metabolic events measured in multiple glands to secretory and electrical events measured in a single gland (Berridge, 1970, 1973, 1975, 1976a,b, 1980; Berridge and Prince, 1972a,b; Berridge and Patel, 1968; Prince et al., 1972, 1973; Berridge and Lipke, 1979; Prince and Berridge, 1973; Berridge et al., 1975a,b; Hansen-Bay, 1978).

The basic electrical and secretory responses to 5-hydroxytryptamine (5HT), the presumed natural secretagogue, are shown in Figure 5.6. Application of hormone leads to an immediate, sustained shift to a more negative transepithelial membrane potential and, shortly thereafter, to an increase in the rate of fluid secretion which is sustained until hormone is removed.

Analysis of this system in terms of the Sutherland criteria demonstrated the following: (1) exogenous cAMP mimicked the effect of 5HT on fluid secretion (Figure 5.6); (2) 5HT addition caused a rise in the cAMP content of isolated glands; (3) the effect of a submaximal 5HT concentration on fluid secretion was enhanced in the presence of the phosphodiesterase inhibitor theophylline; (4) a particulate hormone-sensitive adenylate cyclase was present; and (5) a cAMP-dependent protein kinase was present in gland homogenates. Thus, all the criteria with which to establish the second messenger function of cAMP in the action of 5HT on the fly salivary gland were fulfilled. Nevertheless, a more detailed analysis revealed important differences between the effects of 5HT and exogenous cAMP. The most

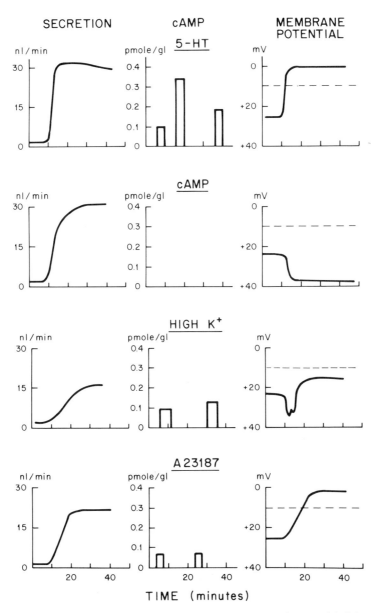

Figure 5.6 Changes in rate of fluid secretion, cAMP content, and transepithelial membrane potential in the fly salivary gland when exposed to, from top to bottom, 5HT, exogenous cAMP, high external K⁺, and the divalent ionophore A23187.

striking was the fact that 5HT caused a shift to a more negative potential but exogenous cAMP caused a more positive one (Figure 5.6) when administered in a dose sufficient to produce the same secretory response as 5HT. Additionally, when the serosal chloride content was lowered, the secretion

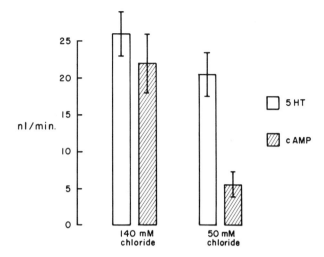

Figure 5.7 Effect of low and high serosal chloride concentration on the rate of fluid secretion induced by 5HT (open bars) and exogenous cAMP (hatched bars). From Prince and Berridge (1973), with permission.

induced by cAMP was inhibited more than was the fluid secretion induced by 5HT (Figure 5.7).

The effect of calcium depletion upon the response to the two agents also differed. In glands depleted of calcium ion and incubated in a calcium-free medium, neither 5HT nor exogenous cAMP induced secretion even though 5HT stimulated cAMP production. In spite of the fact that neither agent induced secretion under these circumstances (no calcium), they both influenced the transepithelial membrane potential. In this case, the potential becomes more positive after addition of either 5HT or exogenous cAMP. When at this point calcium was added to the medium, glands exposed to either 5HT or to exogenous cAMP began to secrete again (Figure 5.8). In the glands exposed to 5HT, there was an immediate reversal of membrane potential from positive to negative but no change in the membrane potential in cAMP-treated glands. Under some conditions, the membrane potential oscillated in cAMP-treated glands, but it never became as markedly negative as in 5HT-treated ones.

These data indicated that there was a calcium-dependent response to 5HT not seen with exogenous cAMP. Examination of the effects of the two agents on cellular calcium metabolism showed that although both stimulate calcium efflux from glands incubated either in media containing or deficient in calcium, only 5HT stimulated calcium influx, indicating a direct effect of 5HT on calcium metabolism not mediated by cAMP. Later experiments by Berridge and Lipke (1979) have extended these observations. They have shown that addition of 5HT causes a marked increase in transcellular calcium transport but that cAMP causes only a small change (Figure 5.9). These findings are consistent with the previous conclusion that 5HT but not cAMP

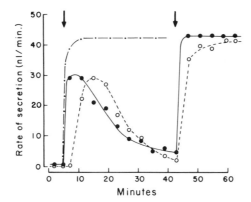

Figure 5.8 Effect of either 5HT or exogenous cAMP on the rate of fluid secretion in fly salivary glands incubated in a medium containing no calcium. The thin monotonic curve represents a typical secretory response to either agent in the presence of calcium. When either hormone or nucleotide was added (left-hand arrow) there was a significant increase in fluid secretion. But, this was not sustained, and by 40 minutes, the rate had returned to nearly the basal value. Addition of exogenous Ca^{2+} (right-hand arrow) at this point caused a prompt increase in rate of fluid secretion to normal stimulated values. From Prince et al. (1972), with permission.

increases the rate of influx of calcium into the cell across its basal membrane. These data showed that Ca^{2+} as well as cAMP had a second messenger function in 5HT action.

This conclusion was tested in several ways. The first employed the ionophore A23187. This substance is known to increase the permeability of biological membranes to divalent cations (Reed and Lardy, 1972). The addition of A23187 caused qualitatively similar changes in fluid secretion and

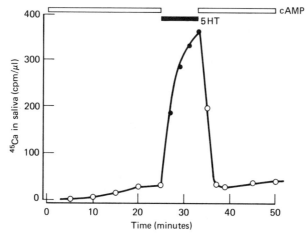

Figure 5.9 Effect of exogenous cAMP (open bars) and of 5HT (solid bar) on the rate of appearance of ^{45}Ca in the saliva of a gland with essentially the same rates of secretion in the presence of cAMP and 5HT. From Berridge and Lipke (1979), with permission.

membrane potential to those seen after 5HT (Figure 5.6), but the rate of increase in fluid secretion was slower and never reached the same maximal value as that seen after 5HT. The change in membrane potential also occurred more slowly, but eventually reached essentially the same value as that seen after 5HT. Even though A23187 mimicked these two effects of 5HT, it caused a fall rather than a rise in the cAMP content of the tissue. It is noteworthy that A23187 had no effect upon potential or secretion in the absence of external calcium and that A23187 stimulated Ca^{2+} influx into and Ca^{2+} efflux from the tissue. Comparable results were obtained by increasing the K^+ concentration in the incubation medium (Figure 5.6). This caused an immediate rise in membrane potential followed by a calcium-dependent decrease associated with an increase in secretion and a very small rise in cAMP concentration. As in the case of A23187, these effects of K^+ depended upon the presence of extracellular calcium.

These results indicate that fluid secretion in the fly salivary gland can be initiated either by a rise in cAMP content without a concomitant increase in calcium entry into the tissue or by an increase in calcium influx into the tissue without a rise or even a fall in cAMP content. One way to explain these data would be to propose that the cAMP and the calcium messages speak to the same intracellular response element to initiate secretion by a final common mechanism. However, this would not explain the fact that the calcium message causes a fall in membrane potential but that the cAMP message causes a rise. Also, it would not explain three other facts: (1) in the absence of calcium, 5HT causes a greater rise in cAMP content than in its presence; (2) the cAMP-dependent secretion does not occur in a calcium-depleted gland even though a cAMP-induced increase in membrane potential is seen; and (3) cAMP induces an efflux of calcium.

These data indicate that the calcium and cAMP messages influence each other and that the messages are not received by the same final response element. From the electrophysiological properties of the gland, it can be concluded that the major response element is the luminal membrane of the cell. The calcium-mediated effect of 5HT on membrane potential is associated with a marked fall in the electrical resistance of the luminal membrane (Berridge et al., 1975) and a lesser fall in the resistance of the basal membrane (Figure 5.10). This change is thought to result from a calcium-induced change in anion (chloride) permeability. In contrast, the accumulated data indicate that cAMP acts to increase the activity of a luminal membrane K^+ pump. Hence, the two messengers influence the behavior of the final response element in a complimentary fashion, operationally similar to the relation between calcium and cAMP in the activation of the phosphorylase cascade (see Chapter 4). Either change is sufficient to activate secretion as long as a minimal change in the second component is maintained; but under physiological circumstances, it is the coordinated action of the two upon the final response element that determines response.

An additional type of evidence showing that 5HT has primary effects upon

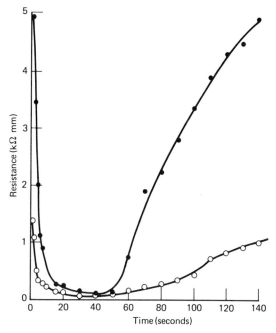

Figure 5.10 Effect of brief exposure (10 seconds) of the fly salivary gland to 5HT on the membrane resistance of the basal (●) and luminal membranes (○). From Berridge et al. (1975), with permission.

membrane function other than that of turning on adenylate cyclase are the results of studies carried out by Fain and Berridge (Berridge and Fain, 1979; Fain and Berridge, 1979) concerned with the hormone-mediated changes in phosphoinositide turnover. They showed that if glands were prelabeled with [³H]inositol, this inositol was largely incorporated into the phosphoinositide fraction of the gland. If such labeled glands were then exposed to 5HT, there was a release of [³H]inositol back into the medium. The onset of this release coincided with the onset of a change in fluid secretion (Figure 5.11) and was associated with a concomitant transcellular movement of calcium. The dose–response characteristic of the three changes to 5HT were similar. The 5HT-induced inositol release had the following characteristics: (1) exogenous cAMP did not cause inositol release; (2) it occurred even if there was no calcium in the external medium; and (3) A23187, which should bypass any natural calcium gating system, caused calcium transport and fluid secretion but did not alter [³H]inositol release. The hormone, 5HT, also inhibited the resynthesis of PI as shown by the fact that it reduced the rate of uptake of labeled [³H]inositol into the glands. This combination of increased breakdown and decreased synthesis led to a progressive depletion of PI which was associated with a progressive fall in calcium transport. When the PI content of the gland was restored, calcium transport returned to normal values.

These data led to two conclusions. The first was that 5HT has a cAMP-

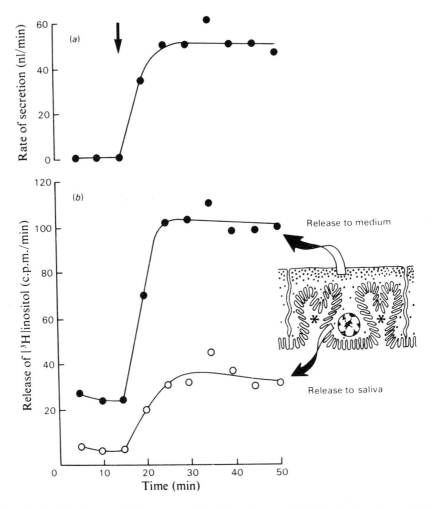

Figure 5.11 Stimulation of fluid secretion (*a*) and breakdown of PI (*b*) in the fly salivary gland in response to stimulation with 5HT. At the point indicated by the arrow, $10^{-8}M$ 5HT was added. From Fain and Berridge (1979), with permission.

independent effect upon membrane function—that of mediating PI turnover directly. The second was that PI turnover is the biochemical counterpart of calcium gating, that is, 5HT opens a gate in a calcium channel which gives rise to an increase in calcium entry into the cell. These studies of Fain and Berridge provide significant biochemical support for the concept, based previously on physiological evidence, that 5HT causes the transduction of more than one primary event in the plasma membrane of the fly salivary gland.

The simplest scheme to account for these observations would be one in which 5HT, interacting with its receptor, gives rise to two independent second messengers, cAMP and calcium, which upon entering the cell could interact with different response elements on the luminal membrane—an activation of a K^+ pump and an increase in chloride permeability, respectively—to bring about the final response. However, this is an incomplete description because it ignores a crucial feature of this control system: the fact that the cAMP and calcium signals interact and by those interactions provide the element of feedback control in the system. These interactions are at least two in number: cAMP causes the mobilization of calcium from an intracellular pool, and calcium either inhibits cAMP synthesis and/or increases its rate of hydrolysis. A more complete model of coordinate synarchic control in the fly salivary gland is that depicted in Figure 5.2.

Several features of this system are worthy of comment. The first is a consideration of the time course of change in cAMP concentration within the cell after hormone addition (Figure 5.6). When 5HT is added, there is an initial three- to fourfold increase in cAMP concentration, but the concentration then falls so that in the chronically stimulated gland it is only 1.5-fold greater than in the unstimulated gland. The threefold rise in cAMP content is sustained if the hormone is added to a calcium-depleted gland, indicating that the fall in cAMP content after the initial rise is calcium dependent. The sequence of events appears to be as follows: 5HT stimulation of adenylate cyclase results in a rise in cAMP concentration which leads in turn to a shift in ratio of calcium influx to efflux across the mitochondrial membrane which, coupled to the 5HT-induced rise in calcium entry, leads to a suppression of cAMP concentration. This represents a negative feedback loop in this control system. As the cAMP level declines, the magnitude of the imbalance between calcium influx and efflux also becomes less. From these data and the known characteristics of the calcium response elements in other cells, one can predict that the steady state shift in cytosolic Ca^{2+} concentration must also be of the same relative magnitude as the change in cAMP content and probably has a similar time course.

Recent studies by O'Doherty et al. (1980) support this view. These workers have impaled fly salivary gland cells with calcium-sensitive microelectrodes and monitored the intracellular Ca^{2+} activity after serotonin addition. Immediately after hormone addition, there is a threefold increase in activity, but this declines rapidly and reaches a value not measurably different than that seen in the unstimulated gland. Nevertheless, transcellular Ca^{2+} flux shows a sustained increase. Furthermore, there is a sustained increase in Cl⁻ permeability of the luminal membrane which decreases rapidly if hormone is removed. Employing a similar method, Berridge (1980) has also studied the response of the fly salivary gland to 5HT. He reported that the resting intracellular (presumably cytosolic) Ca^{2+} concentration was approximately 10^{-7} M and upon maximal stimulation rose to values as high as 10^{-6} M. This hormonally induced rise in cytosolic Ca^{2+} concentration depended upon the presence of extracellular calcium. His data also show that after an initial sharp rise in cytosolic Ca^{2+} concentration occurring immediately after hormone addition, the level declines to a value only slightly above the basal or resting value, even though 5HT is continually present.

Although the above discussion assumes that the site of cAMP action on cellular calcium metabolism is the inner mitochondrial membrane, this point is not completely established. The following points are strongly in favor of this conclusion: (1) There is a large internal calcium pool that can be released by exogenous cAMP and temporarily sustain secretory response. (2) The only pool of sufficient size to participate in this process is that in the mitochondria. (3) The mitochondrial pool becomes depleted when the gland is stimulated by cAMP in calcium-free media. (4) Salivary glands from newly hatched flies contain no calcium phosphate deposits in their mitochondria, and these glands cannot be induced to secrete either 5HT or cAMP in a calcium-free medium. (5) Addition of cAMP to various particulate fractions of homogenized glands causes a reduced uptake of calcium by the "mitochondrial" fraction. (6) In all other tissues in which an effect of cAMP upon mitochondrial calcium exchange has been seen either in intact cells or homogenates, the effect of cAMP is to cause a net shift of calcium out of the mitochondria. (7) In all tissues in which an effect of cAMP upon microsomal calcium metabolism has been demonstrated, the effect of cAMP has been to stimulate calcium uptake by this membrane. The most logical conclusion is that the effect of cAMP upon calcium metabolism in the fly salivary gland is exerted at the level of the inner mitochondrial membrane (see also discussion in Chapter 2).

A recent study by Heslop and Berridge (1980) shows that not only does cAMP regulate Ca^{2+} metabolism in the fly salivary gland, but intracellular Ca^{2+} regulates cAMP metabolism in a complex fashion. Of particular interest is that, following 5HT addition, there is a triphasic change in cAMP concentration in the gland similar to that seen after isoproterenol addition to the rat erythrocyte (see Chapter 4). The initial rise and subsequent fall in cAMP concentration after addition of 5HT to the gland were seen even in glands preincubated in calcium-free media, but the subsequent re-increase in cAMP concentration did not occur in calcium-depleted glands. Addition of Ca^{2+} to the medium at this point induced a triphasic response—an immediate rise followed by a fall within a few minutes, and then a more sustained rise. These data indicate that Ca^{2+} has a complex effect on cAMP metabolism in this tissue which probably involves effects both upon the cyclase and phosphodiesterase and may include effects on the redistribution of calmodulin between membrane-bound and soluble pools as seen in the erythrocyte (see Chapter 4).

In addition to secreting fluid, the fly salivary gland secretes digestive enzymes such as sucrase in response to 5HT. Study of this process reveals certain similarities but also differences between the control of fluid and enzyme secretion (Hansen-Bay, 1978). Enzyme secretion has the following properties: (1) it can be stimulated by 5HT, exogenous cAMP, or A23187; (2) theophylline enhances the rate of 5HT-stimulated enzyme secretion; (3)

removal of calcium from the bathing medium enhances fluid secretion to low but not to high 5HT doses and does not alter the effect of cAMP upon enzyme secretion; and (4) addition of 0.1 mM lanthanum lowers the rate of fluid secretion in a 5HT-stimulated gland but enhances enzyme secretion.

These results have been interpreted to mean that the rate of enzyme secretion is regulated by the intracellular concentrations of both Ca^{2+} and cAMP. However, it would appear that as the intracellular Ca^{2+} concentration increases, the optimal concentration of this ion for mediating enzyme secretion is lower than that for altering anion permeability.

This conclusion raises a second important control characteristic that may have significant implications in the long-term control of cell function in which more than one metabolic process is altered. This characteristic is that different response elements respond optimally to different amplitudes (concentrations) of the same signal. In the case of the fly salivary gland, it is possible to predict that the dual control system employing calcium and cAMP could put out either an enzyme-rich or enzyme-poor solution depending upon the ratios of the two signals. If the same 5HT concentration led to a relatively greater rise in Ca^{2+} than in cAMP, then an enzyme-poor secretion would be manufactured; and if the cAMP rise were relatively greater, then an enzyme-rich saliva would be manufactured. As we shall see, these control characteristics are exploited in the regulation of fluid and enzyme secretion in the mammalian salivary gland (see Chapter 6).

CONCLUSION

In the case of the response of the mammalian renal tubule to PTH and of the fly salivary gland to 5HT, a strong case can be made for the participation of both Ca^{2+} and cAMP as intracellular messengers in the action of these hormones. In each case, the involvement of both limbs of the universal information transfer system is clear. However, even in the case of the fly salivary gland when 5HT regulates fluid and electrolyte secretion, the interplay between Ca^{2+} and cAMP is complex. A full understanding of their relationship in this system as well as many others discussed later will require a greater attention to the time course of change in messenger concentration rather than measurement of these at a single time point.

There are probably other systems in which a similar type of coordinate control of cellular response exists. However, in many mammalian tissues, the relationships between cAMP and Ca^{2+} are more complex. These are discussed in succeeding chapters.

Hierarchical Control

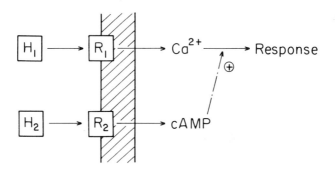

INTRODUCTION

One of the commonest recognizable types of synarchic regulation is one in which the two intercellular messengers, Ca^{2+} and cAMP, regulate cell function in some hierarchical fashion. This type of *hierarchical control* can be achieved by having two receptors, with widely different affinities for the same hormone or stimulus, coupled separately to the Ca^{2+} and cAMP limbs of the information flow pattern, or by having two separate extracellular stimuli coupled separately to the two limbs.

In the first case, at low hormone concentrations, one of the two intracellular messengers would initiate response; and at high concentrations of hormone, the second intracellular messenger would act in some supplementary fashion to enhance cellular response. A specific example of this type is the regulation of steroid hormone production in the zona fasiculata of the mammalian adrenal cortex by the anterior pituitary hormone adrenocorticotropin (ACTH).

In the second type, one extracellular stimulus initiates response by controlling the production of one type of intracellular messenger and thereby provokes a cellular response which can be modified by the action of a second extracellular stimulus regulating the production of the other type of intracellular messenger. An example of this type of regulation in the endocrine system is the control of insulin secretion from the beta cells of the endocrine pancreas by changes in the extracellular concentrations of glucose and glucagon. This example has its counterpart in the nervous system. A prime example is the control of the strength of contraction of a specific muscle in *Aplysia* by cholinergic and serotonergic neurons. Other examples of this type of control operating in neural tissue will also be discussed.

Variations on this type of hierarchical control are seen in mammalian exocrine glands such as parotid and pancreas. These glands secrete both fluid and digestive enzymes. The relative proportion of each constituent can vary considerably. In order to achieve this compositional variability, partially separate means are employed for controlling the fluid production and enzyme secretion. As might be anticipated, the cAMP and Ca^{2+} messenger systems underlie this type of hierarchical control of gland functions. What is particularly striking, however, is that in two different tissues their roles are the obverse. In the parotid, cAMP is the major mediator of enzyme secretion, and Ca^{2+} is the major mediator of fluid secretion. In the exocrine pancreas, Ca^{2+} is the major mediator of enzyme secretion, and cAMP that of fluid secretion. This difference emphasizes, in a most dramatic way, a thesis already alluded to but not overtly formulated. This thesis is that either cAMP or Ca^{2+} can control the activity of a particular type of cellular response element. The validity (or proof) of this statement is inherently obvious from the previous discussion of the control of glycogen metabolism and will become more evident when redundant control is discussed (Chapter 7).

ADRENAL CORTICAL STEROIDOGENESIS—
CORTICOSTEROID PRODUCTION

The mammalian adrenal cortex is divided anatomically into three zones—glomerulosa, fasciculata, and reticulosa. Each produces a different major steroid hormone (aldosterone, a corticosteroid, or androstenedione, respectively). Each responds to different extracellular messengers. The production of aldosterone by glomerulosa cells is controlled by the external K^+ concentration, ACTH, and angiotensin; that of corticosteroids by fasciculata cells is controlled by ACTH; and that of adrenal androgen by the reticulosa cells is controlled by ACTH. In the ensuing discussion, only the regulation of events in fasciculata cells will be considered.

The pathway of corticosteroid production in the adrenal cortex is summarized schematically in Figure 6.1. Several points about this pathway are noteworthy. It is a very complex reaction sequence in which the enzymes participating in this sequence are membrane bound to two separate organelles, the mitochondria (inner membrane) and the endoplasmic reticulum (ER). The initial substrate is stored either as free cholesterol in lipid droplets within the cytosolic compartment of the cell or as cholesterol esters. When steroid hormone production takes place, this cholesterol must be moved to the mitochondria, enter this organelle (matrix space), and undergo metabolic transformation to form an intermediate which leaves the mitochondria. It then undergoes further transformation in the ER and returns to the

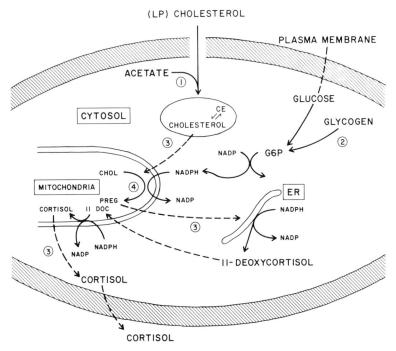

Figure 6.1 Schematic representation of the pathway of steroid hormone biosynthesis in the adrenal cortex. Circled numbers represent intracellular sites of metabolic control: 1 cholesterol synthesis and/or uptake; 2 glycogenolysis; 3 cholesterol transport from cytosol to mitochondria and transport of steroids to cytosol; and 4 conversion of cholesterol to pregnenelone.

mitochondria, where it undergoes its final modification and then leaves this organelle to be secreted by the cell into the extracellular space (Stone and Hechter, 1954; Karaboyas and Koritz, 1965; Simpson and Boyd, 1967; Sulimouici and Boyd, 1968; Wilson and Harding, 1970; Wilson and Harding, 1970; McIntosh et al., 1971; Hall and Koritz, 1965; Hall, 1966; Arthur and Boyd, 1974; Boyd et al., 1975; Dufau et al., 1973).

Although there is evidence that control of steroidogenesis is exerted at several of these steps, there is a general consensus that the major rate-determining step in steroid hormone biosynthesis is the reaction sequence controlling the intramitochondrial conversion of cholesterol to pregnenolone. This conclusion is of considerable interest because, in contrast to the situation in most of the other systems discussed in this monograph, the rise in cytosolic messenger concentration (calcium ion and/or cAMP) leads to a change in function of a response element not in direct contact with the cytosolic compartment of the cell. In the adrenal cortex, these cytosolic messengers apparently activate a system within the inner mitochondrial membrane. The question of how this flow of information takes place is discussed later.

Having indicated that the cholesterol-to-pregnenolone conversion is the important rate-determining step in steroid biosynthesis, it is essential to add that ACTH has multiple simultaneous effects upon adrenal cell function (Garren et al., 1971; Mahaffee et al., 1974). It stimulates corticosteroid production, increases the cAMP content of the gland, enhances calcium uptake into the gland, enhances acetate uptake and cholesterol biosynthesis, increases the conversion of cholesterol esters to cholesterol, increases the breakdown of glycogen, activates the hexose monophosphate shunt, causes a reduction in ascorbic acid content, increases the cGMP content, increases the phosphorylation of a cytosolic protein, increases protein synthesis, and accelerates the rate of transport of cholesterol from cytosol to the side-chain cleavage site within the mitochondria by a mechanism that involves the participation of actin. These multiple effects can all be viewed within the context of our previous discussion (see Chapter 3) concerning the fact that when a hormone excites a cellular response, it usually produces multiple effects on the metabolic processes of the cell in such a fashion as to produce an integrated cellular response. In this example, it not only stimulates hormone synthesis but it provides by several means the precursors—cholesterol and NADPH—necessary for the maintenance of high rates of hormone biosynthesis.

This is another example of the integrative action of a hormone on its target cell. In terms of our discussion, its importance lies in understanding that the intracellular messengers in many cells act simultaneously on several different response elements to initiate and integrate cellular response. However, these are not its only effects. Adrenocorticotropin (ACTH) has, as its name implies, a trophic action of the adrenal gland. In its absence, the adrenal gland atrophies and its capacity to make adrenal steroid falls. Conversely, when there is a chronic excess of ACTH, the gland enlarges greatly, and its capacity to synthesize steroid hormones is markedly increased. These adaptative changes to long-term changes in trophic hormone concentration have time constants of days rather than minutes, as do the immediate responses of the gland to ACTH. As a consequence, the intracellular messengers involved in these long-term responses have not been identified. The present presumption is that they are the same as those involved in controlling the short-term events. In any case, it is important to emphasize that in most of the systems to be discussed, the results to be considered concern the consequences of short-term changes in the strength of extracellular stimuli, but that in the intact organism long-term changes are also common, and these long-term changes have long-term effects on cellular function. The mechanisms by which extracellular stimuli regulate these long-term effects are not known.

Messenger Function of Cyclic AMP

The effect of ACTH on corticosteroid production was historically the second well-defined hormonal system in which cAMP was found to serve as a second messenger (Haynes, 1958; Haynes and Berthet, 1957). The action of ACTH on corticosteroid production was found to fulfill all the Sutherland criteria (Grahame-Smith et al., 1967; Robison et al., 1971; Garren et al., 1971; Hayashi et al., 1979): (1) a hormone-responsive adenylate cyclase was identified in the plasma membrane; (2) a rise in cAMP concentration was seen after ACTH action, and there seemed to be a correlation between the rate of steroid production and the rise in cAMP content; (3) inhibitors of cAMP hydrolysis augmented the effects of submaximal doses of the hormone; (4) addition of large concentrations of exogenous cAMP or dibutyryl cAMP were found to stimulate steroid production; and (5) a cAMP-dependent protein kinase was identified in this tissue. More recently, a correlation has been reported between the extent of activation of this protein kinase and the rate of steroid hormone production (Hayashi et al., 1979; Sala et al., 1979). A very strong case can be made in the adrenal cortex for the original second messenger hypothesis; cAMP is *the* second messenger in hormone action.

Nevertheless, there is considerable evidence that Ca^{2+} also plays a messenger function. When ACTH is added to adrenal tissue incubated in the absence of Ca^{2+}, the rise in cellular cAMP concentration is greatly reduced (Sayers et al., 1972; Haksar and Peron, 1972; Bowyer and Kitabachi, 1974; Lefkowitz et al., 1970). On the other hand, when exogenous cAMP is added to a calcium-depleted gland, there is a stimulation of steroid hormone production, albeit at a reduced rate when compared to a similar gland incubated in the presence of calcium and exposed to the same cAMP concentration (Farese, 1971a,b,c; Bowyer and Kitabachi, 1974). It has been found that ACTH increases calcium uptake into adrenal cells (Leier and Jungmann, 1973), that some of the biochemical responses to ACTH or to cAMP are calcium dependent (Jaanus et al., 1971; Farese, 1971a,b), and that extracellular calcium is essential for steroidogenesis in the intact perfused gland. However, work with various isolated adrenal cell preparation has given variable results concerning the need for calcium so that the importance of calcium as coupling factor or second messenger in ACTH action is ill-defined. Another complication is that when ACTH is added to isolated adrenal tissue or cells incubated in the absence of extracellular Ca^{2+}, there is very little rise in steroid production rate or in cellular cAMP content, indicating that Ca^{2+} is necessary for ACTH-dependent activation of the adenylate cyclase in this tissue. On the other hand, it is evident that Ca^{2+} deficiency influences postreceptor-cyclase events because the ability of exogenous cAMP to stimulate steroidogenesis is significantly reduced in adrenal cells incubated in the absence of extracellular Ca^{2+}. This picture of an apparently clearly defined role of cAMP and an ill-defined role of Ca^{2+} has led most investigators to favor the "cAMP as messenger" concept of ACTH action. However, a major problem exists with this conclusion—the problem of sensitivity of response.

When carefully prepared cells or tissue are incubated with increasing concentrations of ACTH and the cAMP content of the cells and their rates of steroid hormone production plotted as a function of ACTH concentration, there is a dissociation between the effect of ACTH on steroidogenesis from that on cAMP accumulation (Beall and Sayers, 1972; Nakamura et al., 1972; Moyle et al., 1973; Perchellet et al., 1978; Saez et al., 1978; Machie et al., 1972; Bowyer and Kitabachi, 1974; Honn and Chavin, 1977; Sharma et al., 1976; Yanagibashi, 1979; Yanagibashi et al., 1978) (Figure 6.2). The hormone stimulates steroidogenesis at lower concentrations than it stimulates cAMP production. A concentration of hormone sufficient to stimulate hormone production half-maximally has no significant effect upon cAMP production. This discrepancy is even greater with certain ACTH analogs (Moyle et al., 1973). These can induce essentially normal maximal rates of steroid hormone production with little or no change in cAMP content (Figure 6.3). To account for this dissociation, one of three possibilities has been considered: (1) there are spare receptors for ACTH; (2) the cAMP is compartmented within subcellular domains; and (3) a shift of cAMP-dependent protein kinase from nonactive to active form takes place even though there is a barely detectable change in cellular cAMP content.

In the spare receptor hypothesis, it is proposed that occupation of only a few of the surface receptors and consequently activation of only a few adenylate cyclase molecules is sufficient to totally activate the steroidogenesic response. The remainder of the receptors exist more or less as a spare pool, as do all the extra adenylate cyclase molecules. However, this hypothesis does not fit with data in other systems where there is a correlation between receptor occupation, cyclase activation, and cell response.

More difficult to deal with is the hypothesis of protein kinase activation

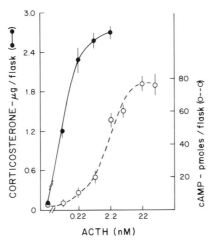

Figure 6.2   Rate of steroid hormone production from (●) and the cAMP content of (○) adrenal glands as function of ACTH concentration. Replotted from Moyle et al. (1973).

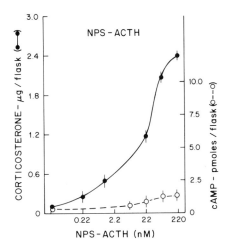

Figure 6.3 Rate of steroid production from (●) and cAMP content of (○) adrenal glands as function of NPS–ACTH. Replotted from Moyle et al. (1973).

without a significant change in cAMP content. The concept here is that the rise in cAMP content is confined to such a small portion of the total intracellular domain that it cannot be detected against the background of basal cAMP content. However, the major contradiction in this hypothesis vis-à-vis the second messenger model is that the generation of a message at the plasma membrane must, if it is to activate an intramitochondrial process, diffuse throughout at least the cytosolic domain. Also, it is exceedingly difficult to test experimentally. On the other hand, its extension—the activation of protein kinase with only a small rise in cAMP—is testable and has been tested. The most thorough study is that recently reported by Sala et al., 1979. The single most significant result from their study is reproduced in Figure 6.4. In this figure, both the amount of receptor-bound cAMP (R·cAMP) and the rate of steroid hormone production are plotted as a function of ACTH concentration. These authors concluded that there is a close correlation between these two parameters. However, this is by no means clear from their data.

A comparison of the data in Figure 6.2 with those in Figure 6.4 shows a similar dissociation between steroidogenesis and cAMP content or receptor-bound cAMP. The results are qualitatively similar. The data presented in Figure 6.4 indicate that the major activation of the protein kinase occurs at ACTH concentrations above those necessary to fully activate steroid hormone production. These new data only reinforce the earlier conclusions concerning a dissociation of the two effects. The logical extension of this line of reasoning is that in spite of considerable circumstantial evidence for the second messenger function of cAMP in ACTH-induced adrenal steroidogenesis, there is a major dilemma. It is a lack of correlation between messenger intensity (concentration) and cellular response. The resolution of this dilemma has been approached in two ways: (1) a search for

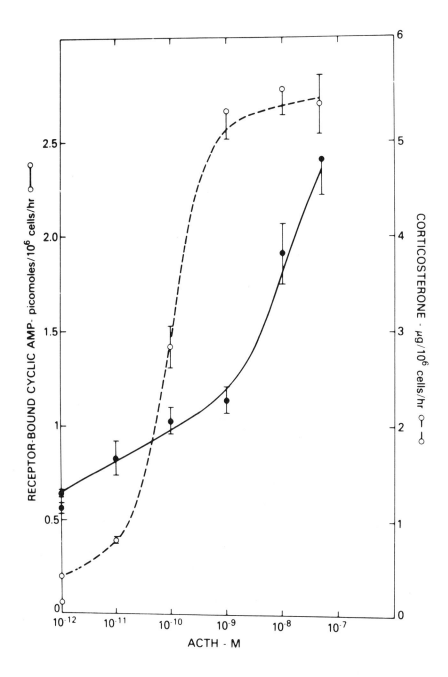

Figure 6.4 Rate of steroid hormone production from (○) and the active protein kinase in (●) the adrenal cortex as function of ACTH concentration in the medium. From Sala et al. (1979), with permission.

other second messengers; and (2) a search for more than one class of ACTH receptors.

ACTH Receptors

Let us first consider the receptor question. In the initial studies, a good correlation between the occupancy of the receptors and the cellular content of cAMP was found but not between receptor occupancy and steroid hormone production. This finding suggested that a second class of receptors might exist with a higher affinity for ACTH than those coupled to the adenylate cyclase. Studies from several different laboratories support the concept of two types of classes of ACTH receptors (Lefkowitz et al., 1971; Wolfsen et al., 1972; McIlhinney and Schulster, 1975; Yanagibashi et al., 1978): a high-affinity low-capacity group ($K_d = 2.6 \times 10^{-10}$ M; $n = 3000$ to 7500 sites per cell) and a low-affinity, high-capacity group ($K_d = 7.1 \times 10^{-9}$; $n = 30,000$ to 58,000) (see Figure 3.5). The latter are thought to be coupled to the adenylate cyclase, the former to some other membrane transducing system giving rise to a different second messenger more closely related to the immediate steroidogenic effect of ACTH.

Messenger Function of Calcium

If we accept the validity of these conclusions, then the question becomes that of identifying this other messenger. Earlier work by Sharma et al. (1976) suggested that this messenger was cGMP. On the other hand, Yanagibashi has presented impressive evidence in support of the involvement of Ca^{2+} as second messenger in ACTH action (Yanagibashi et al., 1978; Yanagibashi, 1979). In studies employing isolated rat adrenal cells, he demonstrated that $ACTH^{1-24}$ at a concentration of 100 pM stimulated Ca^{2+} uptake and steroid hormone production but did not change the cAMP content of these cells. Furthermore, the rate of steroid production and of Ca^{2+} uptake was a function of external Ca^{2+} concentration between concentration of 0.0 and 1.0 mM external Ca^{2+}. There was a direct correlation between steroid production and calcium uptake. In addition, Verapamil blocked both calcium uptake and steroid hormone production.

These data are not yet complete. For example, it would be of interest to correlate ACTH binding to the high-affinity sites, calcium uptake, and steroid hormone production as a function of hormone concentration. On the other hand, these data plus all the previous evidence (Birmingham et al., 1953, 1960; Farese, 1971a,b; Haksor and Peron, 1972; Jaanus et al., 1970) are consistent with a model in which there are two specific ACTH receptors differing in their affinity for the hormone and in the transducing element to which they couple, the high-affinity receptors being coupled to a calcium channel and the low-affinity ones to adenylate cyclase (Figure 6.5). In such a model, low concentrations of hormone regulate hormone production primarily by inducing a rise in cytosolic Ca^{2+} concentration, and higher concentrations of hormone mediate additional intracellular responses by stimulating adenylate cyclase.

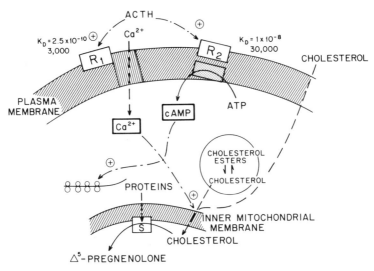

Figure 6.5 Model of ACTH action on the adrenal cortex. See text for discussion.

Additional evidence for a messenger role of calcium in ACTH action comes from the work of Schrey and Rubin (1979). They showed that an early metabolic effect of ACTH upon isolated cat adrenal cells is the stimulation of arachidonic acid incorporation in the 2-position of membrane phosphoinositidylinositol. The effect was dependent upon the presence of Ca^{2+} in the medium and could be reproduced by addition of the calcium ionophore A23187. From other experiments, they concluded that this effect of ACTH was due to a calcium-dependent activation of phospholipase A_2.

Messenger Function of Cyclic GMP

An additional messenger in the adrenal cortex that deserves mention is cGMP. Sharma and associates (Sharma et al., 1976, 1978, 1978; Sharma and Sawhney, 1978; Perchellet et al., 1978; Perchellet et al., 1978; Perchellet and Sharma, 1979) have shown that at low ACTH concentrations which are steroidogenic but do not enhance cAMP concentration, there is a transient rise in cGMP concentration. Thus, a 2.5-fold increase in the concentration of this nucleotide is seen 10 minutes after ACTH addition, but the cGMP concentration is back to control values by 60 minutes even though steroid biosynthesis and secretion continue at a high rate. The secondary fall in cGMP concentration appears to be due to a cGMP-induced activation of a cGMP phosphodiesterase.

The relationship of these changes in cGMP metabolism to those in cellular calcium metabolism is not clear. In other tissues, a soluble (cytosolic) guanylate cyclase is activated by a rise in the Ca^{2+} content of the cell cytosol. Hence, one possibility is that the hormone-stimulated entry of calcium into the cell causes an increase in cGMP by activating guanylate cyclase. If so, then an unresolved question is whether subsequent protein kinase activation and protein phosphorylations are due to cGMP-dependent or calcium-dependent protein kinases. This question requires further evaluation, particularly in the light of the findings of Hayashi et al. (1979) that the increase in cGMP which follows ACTH action is largely, if not entirely, in the extracellular space and not within the cell. The work of Perchellet and Sharma (1979) suggests that cGMP is somehow related to the calcium signaling system. First, in the absence of calcium, ACTH does not cause a rise in the cGMP content of the adrenal cells; and second, the ability of either cGMP or dibutyryl cAMP to stimulate corticosterone production is calcium dependent. These findings support the conclusion that cGMP is intimately related to the calcium signaling system (see Chapter 4).

A similar conclusion has been reached from studies in a variety of other tissues. Nonetheless, at present there is no clear simple or unifying hypothesis that incorporates this conclusion into a general model for the role of cGMP in stimulus–response coupling. In addition, the results obtained by the Sharma group have been obtained largely from studies of the behavior of isolated adrenal carcinoma cells. As such, these cells are clearly abnormal in their growth characteristics, and it is quite possible that other alterations exist such as changes in the nature of the control systems involved in cell response. Thus, the finding that cGMP serves a coupling function in this tissue may reflect the fact that this nucleotide serves a similar role under physiological circumstances, or that its function in this regard is restricted to these particular altered cells.

Messenger Function of Phosphoinositides

The turnover of plasma membrane phosphotidylinositol has been correlated with changes in calcium gating in the plasma membrane of many cells (see Chapter 3). Less attention has been paid to the possible role of polyphosphoinositides (di- and triphosphoinosides—DPI and TPI) in cell function (but see Chapter 3). It is of considerable interest, therefore, that in recent studies Farese and his collaborators (Farese et al., 1979; Farese and Sabir, 1980; Farese et al., 1980a,b) have shown that addition of either ACTH or exogenous cAMP increases the cytosolic concentration of PA, PI, DPI, and TPI (Figure 6.6). The effect appears to be due to an increase in the *de novo* synthesis of PA $\rightarrow$ PI $\rightarrow$ DPI $\rightarrow$ TPI (reactions 1, 3, 4, 5, and 6, Figure 3.9). The effect of either cAMP or ACTH on DPI and TPI synthesis requires the presence of extracellular calcium and is blocked by the prior administration of cycloheximide. Of particular note is the fact that, in contrast to other tissues (Michell and Hawthorne, 1965), the site of synthesis of DPI and TPI in the adrenal is the mitochondria and not the plasma membrane. Using short- and long-acting homologs of ACTH, it was found that the time course of change in DPI and TPI content correlates with the time course of change in steroid hormone synthesis. Furthermore, addition of DPI or TPI but not PI, PA, PC, or PE to isolated adrenal mitochondrial stimulates the conversion of cholesterol to pregnenolone. Also, addition of PI, DPI, or TPI to isolated adrenal tissue increases steroid hormone production, and this effect is not blocked by cycloheximide.

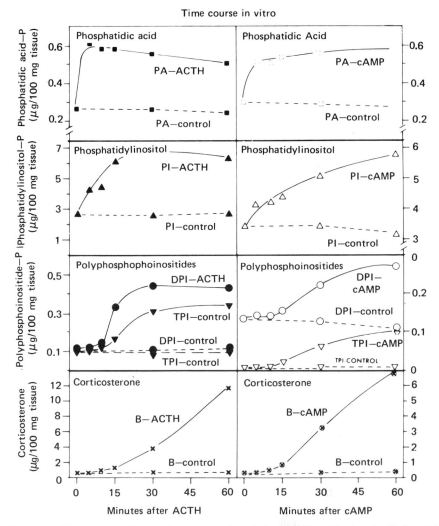

Figure 6.6 Time course of change in concentration of phosphotidic acid, phosphatidylinositol, and polyphosphoinositides (PPI plus TPI) and the rate of corticosteroid production in rat adrenal glands following exposure to ACTH (left) or exogenous cAMP (right). From Farese et al. (1980a), with permission.

These findings have led Farese and colleagues to suggest that DPI and TPI are the proximate regulators of the cholesterol side chain cleavage reaction, the rate-limiting step in steroidogenesis. On the basis of their data, it is possible to suggest that cAMP and/or Ca^{2+} regulate DPI and TPI synthesis at the mitochondrial level and that an increase in these polyphosphoinositides leads to the local activation, within the mitochondria, of side chain cleavage. In this view, mitochondrial reactions regulated by extracellular messengers in the synarchic system are not regulated directly by changes in cAMP or Ca^{2+} within the mitochondrial compartment, but by an effect of cytosolic messengers on DPI and TPI synthesis and the generation thereby of a local messenger which regulates mitochondrial function.

Cytosolic Messengers and Changes in Intramitochondrial Function

As noted above, when ACTH acts upon its target tissue, a number of changes in cellular metabolism ensue. Many of these occur in the cytosolic compartment, for example, increased glycogenolysis and increased hydrolysis of cholesterol esters, or in organelles with direct access to this compartment, for example, increased protein synthesis on ribosomes or steroid hydroxylation in the ER. One specific example is a cytosolic cholesterol ester hydrolase of the adrenal gland which is activated by a cAMP-dependent protein kinase (Boyd et al., 1975). Hence, at least one of the ACTH-regulated steps is in the cell cytosol. Nonetheless, there is general agreement that the major rate-limiting step in steroid hormone synthesis within the mitochondria is the conversion of cholesterol to pregnenolone. This step involves a series of reactions resulting in the cleavage of the cholesterol side chain and is catalyzed by a complex of enzymes involving cytochrome P-450 and located in or on the inner mitochondrial membrane.

Several hypotheses as to the mechanism by which ACTH alters the function of this enzyme complex have been formulated: (1) the second messenger(s) act by increasing the activity of the enzyme system in the mitochondria; (2) they regulate steroidogenesis by controlling the efflux of Δ^2-pregnenolone from the mitochondria; and (3) they act by regulating the supply of cholesterol to the mitochondrial enzyme system (Mahaffee et al., 1974; Bell and Harding, 1974; Boyd et al., 1975; Garren et al., 1965; Mrolek and Hall, 1977a,b). Few data have been developed that support the first two alternatives, but considerable data exist in support of the third.

The data in support of the third hypothesis have come from a variety of studies. First, it has been shown that ACTH activates a cholesterol esterase in the cytosol and that ACTH increases the adrenal content of free cholesterol even though it does not increase hormone production in glands pretreated with cycloheximide (Mahaffee et al., 1974). Second, the hormone increases the uptake of cholesterol into the target cells and the mobilization of cholesterol from cytoplasmic lipid droplets (Boyd et al., 1975). Third, in actively secreting cells, mitochondria are often seen in close proximity to sterol-rich lipid droplets. Additional data in support of this hypothesis have come from two separate studies each of which supplements the data in the other, and each of which will be considered in some detail because of the light they shed on this problem.

The first study was that of Mahaffee et al. (1974). They found that adrenal cortical mitochondria from ACTH-treated hypophysectomized rats produced significantly more Δ^5-pregnenolone than mitochondria isolated from hypophysectomized controls and that this increase in steroid synthesis correlated with an increase in the cholesterol content of the isolated mitochondria. When rats were treated with aminoglutethimide, a drug that blocks the mitochondrial conversion of cholesterol to Δ^5-pregnenolone, and then given ACTH, the accumulation of cholesterol in subsequently isolated mitochondria was greater than in those given ACTH alone.

The second study is that of Hall et al. (1979). In previous work, Mrolets and Hall (1977a,b) had shown that cytochalasin B blocked the steroidogenic effect of ACTH as well as its stimulatory effect of causing a shift of cholesterol from lipid dropets (cytosol) to mitochondria. From these data, they proposed that microfilaments played a critical role in the control of steroidogenesis. To test this hypothesis more directly, Hall et al. (1979) entrapped antiactin antibody (actin is a major protein component of microfilaments) in liposomes which were in turn incubated with Y-1 mouse adrenal tumor cells for 1 hour. During this time, liposomes fused with cell membrane and delivered the antiactin antibody to the cell interior. Upon addition of either ACTH or dibutyryl cAMP, the usual increase in steroid hormone production, either by the intact cells or the mitochondria isolated from them, was completely blocked, as was the accumulation of cholesterol from animals given both ACTH and aminoglutethimide. If the antibody was combined with excess actin before being incorporated into the liposomes, there was no inhibition. The authors concluded that ACTH stimulates steroidogenesis by increasing the transport of cholesterol to the mitochondrial side chain cleavage enzyme by a mechanism which involves actin.

These studies make an extremely strong case for the fact that a major effect of ACTH upon the steroidogenic pathway is that of increasing the supply of available substrate, cholesterol, to the side chain cleavage system in the mitochondria. This appears to involve several steps including the stimulation of uptake of cholesterol from the plasma, the shift of cholesterol from cytosol to mitochondria, and the translocation of the cholesterol across the inner mitochondrial membrane. All of these are events that can be influenced by a cytosolic messenger (Figure 6.6).

REGULATION OF INSULIN SECRETION

The control of insulin secretion from the beta cells of the Islets of Langerhans is achieved by a variation of the type of hierarchical control seen in the adrenal cortex (Floyd, 1966; Curry et al., 1968; Grodsky et al., 1967; Milner and Hales, 1968; Matthews, 1970, 1975, 1979; Dean and Matthews, 1970a,b; Dean and Matthews, 1972; Grill and Cerasi, 1973; Grodsky, 1970, 1972; Grodsky and Bennett, 1966; Hales and Milner, 1968; Montague and Cook, 1971; Montague and Howell, 1973; Sharp et al., 1975; Montague et al., 1976; Unger et al., 1967; Howell et al., 1975; Charles et al., 1975; Gerich et al., 1976; Lambert, 1976; Montague, 1977; Matschinsky and Ellerman, 1973; Matschinsky et al., 1971; Hellman, 1975a,b; Henquin and Lambert, 1974, 1975; Kuo et al., 1973; Malaisse et al., 1973, 1974, 1976, 1977, 1978, 1979a,b; Malaisse-Lagae and Malaisse, 1971; Malaisse, 1973; Matthews and

Sakamoto, 1975; Malaisse, Sener, et al., 1978, 1979; Malaisse, Boschero, et al., 1978; Taljedal, 1978; Grill and Cerasi, 1974; Sugden et al., 1979; Valverde et al., 1979a,b; Karl et al., 1975; Brisson et al., 1972, 1973). In this variation, separate extracellular messengers control the two separate intracellular signaling systems, and these two intracellular signals operate in a strict hierarchical sense. In addition, the calcium signal is generated by a change in the concentration of some intracellular metabolite rather than being directly coupled to a surface receptor for the extracellular messenger.

The control of insulin secretion has been more thoroughly studied than the control of secretion of any other peptide hormone. Two types of control have been recognized: short-term minute-to-minute control determined by the fluctuations in the concentrations of extracellular metabolites and hormones; and long-term changes determined by dietary or physiological status of the organism.

Studies of the short-term control have defined three types of extracellular signals (Table 6.1). The first have been called primary signals of initiators, and the second, secondary signals or potentiators of insulin secretion. The distinction between primary and secondary stimulators is that none of the secondary stimulators will induce insulin release from islets incubated or perfused with a solution lacking a primary stimulator. In most instances this has meant islets incubated in the absence of glucose. Thus, glucagon en-

Table 6.1   Regulators of Insulin Secretion

1. Primary signals or initiators
   a. Glucose
   b. Mannose
   c. Glyceraldehyde
   d. Leucine
   e. Arginine
   f. Sulfanylurea
2. Secondary signals or potentiators
   a. Glucagon
   b. Secretion
   c. ACTH
   d. Pancreozymin
   e. Theophylline
   f. Cholera toxin
3. Inhibitors
   a. Verapamil
   b. Imidazole
   c. Epinephrine
   d. Mannoheptulose
   e. Iodoacetamide
   f. Menadione
   g. Somatostatin
   h. Phenothiazines

hances the rate of insulin secretion at any fixed, submaximal concentration of extracellular glucose but does not stimulate insulin release if extracellular glucose is absent. This physiological distinction between initiators and potentiators of insulin release has its biochemical counterpart. Initiators alter primarily cellular calcium metabolism. Potentiators alter primarily cAMP metabolism.

In addition to these two classes of stimulators, a group of agents have been identified which act as inhibitors of insulin secretion (Table 6.1). These agents can be shown to alter the metabolism of either calcium, cAMP, or glucose or to change the redox state of the cell membrane.

Glucose—Prototypical Initiator

In the absence of extracellular glucose, the intact beta cell releases little insulin. As the glucose concentration is raised from 2.0 to 20.0 mM, there is a dose-dependent increase in insulin secretion (Figure 6.7). The steepest portion of this dose–response curve is between 4 and 10 mM glucose, which is the normal physiological range of plasma glucose concentration. Although there are reports that under some circumstances, glucose addition to isolated or perfused islets causes an increase in intracellular cAMP concentration, the general consensus is that at physiological concentrations of glucose and extracellular Ca^{2+}, there is a variable increase in cAMP content of the islet cells. The major effect of physiological concentrations of glucose upon plasma membrane function is to alter the fluxes of certain ions across this membrane. This effect induces an increase in Ca^{2+} influx and a decrease in both K$^+$ and Ca^{2+} efflux but has little effect on Na$^+$ fluxes. These changes in ion fluxes are the basis of a glucose-induced change in membrane potential and appear to be the basis for a glucose-induced increase in cytosolic calcium ion concentration and, thus, for calcium-dependent insulin release.

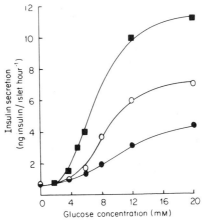

Figure 6.7 Insulin secretion as function of glucose concentration in islet cells of normal sensitivity (○), reduced sensitivity induced by starvation (●), and sensitivity heightened by feeding (■). From Montague (1975), with permission.

It is worth considering these effects of glucose on plasma membrane function in some detail because it represents a prime example of ionic coupling in an endocrine system.

Electrical Events in Stimulus–Response Coupling

The studies of the glucose-induced changes in the electrical activity of the plasma membrane of the islet cell raise the problem of the distinction between excitable and nonexcitable cells as discussed previously (see Chapter 1). The islet cell is normally stimulated by chemical stimuli brought to it by the blood stream. However, it can and is also stimulated by parasympathetic and inhibited by sympathetic nerve stimuli. For the sake of the present discussion, we confine our attention to the physiologically most important chemical stimulus, glucose, and consider specifically whether the response of the beta cell to this stimulus fits the restricted definition of excitability, that is, does it display regenerative ion currents giving rise to action potentials?

The elegant studies of Matthews and colleagues (Dean and Matthews, 1970a,b, 1972; Matthews, 1970, 1975, 1979) have demonstrated that the addition of glucose to pancreatic islet cells causes a slight depolarization of the membrane, but also a train of spike or action potentials (Figure 6.8). There is a dose-dependent increase in the number of cells exhibiting action potentials as the glucose concentration is raised from 3 to 12 mM, that is, in the same range over which there is a glucose-dependent increase in insulin release. This means that as the strength of the extracellular stimulus increases, both the rate of response of already active cells increases and more cells become responsive. This dual phenomenon of recruitment of new units and increased activity of already responding units is the counterpart of what occurs in stimulation of a peripheral or autonomic nerve, that is, the control characteristics are similar. In fact, a valid generalization in discussing how an increasing strength of stimulus increases organ or cellular response is that it does so either by increasing the rate of activity of already operative units or by increasing the number of such units.

An exploration of the characteristics of the current pulses induced by glucose has shown that (1) the current pulses are enhanced by a hyperpolarizing current induced by intracellular current injection and reduced by depolarizing current; (2) current injection evokes a spike potential in the absence of glucose, but not in the absence of extracellular calcium (i.e., these cells are electrically excitable); (3) low extracellular calcium or addition of D600 (a calcium channel blocker) abolishes the spike potentials; (4) low extracellular Na$^+$ concentration or tetrodotoxin (a sodium channel blocker) enhances the spike potentials; and (5) inhibitors of glucose metabolism prevent glucose-induced action potentials. These data show that beta cells exhibit most of the characteristics of an excitable tissue such as peripheral nerve.

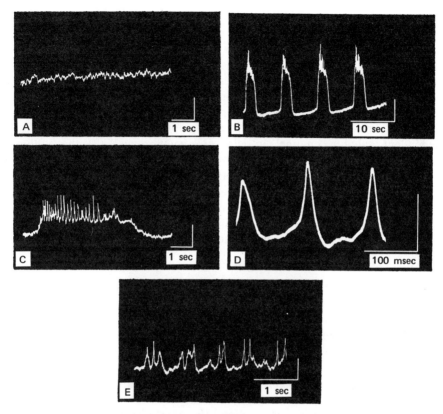

Figure 6.8 Action potentials induced in islet cells by addition of D-glucose. A, Control; B, rhythmic bursts of action potentials induced by addition of 16.6 mM glucose; C, record of a single burst of potentials on a 1-second time scale; D, record showing shape of individual action potentials on time scale of 100 ms; E, action potentials with 27.7 mM glucose. From Dean and Matthews (1970) with permission.

From his data, Matthews (1975) concluded that the spike potentials were primarily calcium currents. He proposed a model to account for these currents and their regenerative nature. In this model, the primary effect of glucose (exerted via one of its metabolites—see below) is to decrease K^+ efflux leading to a depolarization of the plasma membrane sufficient to lower the threshold of a voltage-dependent calcium ion channel and lead thereby to an increase in calcium entry into the cell. The rise in calcium ion content on the inside surface of the cell membrane would in turn increase the K^+ permeability of the plasma membrane and act to repolarize the membrane and close the voltage-dependent calcium channel.

Studies by a number of other investigators provide considerable direct support for this hypothesis (Sehlin and Taljedal, 1975; Malaisse, Boschero et al., 1978; Valverde et al., 1979; Henquin and Lambert, 1975; Atwater et al., 1978; Henquin, 1978a,b; 1980). A direct inhibitory effect of glucose upon

Rb^+ and/or K^+ efflux from isolated islets has been found (Henquin, 1978a,b; Sehlin and Taljedal, 1975). A calcium-dependent increase in efflux of K^+ has also been demonstrated similar to that produced by a rise in cytosolic $[Ca^{2+}]$ in the red cell, many nerve cells, and a variety of exocrine cells (Meech, 1976, 1978; Krnjevic, 1974). Furthermore, Donatsch et al. (1977) have shown that if membrane depolarization is produced by a veratridine-induced increase in Na^+ influx, a voltage-dependent increase in calcium influx is observed. These data all lead to the conclusion that (1) there is a voltage-dependent calcium channel in islet cell membranes; (2) the voltage-dependent calcium channel is opened when the external glucose concentration is increased; (3) the primary effect of glucose which mediates this opening is a glucose-dependent decrease in K^+ efflux; and (4) the regenerative spike potentials seen after glucose addition depend upon the sequential closing of the K^+ channel in the plasma membrane by glucose and upon the subsequent opening of this (or another K^+) channel by Ca^{2+}.

Calcium as Second Messenger

Having established that the islet cells display glucose-induced, regenerative calcium current, two questions arise. The first is whether calcium serves to couple stimulus to response, and the second is the mechanism by which glucose mediates this effect upon plasma membrane function.

Considerable data were obtained by a variety of experimental techniques and under a host of different experimental conditions all of which support the concept that the primary signal generated when glucose acts upon the beta cell is a rise in the Ca^{2+} content of the cell cytosol or at least some domain of this cellular compartment (Lambert, 1976; Montague, 1977; Malaisse et al., 1978). A summary of the salient facts supporting this conclusion is shown in Table 6.2.

Based upon the fact that calcium is the main ion-carrying current during the glucose-induced spike potentials, Matthews (1975) was able to calculate the amount of calcium entering the cell per each spike. This figure was estimated to be 0.1 pmol/cm² cell surface, which, based on certain assumptions, translates into a change in Ca^{2+} concentration just beneath the cell surface of $3.3 \mu M$ per spike potential. This value represents a change in Ca^{2+} concentration sufficient to bring about an activation of known calcium-mediated processes regulated by the calcium receptor protein calmodulin. This protein has been found in high concentrations (20 to $50 \mu M$) in islet cells (Sugden et al., 1979; Valverde et al., 1979).

In addition to these calculations from electrophysiological data, studies of islet cell calcium metabolism have been carried out using isotopic techniques. Glucose addition to incubated islets has two effects upon cellular calcium exchange. It stimulates net calcium accumulation and inhibits calcium efflux. The magnitude of the calcium accumulation is a function of both the glucose and external Ca^{2+} concentration. Furthermore, the extent of calcium accumulation correlates with the magnitude of the insulin released.

Table 6.2   Evidence That Calcium Ion Is Primary Messenger in Glucose-Induced Insulin Release

1. Glucose effect depends upon external calcium
2. At a fixed external glucose concentration, the rate of insulin secretion is a function of the external calcium concentration
3. Glucose stimulates calcium uptake into and calcium efflux from beta cells
4. Glucose induces membrane depolarization and regenerative calcium currents across beta cell plasma membrane
5. There is a correlation between calcium current intensity and rate of insulin release
6. Depolarization by high external K^+ induces Ca^{2+} uptake and insulin release
7. Depolarization by veratridine and Na^+ induces Ca^{2+} uptake and insulin release
8. Calcium ionophore A23187 stimulates Ca^{2+} uptake and insulin release
9. Agents that block the voltage-dependent calcium channel (Verapamil, D-600, cobalt) block calcium uptake and insulin release
10. When physiological concentrations of extracellular calcium and glucose are employed, glucose does not cause an increase in the cAMP content of the beta cell
11. There is a high concentration of the calcium receptor protein calmodulin in beta cells
12. Under pharmacological conditions, insulin secretion can be stimulated without an evident increase in the uptake of calcium by the beta cell; but in all of these conditions, there is evidence for a mobilization of calcium from an intracellular pool
13. The amount of calcium normally taken up by the glucose-stimulated cell is sufficient to increase the Ca^{2+} content of the cytosol into the calcium control range
14. Other primary initiators of insulin secretion stimulate calcium uptake
15. Close structural analogs of glucose that do not stimulate insulin release do not stimulate calcium currents or uptake
16. After glucose addition, there is a rapid fall in the amount of [2-³H]myoinositol recovered from islet phosphoinositol in the prelabeled gland

These data are consistent with and seem to support the data of Matthews (1975) in indicating a glucose-dependent stimulation of calcium uptake by these cells. However, it is difficult to interpret these data in such a straightforward manner because net accumulation of radiocalcium reflects possible changes in both rate of influx into and efflux from the cell, as well as a possible change in the size of exchangeable calcium pools. There is an additional problem in relating total calcium uptake data to cell response because a significant amount of the calcium accumulated during long-term incubations is taken up by the insulin-containing secretory vesicles. All present evidence indicates that the calcium in this pool is not in rapid exchange with that in other subcellular pools. Nonetheless, it represents 75 to 80% of the total calcium accumulated during a long-term incubation.

Studies of the effect of glucose on calcium uptake at early time points after glucose addition are consistent with a glucose-dependent stimulation of calcium entry. Another type of data also supports this conclusion. These data come from studies of the effect of the calcium channel blockers verapamil, D-600 (methoxyverapamil), and cobalt on insulin release and calcium uptake. Verapamil, D-600, and cobalt block the electrical excitability (i.e., glucose-induced spike potentials), calcium accumulation, and insulin release (Devis et al., 1975; Malaisse et al., 1976, 1977; Henquin and Lambert, 1975). Their inhibitory actions can be reversed by an increase in extracellular Ca^{2+} concentration. Conversely, addition of the calcium ionophore A23187 leads to a non-glucose-dependent influx of calcium into the islet cell and a calcium-dependent release of insulin (Karl et al., 1975; Hellman, 1975a,b; Ashby and Speake, 1975). Finally, as noted above (Table 6.2), the phenothiazines have been shown to inhibit insulin release, and Weiss has shown that a major site of action of this class of compounds is inhibition of calmodulin-mediated activities.

Taken *in toto,* these data provide strong support for the concept that calcium is the second messenger in the action of glucose upon the beta cell of the Islets of Langerhans. However, two points of controversy still exist. The first is that in some experiments, a glucose-induced rise in the cAMP content of the islets has been seen when physiological concentrations of extracellular glucose were employed (Charles et al., 1975). The second is that recent data has been interpreted as indicating glucose may not actually induce a change in plasma membrane calcium permeability, but only the release of calcium from a membrane-bound pool (Malaisse et al., 1978).

The first point at issue is whether or not under usual physiological circumstances the concentration of cAMP increases in islets after exposure to physiological concentrations of glucose. The answer is that it does not usually occur, but under some conditions it is seen (Grill and Cerasi, 1974; Charles et al., 1975). This rise depends upon the presence of extracellular Ca^{2+}, and a similar calcium-dependent rise in cAMP content is seen after addition of the ionophore A23187 to isolated islets (Karl et al., 1975). The explanation of this rise is to be found in the fact that calcium stimulates a calmodulin-mediated activation of a particulate adenylate cyclase from the pancreatic islets (Velverde et al., 1979). A logical interpretation of all the observations is that under normal circumstances a small rise in glucose concentration induces a rise in the cytosolic calcium concentration sufficient to activate insulin secretion, but not sufficient to activate adenylate cyclase. If the glucose concentration rises higher, then the rise in cytosolic calcium concentration is sufficient to activate both insulin secretion and adenylate cyclase. If this is a correct interpretation of these data, then two calcium–calmodulin-regulated response elements, both at or near the plasma membrane of the cell and therefore presumably responsive to change in the Ca^{2+} concentration in the same domain within the cell, show a differential sensitivity to activation by changes in Ca^{2+} concentration within this domain.

The second question about the role of calcium in stimulus–response coupling is that raised by Hellman (1975) and Täljedal (1978). They demonstrated that glucose stimulates calcium uptake (as measured by accumulation of radioactive calcium from the medium) into two pools that are distinguishable by subsequent washing of the islets in solutions containing lanthanum. The two pools were defined as the lanthanum-displaceable and nondisplaceable pools. The identity of the latter was considered to be the insulin-containing secretory vesicles. They found that glucose stimulated the accumulation of calcium into both pools and concluded that only the calcium in the displaceable pool is involved in the initial signaling of insulin secretion. These data are consistent with the previous data of others as discussed above. However, Hellman et al. (1976) conclude that since the half-time of exchange of this displaceable pool is of the order of 2 minutes, this pool is not in the cell cytosol but in the plasma membrane. However, Hellman et al. (1976) ignore the considerable physiological data, particularly the studies of Dean and Matthews (1970a,b) in which direct evidence for a change in the calcium permeability of the plasma membrane has been demonstrated (see also Täljedal, 1978).

The final point concerning the relationship between glucose and calcium metabolism in the islet cell relates to the effect of glucose on calcium efflux. When glucose is added to islets prelabeled with radioactive calcium, a biphasic response ensues (Figure 6.9): first a decrease in calcium efflux is seen, followed by a marked increase. However, if insulin secretion is blocked by prior addition of Verapamil, then only the first phase of the response is seen. These data have been interpreted to mean (Malaisse et al., 1978) that the initial decrease in calcium efflux is due to a direct inhibitory action of glucose on calcium efflux and that the subsequent rise in efflux is due to the release of calcium from secretory vesicles during the process of insulin secretion.

Although the above evidence supports the view that glucose initiates insulin release by a stimulation of calcium entry and an inhibition of calcium release across the plasma membrane, there are recent data (Wollheim et al., 1978; Kikuchi et al., 1979) that have raised questions above this simple interpretation. In order to discuss these experiments, it is necessary to reemphasize the fact that the time course of insulin release in response to a sudden elevation in glucose concentration is biphasic (Figure 6.10). Upon initial application of glucose, there is an initial sharp and transient rise in insulin release followed by a fall in rate back toward baseline, and then a slower, progressive, and sustained increase in insulin secretion. The initial increase is seen within 2 to 3 minutes and reaches a peak in 4 to 5 minutes. Likewise, within 1 to 2 minutes of the application of glucose, there is an initiation of action potentials and membrane depolarization (Matthews, 1975). Given this close temporal relationship between the electrical events in the plasma membrane and the time course of insulin release, it is logical to assume that there is some cause-and-effect relationship between them. However, recent experiments employing either Verapamil or low-calcium perfusates appear to argue against this concept. If islets are first exposed to

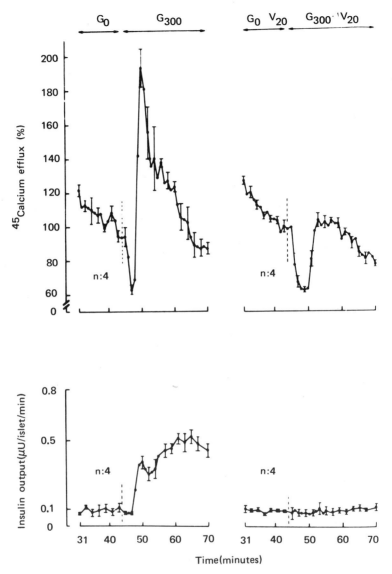

Figure 6.9 Time course of change in insulin secretion (bottom) and in efflux of radiocalcium from prelabeled islets as a function of time before and during glucose perfusion (16.7 mM). On the left, responses from normal islets; on right, the responses in the presence of verapamil (0.02 mM). From Malaisse et al. (1978), with permission.

Verapamil in concentrations sufficient to block glucose-stimulated calcium uptake and then exposed to a high extracellular glucose concentration, the initial or first peak of insulin release occurs but the second is nearly completely abolished (Wolheim et al., 1978). From these results, the authors concluded that the first phase of insulin release depends upon the mobilization of calcium from an internal source.

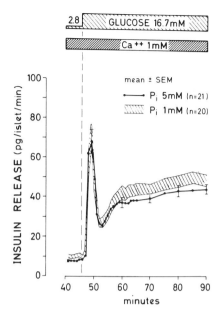

Figure 6.10 Biphasic pattern of insulin release with time from pancreatic islets exposed to glucose. From Kikuchi et al. (1979), with permission.

Employing a different protocol, Kikuchi et al. (1979) came to a similar conclusion. They pre-perfused islets with phosphate which, as shown by Borle (1972), increases the total intracellular calcium content of both the presumptive cytosolic and mitochondrial pools. When the fluid perfusing such "calcium-loaded" islets and control islets was suddenly changed from one containing normal calcium and low glucose to one containing low calcium and high glucose, the initial peak of insulin release was higher in the "calcium-loaded" cells than in the control ones, and the second phase of release was suppressed in both, although more so in the control than in the "calcium-loaded" cells. These data were taken as a further indication that the initial peak of insulin secretion depended upon an intracellular pool of calcium.

There are several difficulties with these conclusions. First, the authors of the first study ignore the fact that Verapamil blocks the voltage-dependent calcium channel in the islet cell membrane but not the Na^+ channel, which is also activated by glucose and through which some Ca^{2+} enters the cell (Donatsch et al., 1977). This small amount of calcium can probably not be measured using $^{45}Ca^{2+}$ uptake measurements because of the rapid exchangeability of the subsurface cytosolic calcium pool. Second, Malaisse et al. (1978) have shown that the addition of glucose to Verapamil-treated islets leads to a transient but significant decrease in the efflux of calcium from these islets. This effect alone may be sufficient to raise the Ca^{2+} concentration just beneath the surface of the plasma membrane sufficiently to induce secretion. Third, if in fact the calcium for first-phase secretion is mobilized from an intracellular pool, that is, a pool separate from the plasma membrane, then one is faced with the additional problem of identifying the signal generated by glucose or one of its metabolites interacting with the plasma membrane which triggers the release of calcium from this pool. Fourth, if one considers a somewhat analogous situation studied by Putney (1979), namely the first messenger-induced change in the plasma membrane permeability to K^+ in the parotid gland, then an alternative explanation of the insulin release data is possible. Putney showed that the change in K^+ permeability by any of three extracellular messengers was Ca^{2+} dependent and biphasic. The first phase but not the second was seen even if the extracellular Ca^{2+} concentration was reduced. However, the first phase was transient and, once evoked in a particular tissue, could not be reinvoked by washing out the extracellular messenger and then reapplying it unless the tissue was reexposed to extracellular calcium.

From these results, Putney concluded that the pool of calcium responsible for the initial phase of the K^+ permeability change was a plasma membrane-bound pool that, once released, could not be replenished without the reexposure of the cell to extracellular calcium. It is quite likely that a similar situation prevails in the case of the islet cell membrane. If so, one would predict that if one exposed Verapamil-treated islets to 16.7 mM glucose for 6 to 8 minutes and then washed away the glucose and repeated the exposure, the first phase of insulin release in response to the second exposure of glucose would be greatly reduced or abolished. Fifth, the studies with the low-calcium media are complicated by an additional problem. It is well known that when the extracellular Ca^{2+} concentration is reduced, there is an increase in the Na^+ permeability of the plasma membrane. Given this fact plus the evidence of Donatsch et al. (1977) that glucose addition alters the Na^+ channel in the islet cell membrane and that a large Na^+ influx can cause a mobilization of calcium from an internal pool, it may well be that the mechanism of insulin release under this nonphysiological circumstance involves a different calcium pool than that participating in the physiological circumstance.

Mechanism of Glucose Action

The mechanism by which glucose induces its effect is still a matter of controversy. On the one hand, it has been proposed that glucose interacts directly with a surface receptor to initiate calcium entry (Pace and Price, 1972; Gerich et al., 1976). On the other hand, it has been proposed that it first enters the cell and undergoes metabolic transformation before exerting its effects (Ashcroft et al., 1973; Ammon and Verspohl, 1976; Zawalich et al., 1977; Malaisse, Hutton, et al., 1979; Sener and Malaisse, 1979; Sener et al., 1978; Malaisse, Sener, et al., 1978; Malaisse, Hutton, et al., 1978). Most recent evidence supports the concept that glucose mediates its effect indirectly.

The evidence in favor of glucose undergoing metabolic transformation is considerable, and this evidence suggests that the signal for insulin release is generated by a metabolite of glucose at or below the triosephosphate level in the glycolytic sequence (Figure 6.11). This evidence is as follows: (1) changes in the rate of glucose oxidation, lactate production, and glucose-6-phosphate concentration show the same dependence on glucose as does insulin release. (2) There is a correlation between rate of hexose utilization by islets and rate of insulin release (Zawalich et al., 1977). (3) When secretion is inhibited by diazoxide or epinephrine, the metabolites of glucose above the phosphoglyceraldehyde dehydrogenase step accumulate. (4) At a concentration of 0.1 mM iodoacetate, an inhibitor of GAPDH, blocks glucose-induced insulin release. (5) Glyceraldehyde initiates insulin release. (6) The effect of glyceraldehyde is blocked by epinephrine or the absence of external Ca^{2+}, and glyceraldehyde stimulates calcium uptake by islet tissue. (7) Menadione and other agents that alter the NADH/NAD ratio block insulin secretion induced by ionophore.

When the menadione concentration is increased in the presence of a fixed glucose concentration (Malaisse, Hutton, et al., 1978), there is a parallel decrease in the amount of oxidized pyridine nucleotide, in the rate of insulin secretion, in the rate of rubidium efflux (a measure of K^+ efflux), and in calcium uptake. These effects of menadione were seen with concentrations that did not alter the rate of the glucose utilization, lactate production, or ATP content of the islet. Menadione increased the flux through the pentose shunt pathway and decreased the cellular content of both NADH and NADPH.

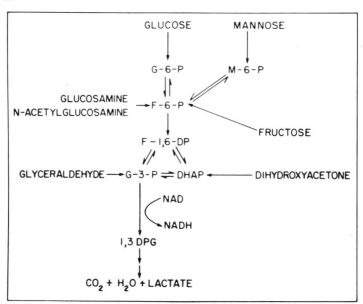

Figure 6.11 The pathways of glucose, mannose, and glucosamine metabolism in the β cell of the pancreas.

Similar results have been found using other agents, for example, NH_4^+, which decrease the concentration of NADH and NADPH. They also inhibit insulin release (Sener, Hutton, et al., 1978). Also, there are circumstances in which insulin secretion can be stimulated in the absence of exogenous nutrients and extracellular calcium. When islets are incubated in calcium-containing buffers containing barium together with theophylline, a release of insulin is seen in the absence of extracellular glucose (Hales and Milner, 1968; Somers et al., 1976; Sener and Malaisse, 1979). Under these conditions, NADH and NADPH concentrations fall. Hence, simply a fall in their concentrations does not inhibit insulin release. In islets treated like this, the addition of glucose causes an augmentation of insulin secretion. This increase in insulin secretion is associated with a dose-related increase in NAD(P)H concentration.

One additional aspect of the mechanism of glucose action is the relationship of glucose-induced calcium entry to glucose-induced alterations in the metabolism of phosphatidylinositol. Clements and Rhoten (1976) have shown that when rat islets are incubated with [2-^{3}H]myoinositol, this compound is rapidly incorporated into phosphatidylinositol. Incubation of these prelabeled islets with sugars, which stimulate insulin release, for example, glucose or mannose, leads to a release of radioactivity from the phosphoinositol pool. Addition of hexoses that do not stimulate insulin release, for example, D-galactose, have no effect upon inositol turnover. In view of the data in other systems (Mitchell, 1975), an attractive possibility is that the PI turnover is involved in the calcium gating. If so, this would represent a situation in which a voltage-dependent calcium gate is coupled to PI metabolism just as are receptor-operated (non-voltage-dependent) calcium channels in other tissues.

Glucagon—Prototypical Potentiator

In contrast to glucose, glucagon alone does not stimulate insulin release, but its addition potentiates the action of a given concentration of glucose. A similar effect is found with phosphodiesterase inhibitors and with secretin, pancreozymin, ACTH, and β-adrenergic agonists. All of these agents cause a rise in the cAMP content of the beta cell (Montague, 1977). Conversely, the drug imadazole, which stimulates phosphodiesterase, causes a fall in cAMP content and a decrease in the rate of glucose-induced insulin release. These results show that in the beta cell, the calcium and cAMP signals are controlled, in part, by different extracellular messengers acting through different surface receptors. Furthermore, the two intracellular signals operate in a hierarchial and complementary fashion (Figure 6.12).

In augmenting the calcium signal, cAMP may act in several ways. It induces the mobilization of calcium from, or blocks the uptake of calcium into, an intracellular pool (Brisson et al., 1972), possibly the mitochondrial pool (Howell et al., 1973, 1975; Sehlin, 1976; Sugden and Ashcroft, 1978;

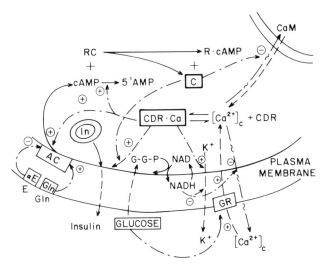

Figure 6.12 Model of the regulation of insulin secretion from beta cells by glucose and other extracellular messengers. A rise in extracellular glucose leads to an increase in islet cell glucose metabolism. This has the consequence of altering the NAD/NADH ratio. A reduction of NAD leads to a decrease in K^+ efflux, which leads to a membrane depolarization opening a voltage-dependent calcium channel in the membrane. This leads to an increase in Ca^{2+} influx into the cell. The increased cytosolic Ca^{2+} associates with calmodulin (CDR) and exerts three effects: it initiates insulin (In) secretion, stimulates K^+ efflux thereby repolarizing the membrane; and, when in sufficient concentration, activates adenylate cyclase (Ac). This enzyme, adenylate cyclase, is also activated by promotors of insulin release such as glucagon (Gln) and inhibited by α-adrenergic agents such as epinephrine (E). A rise in intracellular cAMP has at least two effects: it causes the mobilization of calcium from an intracellular pool and it enhances the effect of calcium CDR on insulin secretion.

Hahn et al., 1979, 1980). In considering the consequences of this effect, it is worth contrasting the situation in the beta cell with that in the fly salivary gland (see Chapter 5). In the latter case, the initial calcium signal is generated at the basolateral cell membrane but acts on the luminal membrane to alter Cl^- permeability. In that case, a rise in cytosolic cAMP was also found to mobilize calcium from an intracellular (mitochondrial) pool, and this was seen as an essential condition for the transmission of the calcium signal from one cell surface to the other in this polar cell. In the case of the pancreatic beta cell, the site of calcium entry across the plasma membrane and its site of action in inducing exocytosis just beneath that membrane do not require the transcellular propagation of the calcium message, hence under some conditions secretion is stimulated by an influx of calcium without an associated rise in cAMP. However, a rise in the cAMP content leads to a mobilization of intracellular calcium into the cytosol, which has the effect of prolonging the calcium signal in both the temporal and spacial domains (Figure 6.12).

In this view, the major effect of cAMP on insulin release is mediated indirectly through an effect on cellular calcium metabolism. It is probable that cAMP also modifies the sensitivity of response elements to the calcium signal and/or alters the response of the plasma membrane calcium channel to a given change in extracellular glucose concentration. At the moment, there is no direct evidence for the first of these suggestions, but this may be due largely to the fact that the final calcium response element(s) regulating secretion has yet to be identified. On the other hand, there are some data that suggest that cAMP may modify the glucose-induced change in plasma membrane function. Before discussing this evidence, it is necessary to consider another class of compounds that influence insulin release—those that inhibit it.

Epinephrine—Prototypical Inhibitor

As noted in Table 6.1, a variety of chemically different compounds can block insulin release. Some, such as Verapamil, do so by blocking calcium entry into the beta cell; others, such as imadazole, do so by lowering cAMP concentrations, and still others, such as mannoheptulose and iodoacetamide, do so by blocking glucose metabolism. However, the most carefully studied natural hormonal agent known to inhibit insulin release is epinephrine. This inhibitory action is mediated through interaction of the catecholamine with an α-receptor upon the cell surface. A major consequence of this catecholamine–receptor interaction is an inhibition of the adenylate cyclase activity with a resultant fall in the intracellular cAMP concentration (Montague, 1977). This fall is associated with a decrease in rate of insulin secretion.

Data discussed above show that a rise in cAMP concentration causes a mobilization of intracellular calcium which, by extending both the temporal and spacial domains of calcium, can account for the enhanced rate of insulin secretion. If this were the sole effect of cAMP, then a fall in the cAMP content of islets should restrict the domains of calcium by allowing for its more rapid uptake into intracellular storage sites. If so, one would not expect to see a significant change in the immediate effects of glucose upon K^+ and Ca^{2+} transport in the cell membrane. However, this is not the case. Prior addition of epinephrine in a dose sufficient to inhibit glucose-induced insulin release also inhibits the initiation of action potentials and the depolarization of the membrane usually seen after glucose addition (Matthews, 1975). These data argue that epinephrine alters the coupling between the glucose metabolite receptor and the fluxes of K^+ and Ca^{2+} across the plasma membrane. It could do so by one of two mechanisms—either as a direct consequence of hormone–receptor interaction in the membrane or indirectly via an alteration in the cellular content of cAMP. Experiments designed to distinguish between these two alternatives have not yet been carried out, but there is some evidence from another line of investigation which suggests indirectly that the effect may be mediated indirectly via cAMP. This line is the study of long-term adaptations of the pancreatic islet to altered nutritional or hormonal states.

Long-Term Adaptation

Up to this point, the data reviewed have dealt almost exclusively with the immediate effects of various stimuli on insulin release from islets prepared from fed animals and involve the nature of the information transfer involved in the minute-to-minute control of insulin secretion. In addition to this type of data, there are data showing that long-term adaptation of the insulin secretory response occurs during starvation or pregnancy (Grand et al., 1973). In the former, a decreased responsiveness is observed; in the latter, an increase (Figure 6.7).

During starvation, the secretory response is markedly reduced (Montague, 1977). The pattern of response to glucose is similar to that seen in tissues from fed animals treated with agents that lower their cAMP content. This adaptations to starvation can be prevented by intermittent administration of small amounts of glucose to the animals. Also, if islets from starved animals are treated *in vitro* with agents that increase their cAMP content, their response to glucose resembles that of islets from fed animals. These results suggest that the cAMP system plays a role in this long-term adaptation. This suggestion is supported by the observation that the cAMP content of islets from starved animals is lower than that from fed animals and that this reduction is due to a decrease in adenylate cyclase activity (Howell et al., 1973; Howell and Montague, 1973, 1975). In contrast, glucose loading of animals leads to an increase in the adenylate cyclase activity and cAMP content of subsequently isolated islets (Howell et al., 1973). Thus, the glucose responsiveness of the insulin secretory system correlates directly with the cAMP content of the tissue. The converse is found in the pregnant animal. The response of the beta cell to glucose is enhanced, and these cells have higher cAMP contents (Green et al., 1973; Montague, 1977) and adenylate cyclase activities than comparable cells from nonpregnant littermates.

Given the fact that starvation (a chronic adaptation) and adrenaline administration (a short-term response) both lead to a concomitant fall in tissue content of cAMP and in the magnitude of the insulin secretory response to a standard change in extracellular glucose concentration, it seems likely that their common mechanism is a cAMP-dependent change in the membrane transduction event mediated by glucose and/or its metabolite(s).

The other conclusion from these studies is that, either directly or indirectly, the extracellular glucose concentration regulates the adenylate cyclase activity of the islets. The effect appears to be a direct one because it is seen when islets are incubated for 24 hours *in vitro* in the presence of high extracellular glucose concentration (Montague, 1977). The nature of the signal mediating this long-term response of the islet cell to glucose is not known.

The fact that the plasma or extracellular glucose concentration appears to regulate the responsiveness of the beta cells to rapid changes in plasma glucose concentration is of considerable interest from the point of control mechanism. As discussed earlier (see Chapter 3), when the concentration of many extracellular messengers increases chronically, there is an adaptive response of the cell called down-regulation, which consists of a reduction in surface receptor number for the particular messenger and hence a decrease in responsiveness of the cell to that messenger. Reasoning teleologically, one can rationalize this phenomenon of down-regulation as a device to protect the target cell from overstimulation by the first messenger. In the case of glucose and the beta cell, we have operationally the complete opposite; namely, a chronic increase in glucose supply and hence in the average plasma glucose concentration alters the responsiveness of the beta cells to abrupt increases in plasma glucose in a positive sense, that is, the higher the basal glucose level, the greater the response to an abrupt increase in glucose concentration. Viewed from the perspective of the control of beta cell function, this arrangement represents a positive feedback loop in this control system and might therefore be considered undesirable from a strictly operational point of view. However, viewed from the perspective of the whole organism, this arrangement makes considerable sense. The main function of insulin is that of a storage hormone. Hence, the larger the glucose load and the higher the basal glucose level, the greater the need for storage. Also, even though a positive feedback of control operates at the level of the beta cell, a negative feedback control operates within the organism because as insulin increases, the rate of glucose disposal increases, leading to a more pronounced fall in plasma glucose and thus to a feedback inhibition of insulin release.

The other point of interest is the time course of the two glucose-mediated effects. The initiation of insulin release follows immediately after a rise in extracellular glucose concentration; and the change in adenylate cyclase occurs over a period of hours or days. Hence, the same extracellular messenger regulates two cellular responses with different time courses. What is not yet known is whether these two responses are mediated by the same intracellular messengers or whether these differ. This is not a trivial question because most of the data concerning stimulus–response coupling deal with immediate cellular responses (microseconds to minutes) and not with long-term changes. The available data favor the view that cAMP and calcium serve to couple stimulus to long-term as well as short-term response, but the data are scanty, and it is possible that there are other second messengers involved in long-term responses of cells to those extracellular messengers that act at the level of the plasma membrane.

EXOCRINE SECRETION IN MAMMALS

Introduction

Of the several exocrine glands in mammals, those most thoroughly studied are the parotid salivary gland and the exocrine pancreas. These have in common the fact that they both secrete digestive enzymes in an isotonic electrolyte solution in response to cholinergic and/or adrenergic stimuli. Yet in spite of their similarities in terms of function and innervation, there are significant differences in the mechanisms by which protein (enzyme) secretion and fluid and electrolyte secretion are controlled. The data concerning these two exocrine glands will be the only reviewed, although recent studies in the lacrimal gland indicate that cholinergic activation of the calcium messenger system plays the predominant function in regulating protein secretion in this tissue (Keryer and Rossignol, 1976; Parod and Putney, 1978). Likewise, mucin secretion from the sublingual gland has been reported to involve the calcium messenger system (Vreugdenhil and Roukema, 1975; Martinez et al., 1976), but a complete analysis of these systems has not yet been carried out.

Parotid Gland

Secretion from the mammalian parotid gland is controlled largely by its autonomic innervation. Both cholinergic and adrenergic nerve fibers innervate the acinar cell. In the cholinergic system, the acetylcholine receptors are muscarinic; in the adrenergic system, both α- and β-receptors are present (Schramm and Selinger, 1975a,b; Leslie et al., 1976). In addition, receptors for a group of undecapeptides, for example, substance P, exist on the surface of the acinar cells. As far as presently known, activation of these receptors produces the same changes in the fluid, electrolyte, and protein secretions as seen after α-adrenergic and cholinergic stimulation.

During adrenergic stimulation, the normal transmitter released is norepinephrine. This agonist binds to two different receptors, α and β, leading respectively to activation of the calcium and cAMP messenger systems. During cholinergic stimulation, acetylcholine is released and activates the calcium messenger system. Unfortunately, few data are available concerning the mechanism by which the two messenger systems interact or concerning the nature of the response elements whose activity they control. A calcium–calmodulin-activated phosphodiesterase has been identified in this tissue but seems to be a small percentage of the total phosphodiesterase present (Butcher and Putney, 1980).

It is of interest that, just as in the liver (see Chapter 7), so in the parotid gland either activation of β-adrenergic, cholinergic, or α-adrenergic receptors or application of A23187 leads to an increase in glycogenolysis (Herman and Rossignol, 1975; Rossignol et al., 1977); the cholinergic and α-adrenergic activation requires external calcium and is not associated with an increase in cAMP. The β-adrenergic activation is associated with a rise in cAMP content. Dual activation of glycogenolysis by the two separate messenger systems is, therefore, of common occurrence and is not confined to liver (see Chapter 7) and muscle.

The difficulties in defining the actions of the messengers and their interactions are several. First and foremost is that the molecular events underlying either fluid or protein secretion are not known. Second, it has not been possible to study transcellular ion and water fluxes in this tissue because of its complex structure; hence, most studies have employed either slices or isolated acinar cells. In the case of protein secretion, this does not represent a major problem because the isolated cells maintain their polarity and all evidence indicates that protein secretion occurs by exocytosis across the luminal cell membrane in the isolated cells, as it does in the intact gland (Bdolah and Schramm, 1962, 1965). However, the situation with fluid and electrolyte secretion is not so clear. When the gland is stimulated *in vivo* by α-adrenergic or cholinergic mediators, a copious protein-pool saliva is produced. Initially, this saliva has a high K^+ content, but later it has a high Na^+ content (Burgen, 1956). This type of secretory response is associated with the formation of multiple, small intracellular vesicles in the acinar cells. When the same agents are added to isolated acinar cells, there is a marked increase in K^+ (Batzri et al., 1973) and Na^+ influx (Putney and Parod, 1978) into the cells and the same change in intracellular vesicle numbers (Schramm and Selinger, 1974, 1975). However, what is not known is the site of these altered ion flows, that is, do they occur on the luminal and/or basolateral membranes of the cell? Nonetheless, they are taken to represent the cellular counterpart of fluid secretion in the intact tissue.

The central question that has been addressed in this tissue is the nature of the receptor-mediated events, and how the messengers generated regulate fluid and electrolyte secretion on the one hand and amylase secretion on the other. From the work of Schramm, Selinger, Butcher, Putney, Peterson, and others, it is clear that occupation of β-adrenergic receptors leads to the generation of cAMP, and that occupation of α-adrenergic, cholinergic, or peptide receptors leads to an increase influx of calcium into the cell (Batzri and Selinger, 1973; Batzri et al., 1971, 1973; Butcher, 1975, 1978a,b, 1979, 1980; Butcher et al., 1975; Butcher et al., 1976; Butcher and Putney, 1980; Durham et al., 1974, 1975; Feinstein and Schramm, 1970; Haddas et al., 1979; Marier et al., 1978; Miller and Nelson, 1977; Parod and Putney, 1978; Petersen, 1976, 1978; Petersen and Iwatsuki, 1978; Petersen and Pedersen, 1974; Petersen et al., 1977; Putney, 1976, 1977, 1979; Putney et al., 1977, 1978; Roberts and Petersen, 1978; Radich and Butcher, 1976; Salomon and Schramm, 1970; Schramm and Selinger, 1975; Selinger et al., 1973, 1974; Strittmatter et al., 1977; Yong, 1979; Rossignol et al., 1977).

When only the β-adrenergic response is elicited, a protein-rich solution is secreted. The counterpart of this in the isolated cell is a marked stimulation of protein release but only a minor increase in K^+ efflux. Amylase release by β-agonists fulfills all the Sutherland criteria: (1) a β-agonist-stimulatable adenylate cyclase is present on the plasma membrane; (2) inhibitors of PDE enhance the response; (3) the rise in cAMP concentration either precedes or occurs concurrently with enzyme secretion; (4) the effects can be mimicked by exogenous application of a variety of cAMP analogs; and (5) the tissue contains both cAMP-dependent protein kinase I and II (Butcher and Putney, 1980). Thus, it would appear that the case for the primary messenger function of cAMP in this response is clear. However, there are two aspects of the response which indicate that the situation may be more complicated. These are that low agonist concentrations produce a response without a detectable increase in cAMP content and that calcium ion is required for the action of cAMP on enzyme secretion (Butcher and Putney, 1980).

The first of these is a recurrent theme in the analysis of tissue responses to agonists thought to act via the cAMP messenger system. The usual explanation given for this apparent discrepancy is that hormone stimulation increases cAMP production sufficient to activate cAMP-dependent protein kinases but not sufficient to increase the total tissue content of cAMP. In a recent review, Levitski (1976) has pointed out that in many tissues there is a large reserve of receptor-cyclase units on the cell membrane. He estimates that occupation of less than 0.1% of the receptors is probably sufficient to bring about a detectable response to the agonist. Methods for approaching this problem by measuring the ratio of total to cAMP-dependent PK activities in cell homogenates after agonist action have been developed. Such experiments have not yet been reported for the parotid gland. However, in view of previous evidence that the catalytic subunits of PK, once freed of the regulatory subunit, can translocate to other intracellular sites raises the intriguing possibility that a small localized rise in cAMP content next to the plasma membrane could lead to the generation of free catalytic subunits which could then diffuse into the cell and activate response elements even though a detectable change in cAMP content was not measurable. On the other hand, it is equally possible that some consequence of hormone–receptor interaction could lead to an alteration in the sensitivity of holoenzyme to dissociation by cAMP.

Complicating this issue in the parotid gland are recent studies showing that adenylate cyclase is present on all the plasma membrane surfaces including the luminal membrane (Durham et al., 1975). If substantiated, this finding must change our thinking about these systems because it is possible that the neurotransmitter, rather than acting exclusively on the basolateral membrane, may diffuse across the cell and causes the production of cAMP at the luminal surface. The cAMP so generated could have a special role in mediating exocytosis.

The second question concerns the role of calcium ion in mediating protein secretion in this tissue. When the calcium messenger system (see below) is activated by α-adrenergic or cholinergic stimulation, a copious enzyme-poor saliva is produced and a net uptake of calcium into the cells occurs (Kanagasuntheram and Randle, 1976). Likewise, *in vitro* cholinergic stimulation causes some protein secretion but less than 15% of that seen with β-agonists. On the other hand, *in vivo* cholinergic stimuli enhance β-agonist-stimulated protein secretion while, at the same time, causing a fall in tissue cAMP content (Butcher et al., 1976; Emmelin and Gjörstrup, 1976; Harper and Brooker, 1977).

Furthermore, if cells are depleted of calcium, protein secretion in response to β-agonist and cyclic nucleotide analogs is markedly reduced, indicating that a minimum level of tissue calcium is essential for activating protein secretion (Butcher and Putney, 1980). A reduction in calcium causes a decrease in the cAMP response to a given concentration of agonist (Butcher, 1978). Hence, part of the decrease in response may be due to the decrease in cAMP concentration, but the fact that a decreased protein secretory response is seen after addition of cAMP analogs indicates an additional site of calcium involvement. This may be more than a passive involvement because cAMP and β-adrenergic agonists have been shown to induce an efflux of calcium from prelabeled acinar cells possibly from the mitochondrial pool (Butcher, 1980; Kanagasuntheram and Randle, 1976; Putney et al., 1977; Randle et al., 1979). Of particular interest is the recent study of Butcher (1980) in which he demonstrated that both isoproterenol and monobutyryl cAMP induced the mobilization of a pool of radiocalcium from prelabeled parotid cells that was different than the pool mobilized by carbachol, phenylephrine, or substance P.

From these data, Butcher and Putney (1980) have concluded that calcium has one of two possible messenger roles in the control of protein secretion. Either it is the proximate message and the role of cAMP is to mobilize calcium from an intracellular source and thus provide messenger calcium in the appropriate intracellular domain, or cAMP and calcium act in some concerted fashion to control the process.

In concluding any discussion of the role of calcium in regulating protein secretion, it is worthwhile pointing out that the studies in isolated cells have their counterpart in the intact tissue. Early work suggested that parasympathetic stimulation of the intact gland (Schneyer et al., 1977) leads to the secretion of a fluid rich in calcium and poor in amylase, but that sympathetic stimulation leads to one rich in amylase and relatively poor in calcium (Schneyer, 1976). When the effects of direct electrical stimulation of the sympathetic innervation of the gland in the presence of selective adrenergic blocking agents were studied, the pattern of response was different depending upon the type of blocking agent. Blockade of α-receptors had little effect on amylase and calcium secretion, but blockade of the β-receptors caused a marked reduction in both calcium and amylase secretion. These results imply that β-receptor activation leads to an increase in calcium secretion and are, therefore, consistent with the view that cAMP mobilizes calcium from an intracellular pool.

When either a cholinergic or α-adrenergic response is elicited *in vivo,* there is a secretion of a protein-poor solution. The *in vitro* counterpart of this is a marked efflux of K^+ from the cell (Schramm and Selinger, 1974), no change in tissue cAMP content, and a small increase in amylase release. The potassium efflux and amylase release are seen only when calcium is present in the external medium (Putney, 1979; Watson et al., 1979). These agonists increase the influx of $^{45}Ca^{2+}$ into the tissue, and a similar effect upon K^+ efflux and amylase release is seen if A23187 is added to the tissue in the presence of extracellular calcium (Selinger et al., 1974). Receptor activation leads to an increase in PI turnover (Jones and Michell, 1974, 1975, 1976, 1978; Oron et al., 1975), which is not dependent on the presence of external calcium (Keryer et al., 1979) and is not seen when A23187 induces a calcium-dependent fluid secretion (Rossignol et al., 1977; Jones and Michell, 1975). These facts have been interpreted as indicating that these receptors mediate a change in calcium influx into the tissue as well as an initial release of Ca^{2+} from the plasma membrane (Putney, 1976, 1979) and that the subsequent increase in intracellular calcium leads to an increase in membrane permeability to K^+ (and Na^+). The exact relationship of these changes in ionic fluxes to fluid secretion is not known. Nor are there any significant data concerning the calcium–calmodulin response elements with the cell.

From the point of view of our central thesis, the parotid represents another example where hierarchical control of cell function is achieved by the interaction of the calcium and cAMP messenger systems. By having additional extracellular messengers (other than norepinephrine) which modulate the function of only one of these systems, a fine control of the two complementary functions of the cell—fluid and protein secretion—is achieved.

Exocrine Pancreas

The control of secretion in pancreatic acinar cells is mediated both by direct cholinergic innervation (acetylcholine muscarinic receptors); indirectly by several gut hormones (Blair et al., 1977; Christophe et al., 1977) including pancreozymin, vasoactive intestinal peptide, secretin, and gastrin; and by several other agents including bombesin and caerulein (see Case, 1978; and Schulz, 1980, for an extensive review).

At first glance, a discussion of the neurohormonal control of secretion from the exocrine pancreas would not appear to fit in a discussion of hierarchical control of cell function by cAMP and calcium, because much of the available evidence has been taken to indicate that calcium is the sole intracellular messenger coupling response to extracellular stimuli in this tissue. The case for a messenger function for calcium is quite strong and is discussed below. Nonetheless, even in this tissue there is evidence that cAMP also serves a messenger function (Scratcherd and Case, 1973; Case, 1973a,b; Kempen et al., 1974, 1977; Christophe et al., 1976; Gardner et al., 1975, 1976, 1977; Gardner and Rottman, 1979; 1980; Robberecht et al., 1974; Heisler et al., 1972; Fast and Tenenhouse, 1976; Schulz, 1975; Chu et al., 1976; Lambert et al., 1975).

There is no doubt that calcium is intimately involved in the process of stimulus–response coupling in the exocrine pancreas (Case, 1973, 1978; Goebell, 1976; Gardner and Hahne, 1977; Fast and Tenenhouse, 1976; Williams and Lee, 1974; Poulsen and Williams, 1977; Scheurs et al., 1976; Christophe et al., 1976; Williams et al., 1976; Chandler and Williams, 1974, 1977; Scheele and Haymovits, 1979; Schulz, 1980). The activation of the muscarinic receptors does not lead to an immediate increase in the calcium permeability of the plasma membrane as in the parotid. When a brief pulse of acetylcholine is applied to the intact acinar cell, there is a reduction in the membrane potential (Petersen, 1976) due primarily to an increase in the Na^+ conductances of the membrane. However, calcium uptake is not an immediate consequence of Ach–receptor interaction. The initial burst of enzyme secretion occurs in the absence of extracellular calcium (Scheele and Haymovits, 1979; Schulz, 1980). Nonetheless, it appears to be calcium dependent (Case and Clausen, 1973). In the presence or absence of extracellular calcium, Ach addition to cells prelabeled with radioisotopic calcium leads to a marked efflux of calcium (Figure 6.13) which has a time course similar to that of the initial phase of secretion (Case and Clausen, 1973; Matthews et al., 1973; Heisler, 1974; Chandler and Williams, 1974; Williams and Chandler, 1975; Gardner et al., 1975; Clemente and Meldolesi, 1975a,b; Kondo and Schultz, 1976; Schulz, 1980). Both from electrophysiological (Iwatsuki and Petersen, 1977a,b; 1978) and *in vitro* calcium flux studies (Scheele and Haymovits, 1979; Schulz, 1980), it has become quite clear that for sustained enzyme secretion to occur, extracellular calcium is required, and that during this phase of the secretory response there is an increase in the calcium conductance of the plasma membrane (Petersen and Iwatsuki, 1978; Schulz, 1980). Secretion can be induced by A23187 in the presence of extracellular calcium. Recent work by Petersen and Iwatsuki (1978) has shown that in both the early and late phases of secretion there is electrical uncoupling between adjacent acinar cells which is taken as evidence that enzyme secretion is associated with, and is probably mediated by, a rise in the calcium ion content of the cell cytosol. If so, a problem of first importance is that of determining the source of the calcium responsible for the initial increase in cytosolic calcium. Since this occurs in the absence of

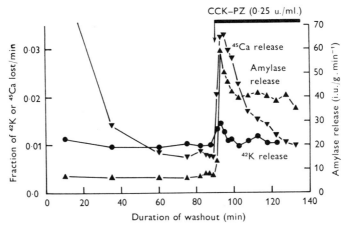

Figure 6.13 Changes in the rate of Ca^{2+} efflux, K^+ efflux, and amylase release from the exocrine pancreas in response to cholecystokinin–pancreozymin (cck-pz). From Case and Clausen (1973), with permission.

extracellular calcium, the source must clearly be within the cell. Two pro-
posals have been made. Petersen and Iwatsuki (1978) and Schulz (1980)
favor the view that the calcium is released from a plasma membrane pool.
Others have proposed a mitochondrial origin (Renckens et al., 1978). In this
regard, the findings of Carafoli and Crompton (1976) and later Argent et al.
(1976) that Na^+ can induce an increase in the efflux of calcium from the
mitochondria of certain tissues, including the pancreas, have led to the
suggestion that the Ach-induced entry of Na^+ into the acinar cell is the signal
leading to calcium release. However, there is considerable evidence to show
that the increase in Na^+ conductance of the plasma membrane is a consequence of a rise in the Ca^{2+} concentration in the cell cytosol (Schulz, 1980).
The best evidence that the calcium initially released by secretagogues comes
from a plasma membrane pool is that summarized by Schulz (1980). This
includes the following: (1) There is sufficient calcium bound to this membrane to account for the amount released. (2) When extracellular calcium is
removed, there is still an initial release by Ach; but if the neurotransmitter is
removed and then reapplied, there is not a second pulse of calcium release.
However, if atropine, an antagonist of the action of Ach on muscarinic
receptors, is added and then washed away and Ach is reapplied, there is a
second pulse of calcium release. (3) The addition of atropine to cells pre-
loaded with calcium and treated with Ach leads to a rapid reaccumulation of
calcium into the "trigger" pool of calcium.

These available data suggest the following model for stimulus–response
coupling in the exocrine pancreas stimulated by acetylcholine. Interaction of
Ach with its muscarinic receptor leads to a release of plasma membrane
bound calcium. The consequent rise in cytosolic calcium concentration has
at least four consequences: (1) it initiates exocytosis (enzyme secretion) by
a largely unknown mechanism that may include a calcium-induced fusion of
zymogen gianule membrane with plasma membrane (Milutinovic et al.,
1977); (2) it increases the Na^+ conductance of the basolateral membrane
(Petersen, 1976; Schulz and Heil, 1975; Schulz, 1980), leading to a depolarization of this membrane and a decrease in its electrical resistance (Petersen,
1976); (3) it leads to an electrical uncoupling of adjacent cells (Petersen and
Iwatsuki, 1978); and (4) it causes an increase in glucose transport into the
cell.

A further consequence of these events is an increase in the permeability of
the basolateral plasma membrane to calcium. This is associated with an
increased turnover of phosphatidylinositol (Hokin and Hokin, 1955, 1956;
Michell et al., 1977). There are two possible explanations for this secondary
increase in plasma membrane calcium conductance after Ach action: The
first is that calcium conductance increases as a delayed consequence of
Ach–receptor interaction, that is, it is mediated by a direct coupling to the
receptor. The second is that the calcium conductance increase results from
the opening of a voltage-dependent calcium channel. In the latter case, one
would have a sequence of calcium release from the plasma membrane, a rise

in cytosolic calcium leading to an increase in the Na^+ conductance of the plasma membrane, and a depolarization of this membrane with the opening of a voltage-dependent calcium channel. On the basis of the available data, this sequence appears the most satisfactory. However, the recent studies by Marshall et al. (1980) indicate that the control of events at the plasma membrane is considerably more complex than just outlined. They found that after carbamoylcholine (a long-acting analog of acetylcholine) addition to mouse pancreatic tissue, there is, as previously discussed, an increase in phosphatidylinositol breakdown. If the membrane lipids are labeled with [^{14}C]arachidonic acid by preincubation with carbamylcholine, then treated with atropine to block the further action of this agonist, washed, and then exposed to a different secretagogue, caerulein, acting via a different receptor, amylase secretion is increased and PI breakdown is seen. Of particular interest is the rapid disappearance of a considerable part of the [^{14}C]arachidonate incorporated into the membrane PI. Approximately half of this appears in phosphatidic acid and the other, in prostaglandin E_2. Application of PGE_2 to the tissue in the absence of secretagogues evokes amylase secretion, and the secretion induced by caerulein is blocked by inhibitors of prostaglandin synthesis. Since arachidonate is the precursor for PGE_2 synthesis, these authors suggest that PGE_2 may either serve as a coordinate messenger with Ca^{2+} or, more likely, that a secretagogue-induced breakdown of PI leads to a release of arachidonate and an increase in the synthesis of PGE_2 which acts to open the calcium channel and possibly plays a major role in inducing the increase in the calcium conductance of the plasma membrane.

Two aspects of the effect of the rise in cytosolic calcium ion concentration in this tissue are worthy of further comment: (1) its effect on electrical uncoupling and (2) its possible role in membrane fusion.

The work of Loewenstein and Rose discussed previously (see Chapter 4) has established that in many epithelial tissues, there are low-resistance pathways between adjacent cells via so-called gap junctions (cell membrane-to-cell membrane junctions of a particular type). Normally, these are freely permeable to ions and small molecules. However, their permeability is markedly reduced when the Ca^{2+} concentration of the cell cytosol increases. Based on these facts and the fact that a rise in Ca^{2+} concentration was postulated to serve as the factor coupling stimulus to response in the exocrine pancreas, Petersen and Iwatsuki (1978) measured the electrical coupling between acinar cells before and after exposure to Ach. They found that Ach caused adjacent cells to become uncoupled and to remain so during prolonged exposure to neurotransmitter. Both sustained uncoupling and sustained enzyme secretion required extracellular calcium. From these results, they concluded that when these cells are activated, there is not just an early transient rise in the Ca^{2+} content of the cell cytosol but a sustained increase as long as the stimulus acts.

Although one of the commonest effects of a rise in cytosolic calcium ion concentration is that of inducing the secretion of an enzyme, hormone or neurotransmitter packaged in a secretory granule, the mechanism by which calcium regulates these exocytotic events, is not established. Two possible roles have been considered: (1) Ca^{2+} controls the function of microtubules and/or microfilaments that are involved in moving the secretory granules to the cell surface; and/or (2) Ca^{2+} triggers the fusion of the granule membrane with the plasma membrane of the cell. The data concerning the first of these are confusing and contradictory and will not be considered here. The data concerning the second are also not complete, but one interesting study deserves comment. Milutinovic et al. (1977) showed that if the calcium concentration in the medium was raised to values between 10^{-6} and $2 \times 10^{-5}\ M$, an aggregation of pancreatic zymogen granules with a plasma membrane function from the pancreas would occur *in vitro*. The interaction was specific for the luminal plasma membrane; it was not seen when contraluminal membrane was employed. Since these concentrations of calcium are in the range one would predict after gland stimulation, this calcium-mediated membrane-to-membrane fusion may represent one of the mechanisms by which calcium mediates exocytosis.

Although the major messenger system mediating the pancreatic secretory response appears to be the calcium system, there is increasing evidence that the cAMP messenger system is also involved. In particular, secretin and VIP, which have no effect upon the membrane potential of acinar cells, have been found to stimulate adenylate cyclase causing a rise in cAMP and marked fluid secretion (Robberecht et al., 1974; Kempen et al., 1974, 1977a,b; Svoboda et al., 1976; Beauduin et al., 1974; Depont et al., 1979; Gardner and Jackson, 1977). The fluid secreted is poor in protein. The administration of secretin or VIP to lobules or glands exposed to Ach leads to a marked enhancement of both protein and fluid secretion. Similarly, Heisler et al. (1972) showed that cAMP or dibutyl cAMP added to pancreatic fragments induced amylase release and enhanced the magnitude of enzyme secretion even to maximally effective concentrations of carbachol. Equally interesting are the observations of Gardner and Rottman (1979) showing that treatment of dispersed pancreatic acini with cholera toxin leads to a significant rise in cAMP content and in amylase secretion. The time courses of the two responses are similar. Of interest is that pretreatment with cholera toxin greatly enhances the rate of amylase secretion caused by carbachol or cholecystokinin.

Thus, there is significant evidence that the cAMP messenger system modulates the secretory response in the pancreas in some hierarchical fashion. The question is that of deciding its site of involvement. It is clear that VIP and secretin act on ductal cells; but in some species, possibly many, they also act on the acinar cells (Case, 1978; DePont et al., 1979; Gardner and Jackson, 1979). Since the rate of protein secretion is critically dependent upon the rate of fluid secretion, the finding that secretin enhances the effect of Ach does not necessarily imply that the secretin is acting on enzyme secretion. It may regulate principally fluid and electrolyte secretion. One of the difficulties in clearly defining its role on acinar function is that the available physiological data imply that the cAMP messenger system is coupled principally to the processes of fluid and electrolyte, rather than enzyme, secretion, and evaluation of fluid and electrolyte secretion in dispersed acinar cells is not possible. At present, one can only conclude that a rise in cAMP concentration in ductal cells, and probably in acinar cells as well, in some undefined manner stimulates fluid and electrolyte secretion. A rise in cAMP concentration may also alter the calcium domain within the acinar cell (Heisler et al., 1972) or alter the sensitivity of calcium response elements to the calcium message, and may therefore also influence enzyme secretion.

Although important in an experimental sense, the distinction as to the site of secretion is relatively unimportant in an operational sense. The fact is that the two messenger systems operate in a hierarchical sense in this tissue just as they do in the parotid to regulate the overall secretory process. However, the systems in the two tissues appear to operate as mirror images of one another (Table 6.3). In parotid, cAMP is primarily responsible for modulating enzyme secretion, and calcium for fluid and electrolyte secretion. The opposite is true in the pancreas. This striking difference appears startling at first glance. However, viewed in the present context of our knowledge of cAMP and calcium response elements, it is not so unusual. Both messengers can control the activities of common response elements in the same tissue, so it is entirely logical that one is of major importance in controlling a common response element in one tissue and the other, in controlling it in a second tissue.

Table 6.3   Contrasting Control Mechanisms Involved in the Regulation of Secretion in Parotid Gland and Pancreas[a]

Parotid				Pancreas	
Catecholamine	Ach			Ach	VIP Secretin
Beta Alpha	Muscarnic	*Recognition*	Muscarinic		Peptide
cAMP Ca²⁺		*Second messenger*	Ca²⁺		cAMP
Ensyme secretion	Fluid + electrolyte	*Response system*	Enzyme secretion		Fluid + electrolyte
Secretion		*Final Result*	Secretion		

[a]Modified from Schramm and Selinger (1975).

The possible role of cGMP in regulating fluid and protein secretion has not been discussed in detail. There is considerable evidence that the agents that induce enzyme secretion in this tissue do so by causing an increase in cytosolic calcium and that the rise in cytosolic Ca^{2+} content is associated with a rise in the cGMP content of the tissue (Case, 1978). Earlier work (Haymovits and Scheele, 1976) had suggested that cGMP was an intracellular mediator of stimulus–response coupling in these cells. However, recent studies by Gardner and Rottman (1980) have led to the conclusion that cGMP is not the direct mediator of the secretory events in this tissue.

Gastric Parietal Cells

Another intestinal organ in which a hierarchical control of cell function is evident is the gastric mucosa. This is a complex tissue composed of many cell types including two types of mucus-secreting cells; parietal cells responsible for acid secretion; chief cells responsible for the secretion of pepsin; and enterochromaffin cells, which are a heterogeneous group of endocrine cells responsible for the secretion of serotonin, gastrin, and gut glucagon. The present discussion will concern only the control of acid production by the parietal cells.

These cells respond to three different secretagogues—acetylcholine (muscarinic receptor), histamine (H_2 receptor), and gastrin. There is considerable evidence from *in vivo* experiments employing either intact animals or animals with exteriorized gastric mucosa that the three secretagogues potentiate the actions of one another in stimulating acid secretion (Grossman, 1974; Gillespie and Grossman, 1969; Grossman, 1967; Johnson and Grossman, 1969; Konturek and Oleksy, 1967; Cooke, 1970; Brooks et al., 1970; Dinbar and Grossman, 1972; Kowalewski and Saab, 1972; Kowalewski and Kolody, 1972). However, the nature of their interaction has been a subject of considerable uncertainty because administration of atropine, a muscarinic antagonist, blocks not only the effect of acetylcholine or vagus (cholinergic) nerve stimulation but blocks the effects of gastrin and histamine as well (Hirschowitz and Sacks, 1969; Konturek et al., 1968; Hirschowitz and Hutchinson, 1977). Conversely, the histamine antagonist metiamide blocks the effects of not only histamine but those of both gastrin and acetylcholine. (Grossman and Konturek, 1974; Carter et al., 1974).

These findings have led to the construction of various models in which one of the three agents is the final common pathway by which parietal cell function is controlled, for example, in one model histamine is the proximate mediator of parietal cell acid secretion, and both gastrin and acetylcholine act by increasing histamine release. However, not all the data are consistent with any model of this type. On the other hand, it is possible that part of the interrelationship between these three agents involves regulating the local concentration of one or both of the others. Another aspect of their interrelationship, and the one most germane to our discussion, is their interaction at the cellular level, particularly the possible roles of calcium and cAMP in mediating their actions.

Considerable progress has recently been made in defining these interactions by the use of an isolated cell preparation from canine gastric mucosa that is enriched in parietal cells (approximately 65% of the cells are parietal cells). Using this preparation, Soll and coworkers (Soll, 1978a,b; 1980a,b, 1981; Soll and Wollin, 1979; Wollin et al., 1979) have shown that (1) when stimulated with any of the three secretagogues, these cells undergo the same morphological change (the appearance of prominent canaliculi lined with microvilli) that is seen in parietal cells *in vivo;* (2) either oxygen consumption or the uptake of [^{14}C]aminopyrine into the cell can be employed as a valid biochemical marker for the acid secretory process; (3) all three secretagogues stimulate both oxygen consumption and [^{14}C]aminopyrine uptake; (4) the action of histamine, but not that of either carbamylcholine or gastrin, is blocked by H_2-receptor antagonists such as metiamide and cimetidine; and (4) the action of carbamylcholine, but not that of gastrin or histamine, is blocked by atropine, a muscurinic receptor antagonist.

Soll concludes from these data that the parietal cell possesses specific receptors for each of the agonists and that each agonist can stimulate acid secretion directly. He has also shown that these secretagogues interact in a complex way in regulating acid secretion in these isolated cells, for example, carbamylcholine potentiates the response of a given dose of histamine and a low level of histamine potentiates the effect of a given dose of carbamylcholine. From these data he concludes that part of the explanation for the observed interaction of these agents *in vivo* is that they act in a complex and interrelated fashion to regulate parietal cell function.

The effect of histamine, but not that of the other two secretagogues, is mediated by activation of adenylate cyclase: (1) histamine addition causes an increase in the cAMP content of parietal cells; (2) isomethylbutylxanthine (IBMX), a phosphodiesterase inhibitor, potentiates the effect of submaximal doses of histamine upon the increase in both cAMP concentration and O_2 consumption; (3) H_2-receptor antagonists block the histamine-induced rise in cAMP content; (4) a histamine-sensitive adenylate cyclase is present in the particulate fraction of canine gastric mucosa (Dozois et al., 1977); (5) low doses of PGE block both the histamine-induced rise in cAMP concentration and in O_2 consumption; and (5) cAMP analogs mimic the effects of histamine. In contrast, neither gastrin nor carbamylcholine causes a change in parietal cell cAMP content, nor are their effects on O_2 consumption increased by IBMX. Of particular interest, even though both gastrin and carbamylcholine potentiate the action of histamine on O_2 consumption and [^{14}C]aminopyrine uptake, they do not potentiate the effect of histamine on cAMP content. Thus, their potentiating effect is mediated at a step beyond cAMP generation.

The effect of carbamylcholine upon [^{14}C]aminopyrine (AP) uptake is markedly dependent on the extracellular calcium concentration (Soll, 1981). At 0.1 mM extracellular Ca^{2+}, 10 μM carbamylcholine has practically no effect on [^{14}C]-AP accumulation; but at 1.8 mM extracellular Ca^{2+}, the same concentration of carbamylcholine produces a maximal effect. In contrast, the effect of 10 or 100 μM histamine is only reduced approximately 20 to 30% when the Ca^{2+} concentration is reduced from 1.8 to 0.1 mM. The response to a standard dose of carbamylcholine is a nearly linear function of extracellular Ca^{2+} concentration between 0 and 2.0 mM Ca^{2+}. Addition of 10 μM lanthanum, an inhibitor of the calcium channel in the plasma membrane, causes an 83% reduction in the response to carbamylcholine but only a 12% reduction to histamine. Carbamylcholine, but not histamine, cause a three- to fourfold increase in the rate of $^{45}Ca^{2+}$ uptake into the isolated cells. The effect of carbamylcholine on calcium uptake is dose dependent, and the same doses which enhance [^{14}C]-AP uptake, a measure of acid secretion, also enhance calcium uptake. Atropine blocks both responses. No effect of any of the secretagogues upon calcium efflux is seen. These data indicate that cholinergic agents stimulate acid secretion by a calcium-dependent, cAMP-independent process and that a major source of messenger calcium is the extracellular calcium pool.

It appears, therefore, that the parietal cell of the gastric mucosa represents another target cell in which separate extracellular messengers activate the separate limbs of the synarchic messenger system to achieve aspects of both *hierarchical* and *redundant* control of cell response: hierarchical in the sense that the response of the cell to either secretagogue potentiates its response to the other; redundant in the sense that either secretagogue acting alone stimulates acid production.

The molecular or cellular basis for the hierarchial interaction between the two messengers is not known. However, based on the nature of these interactions in other tissues, it is possible to suggest several possible alternatives: (1) The two messengers regulate the phosphorylation of the same response element at different sites, with each phosphorylation leading to an enhanced activity of this element; (2) One of the two messengers controls the phosphorylation of a response element in the other limb in such a way that the sensitivity of this element to its messenger is increased; and/or (3) the rise in cAMP content increases the intracellular calcium domains.

An intriguing but unresolved question relates to the mechanism of action of gastrin. This secretagogue produces neither a rise in the cAMP content of the cell nor an increase in the rate of calcium uptake into the cell, although its effects are suppressed to approximately 30% of maximal in cells incubated in the absence of extracellular calcium. It is possible that this hormone also mediates its effect on the calcium messenger system, but by a mechanism different from that of acetylcholine. It may alter the intracellular distribution of calcium, for example. However, to date at least, gastrin has not been shown to promote calcium efflux from the tissue. Hence, the mechanism of its action remains to be elucidated.

MUSCLE CONTRACTION AND NEUROSECRETION

Introduction

In reviewing the historical development of concepts concerning cell regulation, it was pointed out that two distinctions were made that seemed to separate neuromuscular systems from metabolic systems. The first of these was the separation of these tissues into excitable and nonexcitable systems, respectively. The second was the concept that ionic extracellular messengers give rise to ionic intracellular messengers and chemical extracellular messengers give rise to chemical intracellular messengers (see Figure 1.5). However, these distinctions break down repeatedly and in many cases obscure the fact that the similarities in the control properties of excitable and nonexcitable tissues far outweigh their differences.

There are numerous examples of chemical extracellular messengers giving rise to ionic intracellular messages. Furthermore, in the pancreatic beta cell membrane, action potentials, the *sine qua non* of the excitable cell, are routinely observed when these cells are activated to secrete insulin in response to a change in the concentration of extracellular glucose. The counter example of this situation is a type of slow striated muscle, a tissue usually classified as excitable, which undergoes contraction in response to neural stimulation even though such stimulation does not cause the initiation or propagation of an action potential in the muscle cell membrane. In spite of this electrical inexcitability, calcium ions couple excitation to contraction in this type of muscle as they do in a truly "excitable" mammalian skeletal muscle. An example of the nonexcitable muscle of this type is the accessory redula closer (ARC) muscle of *Aplysia*. It receives a dual neural innervation that when stimulated generates different intracellular messengers and acts in a hierarchical fashion to control response, that is, contraction.

Another type of excitable tissue, in the classic use of the term, is nerve. The principal messenger that couples stimulus to response, that is, neurosecretion, in most nerves is calcium ion (Katz, 1966). In view of the importance of calcium in neural function and synaptic transmission, it is not surprising that the calcium receptor protein calmodulin, is also found in nervous tissue. It is of particular interest that in addition to its expected presence in presynaptic termini, calmodulin is found as a membrane-associated protein in the postsynaptic densities isolated from the canine cerebral cortex (Cohen et al., 1977; Blomberg et al., 1977; Grab et al., 1979). The role of calmodulin at this locus is not known, but its presence in this location suggests that the voltage-dependent entry of calcium into the cell body of a neuron may play a messenger role in the regulation of cell function in addition to its well-established role in regulating neurosecretion at another portion of the neuron, the presynaptic terminus. The only presently available insight into the possible role of calmodulin regulating synaptic transmission is the discovery that the calcium-dependent phosphorylation of specific synaptosomal membrane proteins (DeLorenzo, 1976; DeLorenzo and

Freedman, 1977a,b; Krueger et al., 1977) is mediated by calmodulin (Shulman and Greengard, 1978a,b).

From the point of view of the main thesis under consideration in this monograph, the most important question is whether or not cAMP also plays a messenger role in this tissue, and of equal interest is the question whether the calcium and cAMP messenger systems interact in regulating nerve cell function. The answers to these two questions are that cAMP does have a prominent messenger role in neural tissue and that in performing this role it interacts in several ways with the calcium messenger system.

One need only recall that two of the major discoveries linking the calcium system to the cAMP system at the molecular level have been made in mammalian brain tissue: (1) the role of calmodulin as a key regulatory subunit of cyclic nucleotide phosphodiesterase (Cheung, 1970; Kakuichi et al., 1971) and (2) the role of calmodulin as a key regulatory modifier of adenylate cyclase (Brostrom et al., 1975, 1978). Calcium-dependent adenylate cyclases have also been found in isolated glial tumor cells (Brostrom et al., 1979). Furthermore, there is evidence that cAMP regulates calcium metabolism in neurons and that both cAMP- and calcium-dependent protein kinases may phosphorylate the same protein substrate in neural tissue (Huttner and Greengard, 1979). This latter finding is of considerable interest because the properties of the system are similar to those seen with cAMP- and calcium-dependent phosphorylation of glycogen synthetase (see Chapter 4). In the case of the neural membrane protein, protein I, its phosphorylation can be catalyzed either by a cAMP- or calcium-dependent protein kinase, but different sites on the protein are phosphorylated in response to the two messengers.

In spite of these various discoveries, it has proven difficult to define the interrelated roles of calcium and cAMP in the central nervous system of higher animals, largely because of the extreme complexity of this tissue. Hence, a search for simpler systems has led to an evaluation of the interrelated roles of calcium and cAMP in restricted parts of the nervous system. The examples to be discussed include presynaptic facilitation, regulation of acetylcholine release at the neuromuscular junction, and acetylcholine release in the abdominal ganglion of *Aplysia*.

Neural Control of ARC Contraction

A primitive behavioral response, that of feeding in *Aplysia californica,* has been studied by Kupfermann and associates (Cohen et al., 1978; Weiss et al., 1975; Weiss et al., 1975, 1978, 1979; Kupfermann et al., 1979; Weiss and Kupfermann, 1977). An aspect of this feeding behavior is a sustained rhythmic biting. Kupfermann et al. (1979) have examined the properties of the motor system which underlies this biting response. It is carried out by the buccal muscle mass, an organ that moves a specialized apparatus, the radula, capable of biting off and ingesting seaweed. One component of this mass, the accessory radula close muscle (ARC), can be isolated easily from the other muscles without interfering with its innervation. It has two types of efferent nerve types which innervate it—cholinergic and serotonergic neurons.

There are two separate motor neurons each of which sends multiple branches to each muscle cell. These are both cholinergic and arise in the buccal ganglion. When stimulated, they produce a graded depolarization of the muscle cell membrane, but no action potentials are seen. There is a close correlation between the magnitude of the muscle membrane depolarization and the degree of muscle contraction (Figure 6.14). It is presumed that Ca^{2+} serves to couple stimulus to response in this muscle, but the source of this calcium is not known.

In addition to this motor innervation, the muscle receives axonal branches from the metacerebral cell (MCC), a serotonergic neuron located in the cerebral ganglion. Stimulation of the MCC does not cause any change in the contractile state of the resting muscle nor a change in its resting membrane potential. Nor does contraction of the muscle by electrical depolarization lead to any electrical activity in the MCC, indicating that the MCC does not serve as a sensory cell in some reflex behavioral arc. However, if the MCC is stimulated for a brief period and then one of the motor neurons is stimulated, the resulting contractions induced by the motor nerve are greater than seen when the motor nerve is stimulated without prior MCC stimulation (Figure 6.15). In other words, MCC stimulation causes a potentiation of the effect of a standard motor nerve stimulation.

The effect of MCC stimulation is primarily on the function of the muscle cell itself and is not an indirect one on motor nerve function; the greater the magnitude of MCC stimulation, the greater the potentiation of the subsequent response to motor neuron stimulation. Thus, the effect is not an all-or-none one, but is a graded one related to the magnitude of the serotonergic stimulus.

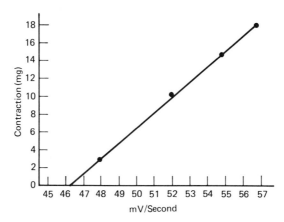

Figure 6.14 Degree of contraction as function of the degree of depolarization junctional end plate potential. From Cohen et al. (1978), with permission.

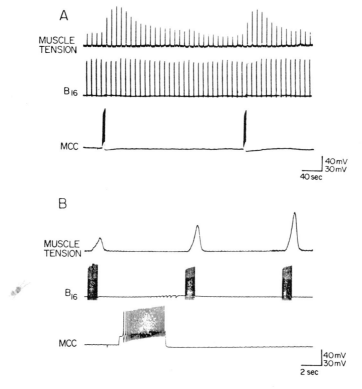

Figure 6.15 Effect of the stimulation of an MCC on the tension developed by aplysia muscle in response to the stimulation of a motor neuron (B16) to that muscle. A, Muscle tension (upper trace), electrophysiological response of motor neuron B16 (middle trace), and periodic stimulation of metacerebral cell (MCC) (lower trace) are recorded. Note that muscle tension increases after prior MCC stimulation. B, Expanded trace (on a time scale) of second period of MCC stimulation shown in A. From Kupfermann et al. (1979), with permission.

As noted, the neurotransmitter released at the MCC synapses in the muscle is serotonin. Direct application of this substance to the muscle potentiates the contractile response to motor nerve stimulation without altering the membrane potential. Either serotonin application or MCC stimulation leads to an increase in the cAMP content of the muscle (Figure 6.16). Phosphodiesterase-resistant analogs of cAMP produce a potentiation similar to that produced by serotonin, and inhibitors of PDE enhance the effect of MCC stimulation. This means that a rise in the cAMP content of the muscle cell leads to a potentiation of the contractile response of this muscle to a standard stimulus delivered either by motor nerve stimulation or by the direct application of acetylcholine to the muscle.

On the basis of the interrelationships known to exist between calcium and cAMP in other systems, one of several possibilities might account for this effect of cAMP: (1) it is possible that a cAMP-dependent phosphorylation of a calcium receptor protein could alter its sensitivity to the calcium signal; (2)

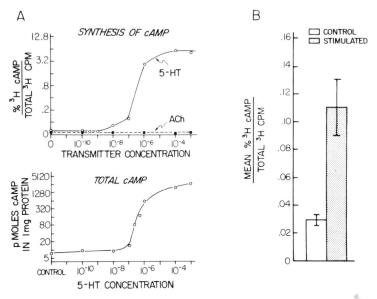

Figure 6.16 Effect of acetylcholine (○) and serotonin (○) on the rate of cAMP synthesis (upper graph) and total cAMP content (lower graph) (A) and the rate of cAMP synthesis in control and 5HT-stimulated muscle (B). From Kupfermann et al. (1979), with permission.

cAMP might alter the temporal and/or spatial distribution of calcium in the cell cytosol by altering the release of calcium from or uptake into an intracellular calcium pool; or (3) cAMP might have both kinds of effects. The biochemical tools are at hand to examine these possibilities.

From the point of view of our dominant thesis, this invertebrate system represents another example of the theme that an understanding of the control of cell function by membrane transducing systems requires a knowledge of the role of both calcium and cAMP in modulating cell function. This system also illustrates the fact that some synapses are electrically silent and give rise to a chemical rather than an ionic intracellular message.

This neuromuscular control complex is organized in an operational sense exactly as is the metabolic control of insulin output from the beta cell of the endocrine pancreas. Two separate neural inputs are coupled respectively to the calcium and cAMP messenger systems in *Aplysia* muscle, whereas two humoral inputs are coupled respectively to these systems in the beta cell (see Figure 6.12). A rise in intracellular Ca^{2+} concentration initiated either by a cholinergic neurotransmitter in *Aplysia* or by glucose in the pancreas is the immediate and required signal that initiates cell response—contraction or secretion. A second neural input from a serotoninergic neuron activates a postsynaptic receptor coupled to adenylate cyclase to potentiate contraction, whereas a second humoral input, for example, glucagon, activates adenylate cyclase and potentiates insulin secretion. The consequent rise in cAMP is unable to initiate contraction, just as a rise in cAMP in the absence of a calcium signal is unable to initiate secretion in the pancreas. However, just as in the pancreas, so in the *Aplysia* muscle the rise in cAMP potentiates the response to a given calcium message by prolonging the spatial and temporal domains of the calcium signal and/or by altering the sensitivity of the response element to calcium.

The similarity of the two systems can be extended further. In the pancreas, glucagon is one of the agents that activates adenylate cyclase; and it also increases plasma glucose, so in a sense it has a central effect on the system of controls that regulate the calcium messenger system. In *Aplysia* muscle, the metacerebral cells send axons not only directly to the muscle but also the cell bodies of the motor neurons in the buccal ganglion. Presumably these axons are also serotoninergic and activate postsynaptic receptor coupled to adenylate cyclase. Activation of these produces a slow depolarization of the membrane of the motor neurons, thereby lowering its threshold to activation by other synaptic inputs. This means that there is enhancement of messenger production in the system controlling the generation of the calcium in the effector organ, the muscle.

Ironically, the only feature of the two control systems that is different is that in one, the β cell—a metabolic system—a critical component of the primary response is regenerative action potentials, that is, excitability by the restricted definition; whereas in the other—a neuromuscular system—there are no action potentials but only a depolarization, that is, nonexcitability, during the generation of the primary response.

Modulation of Presynaptic Events By Cyclic AMP

Given the widespread occurrence in neural tissue of the enzymes involved in regulating cAMP metabolism, the fact that calcium ions regulate both adenylate cyclase and phosphodiesterase, and the fact that calcium couples excitation to neurosecretion at nearly all synapses, there can be little doubt that cAMP and calcium interact in regulating neural function. However, because of the difficulties of identifying populations of cells in neural tissue that can be studied in isolation, progress in defining the interrelated roles of cAMP and calcium has not been rapid.

It is now generally accepted that at all chemical synapses so far studied, it is Ca^{2+} that couples excitation to neurotransmitter release. Thus, the function of the calcium messenger system is well defined at this anatomical point in the nervous system. It is equally clear that excitation of most nerve bodies and axons leads to a transient influx of calcium. Less clear is the function of this calcium influx. One clearly defined function is that of increasing K^+ permeability and thus of hyperpolarizing (Meech, 1976) or repolarizing the nerve membrane. It is likely that it serves another as yet to be defined function. The situation with cAMP is less clear. From the onset, two possible sites of action have been considered: regulation of presynaptic or postsynaptic events. There is evidence supporting the view that cAMP modulates events at both sites.

The fact of greatest significance is that even though synaptic transmission involves a depolarization of the presynaptic terminus, leading to the influx of calcium via both the Na^+ channel and voltage-dependent calcium channel, other neural and humoral inputs to this region of the cell can modify the amount of neurotransmitter released in response to a given stimulus (Langer, 1977). Among these modulators of neurotransmitter release are cAMP, its various analogs, and drugs which alter its metabolism. Other modulators such as encephalins, dopamine, serotonin, and noradrenaline appear to act by interacting with putative presynaptic receptors. Some at least exert their effect by controlling the activity of membrane-bound adenylate cyclase. The problem is that numerous of these agents inhibit neurotransmitter release in some systems and enhance it in others (Weiner, 1979). Many of these studies have involved an analysis of events in part of the central nervous system. Contradictory results are difficult to interpret because of possible multiple inputs into the system under study. On the other hand, there are several studies in more isolated synapses in which the data are somewhat clearer.

Norepinephrine Control of Norepinephrine Release

Weiner et al. (1978) and Weiner (1979) have studied neurotransmitter release in the isolated vas deferens–hypogastric nerve preparation of the guinea pig. Norepinephrine release is associated with an increase in tyrosine hydroxylase activity, and the activity of this enzyme can be increased by the activity of a cAMP-dependent protein kinase. Furthermore, 8-methylthio-cAMP treatment leads to an increase in the activity of this enzyme and a modest increase in the amount of norepinephrine released in response to a standard nerve stimulation. The α-adrenergic antagonist phenoxybenzamine potentiates the release of neurotransmitter. These data are consistent with a model in which adenylate cyclase is activated by neural stimulation and the resultant increase in cAMP leads to the activation of tyrosine hydroxylase (i.e., increased neurotransmitter synthesis) and to an increase in neurotransmitter release. The resultant increase in amount of norepinephrine released would, by interacting with α-receptors on the presynaptic membranes, act as a negative feedback modulator of neurotransmitter release either by inhibiting adenylate cyclase and/or blocking Ca^{2+} entry.

Aside from the specific system under study, this proposal raises an extremely important point. Throughout our discussion, an attempt has been made to call attention to data that argue for a commonality of control properties between neural "excitable" and metabolic "nonexcitable" tissues. In particular, evidence has been discussed invalidating the models of the ionic extracellular messenger giving rise exclusively to an ionic intracellular messenger in excitable tissues and of the chemical extracellular messenger giving rise exclusively to chemical intracellular messengers in nonexcitable tissues. The final evidence which would completely invalidate these distinctions and establish the universality of the calcium and cAMP messenger systems would be the demonstration that in neural cells the depolarization of the cell membrane is coupled to the activation of adenylate cyclase.

A second system that has been studied is stimulation of sympathetic neurons in the cat spleen. In this system, it was shown (Cubeddu et al., 1975) that the output of both norepinephrine and dopamine-8-hydroxylase caused by a standard electrical stimulation of the nerve was enhanced by perfusion of the spleen with either cAMP analogs or phosphodiesterase inhibitors. However, none of these drugs induced neurosecretion in the absence of nerve stimulation. These results indicate that cAMP is probably not directly responsible for the release of neurotransmitter but that it facilitates in some undefined manner the neurosecretory process.

This system represents only one of several norepinephrine synapses which have been analyzed in this fashion. Langer (1977) has recently summarized the results obtained in a number of others. It has been found that these noradrenergic synapses possess both α- and β-receptors on the presynaptic membrane. The β-receptors are thought to be coupled to adenylate cyclase, respond to low concentrations of norepinephrine, and when activated lead to enhanced norepinephrine release, that is, positive feedback. The α-receptors respond to higher concentrations of norepinephrine (approximately 100-fold greater) and produce an inhibition of norepinephrine release.

It is not clear by what mechanism the α-receptor activation leads to inhibition of release. Langer suggests that a direct inhibitory effect upon calcium entry is responsible; but in view of the findings in other tissues that α-receptor activation inhibits adenylate cyclase activity, inhibition of adenylate cyclase activity could also account for α-adrenergic inhibition of neurosecretion, in analogy to the situation in the β-cell of the pancreas. The point to be made is that there is now widespread evidence showing that cAMP modulates presynaptic events in a large number of synapses. These synapses can be other than those secreting norepinephrine.

Acetylcholine Release at the Neuromuscular Junction

Another peripheral synapse in which the role of cAMP in neurotransmitter release has been analyzed is the neuromuscular junction. This is a cholinergic (nicotinic receptor type) synapse. The studies dealing with the possible role of the cAMP messenger system in neurosecretion at this synapse has recently been reviewed by Standaert and Dretchen (1979). From these studies, the evidence, though far from complete, strongly supports the conclusion of these authors and of Wilson (1974) and of Miyamoto and Breckenridge (1974) that cAMP has no role in the regulation of postsynaptic events but does play one of several roles in modulating presynaptic events—both immediate and long-term adaptive changes to environmental stimuli.

When the motor nerve to the cat soleus muscle was stimulated supramaximally once every 2.5 seconds and isometric muscle tension recorded, the intravenous injection of dibutyryl cAMP (DBcAMP) caused a transient increase in the force of muscle contraction. However, if a denervated muscle was stimulated directly and DBcAMP applied, there was no enhancement of the electrically induced tetanus. Furthermore, application of DBcAMP was shown to produce stimulus-bound repetitive activity in the muscle as a consequence of either increasing or prolonging the influx of ions (probably calcium) into the nerve endings. The injection of DBcAMP into a preparation in which the muscle was not being stimulated led to an immediate increase in the frequency of miniature end plate potentials without affecting their amplitude or changing the resting membrane potential of the end plate. Likewise, if muscle contraction was blocked by tubocurare and the nerve stimulated electrically, cAMP analogs increased the end plate potentials, indicating an enhanced release of neurotransmitter and increased mobilization of acetylcholine from releaseable stores (Wilson, 1974). Similar results have been found using the phosphodiesterase inhibitor SQ 20,009 (Jacobs and McNiece, 1977) and theophylline (Wilson, 1974).

Standaert and Dretchen (1979) have tested a wide variety of agents known to influence one of the components of the cAMP messenger system (cyclase, phosphodiesterase, or protein kinase) upon the response of the soleus muscle to neural stimulation. On the basis of their results, they concluded that cAMP plays an important physiological role in regulating events at this presynaptic terminus. At least one of its effects is to promote the influx of calcium into the nerve ending, leading to an increase in frequency of miniature end plate potentials in the unstimulated nerve and to a larger quantal content and larger end plate potential during stimulation. This proposed role of cAMP in facilitating calcium entry is similar to that thought to occur in cardiac muscle (see Chapter 9). However, their results could equally be explained by a cAMP-dependent prolongation of the spatial and/or temporal domain of the calcium message within the presynaptic terminus.

Standaert and Gretchen (1979) raise as an interesting possibility that the early entry of calcium through the Na^+ channel is responsible for the activation of adenylate cyclase in the presynaptic membrane. They also point out that the cAMP may play regulatory roles other than altering neurotransmitter release at this synapse such as controlling the reuptake and/or synthesis of neurotransmitter.

From the point of view of our thesis, the key point to be made about the properties of this identifiable synapse is that there is substantial evidence to support the view that the cAMP messenger system as well as the calcium messenger system play a role in regulating the process of neurosecretion and that the relationship between the two messenger systems appears to have many operational similarities to their relationships in other tissues.

Acetylcholine Release in the Abdominal Ganglion of *Aplysia*

Studies by Brunelli et al. (1976), Castellucci et al. (1970), Castellucci and Kandel (1976), Shimahara and Tauc (1976), and Klein and Kandel (1978) have shown that in the nervous system of *Aplysia californica,* behavioral sensitization of the gill-withdrawal reflex involves presynaptic modulation of voltage-dependent Ca^{2+} currents in presynaptic termini of sensory neurons innervating both central internervous and motor neurons which directly control the withdrawal response.

The gill-withdrawal reflex is a defensive reflex to tactile stimuli. Behavioral sensitization is a prolonged enhancement of this behavioral response to a tactile stimulus as a consequence of the presentation of a second, usually noxious, stimulus to the organism (Pinsker et al., 1973). If an animal is given four days of training consisting of four brief noxious stimuli each day, the sensitization of the animal's response to a tactile stimulus can last up to three weeks.

Castellucci and Kandel (1976) have provided electrophysical data showing that a major anatomic site at which sensitization of the gill-withdrawal reflex occurs is at the level of the presynaptic termini of the sensory neurons that innervate the motor neurons arising in the abdominal ganglion. They suggest that the sensitization, that is, an increase in response to a standard stimulus, results from an increase in the amount of transmitter released from the sensory neuron synapses impinging on motor neurons, a process known as presynaptic facilitation.

Brunelli et al. (1976) in investigating this system found that serotonin enhances synaptic transmission between sensory and motor neurons. This effect of serotonin is blocked by application of the serotonin antagonist cinserine. This compound has no effect by itself but blocks the facilitatory effect of serotonin. Application of dibutyryl cAMP also enhances synaptic transmission. These authors concluded that presynaptic facilitation involves one or more serotonergic neurons which act by increasing the intracellular cAMP content of the presynaptic termini of the sensory neurons. Support for this conclusion comes from the work of Drummond et al. (1980) who showed that serotonin and several cAMP analogs produce a hyperpolarization of a specific neuron, R15, in the abdominal ganglion of *Aplysia*. The rise in cAMP is thought to lead to an increase in the amount of neurotransmitter released in response to a given rate of stimulation of the sensory neuron. Thus, this system represents yet another presynaptic locus in which the cAMP system modulates the effect of the calcium messenger system in controlling neurotransmitter release.

Klein and Kandel (1978) have used electrophysiological methods in an effort to define the mechanism by which cAMP induces facilitation in this presynaptic terminus. They were unable to study the properties of the presynaptic sensory nerve endings directly, but studied instead the cell bodies of these sensory neurons. They showed that the duration of the action potentials measured in the cell body after 5HT treatment was similar to the duration of the excitatory postsynaptic potential measured postsynaptically in the motor neuron. The latter was used as a measure of the duration of transmitter release. From these findings they concluded that ionic changes in the cell body mirror those taking place in the region of the synaptic termini.

The action potential in the cell bodies of these neurons is complex but can be shown to have inward Na^+ and Ca^{2+} currents and an outward K^+ current. The Ca^{2+} current can be measured when the opposing K^+ current (K^+ efflux) is blocked by tetraethylammonium. Under these conditions, stimulation of the nerve, application of 5HT or 1BMX, or intracellular injection of cAMP prolongs the plateau of the action potential (Figure 6.17). This prolongation of the plateau of the action potential parallels the increase in transmitter release measured indirectly by measuring the amplitude of the monosynaptic excitatory potentials of postsynaptic motor neurons. Thus, a serotonin-mediated increase in the cAMP content of the neuron appears to facilitate presynaptic release of acetylcholine by increasing the voltage-sensitive Ca^{2+} current in the presynaptic termini of the sensory neuron (Figure 6.18).

The mechanism by which control of the calcium channel is achieved has been studied by Shapiro et al. (1980). The effect of cAMP apparently is to alter the properties of one or more K^+ channels in the membrane such as to decrease the rate of K^+ efflux from the cell. This, in turn, prolongs the duration of the period of membrane depolarization, which means that the voltage-dependent calcium channel remains open for a longer period of time and a greater influx of calcium occurs leading to a greater release of neuro-

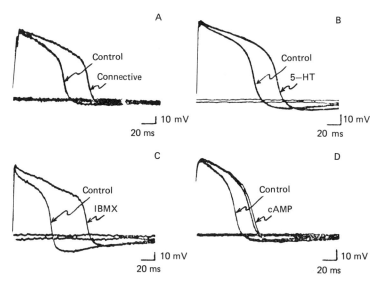

Figure 6.17 Prolongation of the action potential by stimulation of the connective neurons (A), application of 5HT (B), or pretreatment with the phosphodiesterase inhibitor IBMX (C) or with cAMP. From Klein and Kandel (1978), with permission.

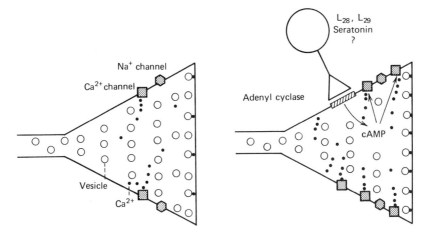

Figure 6.18 Model of the relationship between cAMP and Ca^{2+} as interrelated second messengers in the control of neurosecretion in sensory neurons of the abdominal ganglion of *Aplysia*. The concept is that directly or indirectly an increase in cAMP concentration in the presynaptic terminus causes a prolongation of the period of time during which the voltage-dependent calcium channel is open thereby prolonging the duration of the calcium message. From Klein and Kandel (1978), with permission.

transmitter. These authors have also presented evidence in support of the concept that intracellular calcium regulates the activation of the calcium channel in the synaptic membrane. This means that three factors determine the state of the calcium channel: (1) membrane potential, (2) intracellular calcium, and (3) intracellular cAMP. It seems quite possible that the latter two agents exert their effects by controlling the phosphorylation of membrane proteins related to membrane ion channels.

These results indicate that gating of an ion channel in the plasma membrane (in this case a K^+ channel) is regulated both by chemical and electrical means. This is similar to the situation in the heart (see Chapter 9) and is the counterpart of the observations that in some membranes adenylate cyclase can be activated by both chemical (neurotransmitter) and ionic (calcium–calmodulin) means.

A point to be emphasized is that cAMP acts in this tissue much as it is thought to act in the mammalian heart (see Chapter 9). In both, a rise in the intracellular cAMP content has little effect on the resting membrane potential; it specifically modifies the properties of the voltage-sensitive calcium channel. The only difference is that it is long lasting in the neuron but not in the heart. The consequence of this modification is to increase the temporal and possibly spatial domain of the calcium signal. Such an effect does not rule out the possibility that cAMP in these nerve terminals may also act to (1) alter the intracellular distribution of calcium, (2) alter the sensitivity of calcium response elements to calcium as it appears to do in the heart, or (3) alter the phosphorylation of a membrane protein by activating a protein kinase.

In regard to the latter point, the recent findings of Huttner and Greengard (1979) are of considerable interest. They have found a specific protein in mammalian brain synaptosomes, protein I, that undergoes phosphorylation when either a change in calcium or cAMP concentration occurs, just as in the case of glycogen synthase (see Chapter 4) the sites of phosphorylation of protein I are different when calcium rather than cAMP is the messenger. Hence, in the nervous as well as the endocrine system, phosphorylation of the same protein can be induced either by a calcium-dependent or a cAMP-dependent protein kinase; but when this occurs, the sites of phosphorylation differ. Nevertheless, if the analogy holds, then a similar change in neuronal function should occur after phosphorylation of either site just as happens in the case of glycogen synthase (see Chapter 4) or phospholamban (see Chapter 9).

CONCLUSION

A consideration of the data obtained from studying these various presynaptic loci leave little doubt that the cAMP messenger system plays a significant role in modifying or facilitating the calcium messenger-mediated release of various neurotransmitters. This modulatory role of the cAMP messenger system is undoubtedly widespread and provides evidence for the essential unity of cellular control mechanisms in neural (excitable) and nonneural (nonexcitable) cells. The same hierarchical relationship found between the calcium and cAMP messenger systems in endocrine and exocrine secreting tissues is found in many neurosecretory tissues.

In a broader sense, the data reviewed in this chapter indicate that one of the most common variants of the synarchic messenger system is one in which the calcium and cAMP limbs of this system are organized in a hierarchical fashion. A particularly common mode of organization appears to be one in which calcium serves as the basic factor involved in initiating cellular response, and cAMP serves to modify the calcium messenger system in a positive way either by increasing the spatial and/or temporal domains of the calcium message and/or altering the sensitivity of calcium response elements to calcium.

7

Redundant Control

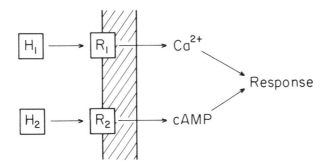

INTRODUCTION

A common type of synarchic regulation is one in which the calcium and cAMP messenger systems coexist in the same cell, are regulated separately by different extracellular stimuli, and yet control the same response elements within the cell leading to the same final common cellular response. This type of *redundant control* of cell function is seen in the hormonal control of aldosterone secretion from the zona glomerulosa of the adrenal cortex, the hormonal regulation of hepatic glucose production, and the neural and humoral regulation of fluid and electrolyte secretion in the small intestine.

ALDOSTERONE PRODUCTION

The production of aldosterone by the cells of the adrenal glomerulosa is under the control of three major extracellular stimuli: ACTH, K^+, and angiotensin II (AII) (Rosenkrantz, 1959; Davis, 1961; Kaplan, 1965; Ganong et al., 1966; Aquilera and Catt, 1978; Muller, 1971; Saruta et al., 1972; Williams and Dluhy, 1972; Boyd et al., 1973; Fredlund et al., 1975; Tait and Tait, 1976; Peach, 1977; Douglas et al., 1978; Machie et al., 1978; Sharma et al., 1978; Fujita et al., 1979; Fakunding et al., 1979; Aquilera and Catt, 1979; Foster et al., 1981; Fakunding and Catt, 1980). When ACTH acts upon isolated glomerulosa cells, there is a rise in their cAMP content; but when either K^+ or AII act, no change in cAMP concentration is seen even though these latter

235

agents provoke a similar increase in rate of aldosterone biosynthesis. Evidence from several different laboratories demonstrates that in the case of both AII and extracellular K^+, Ca^{2+} serves as a major messenger in coupling stimulus to response. Thus, in this tissue there are two pathways by which information flows into the cells to initiate the same cellular response.

Before accepting this conclusion, it is necessary to consider whether or not ACTH and angiotensin II or K^+ control cell responses at the same or different steps in the sequence of metabolic reactions involved in steroid hormone production. As discussed previously (see Chapter 6), a substantial body of evidence exists pointing to the step between cholesterol and pregnenolone as the major one regulated when ACTH acts in the zona fasiculata to enhance corticosteroid production. Aquilera and Catt (1979) have shown that addition of ACTH to isolated glomerulosa cells also leads to a marked stimulation of pregnenolone synthesis at this step. Hence, in both zones of the adrenal, ACTH acts on the same key metabolic step in steroid biosynthesis even though the ultimate product is different. Similarly, Aquilera and Catt (1979) found that after either AII or K^+ addition to glomerulosa cells, pregnenolone biosynthesis was stimulated. In addition, all three extracellular stimuli activated a later step in the pathway of aldosterone biosynthesis, but their effects varied in cells from different species. These results provide evidence that the two hormones ACTH and AII regulate the same steps in the pathway of aldosterone biosynthesis, even though they employ different intracellular messengers in doing so.

That calcium is the messenger in AII and K^+ action is supported by several lines of evidence (Fakunding et al., 1979; Machie et al., 1978; Fakunding and Catt, 1980; Foster et al., 1981): (1) the effect of AII and K^+ upon aldosterone production is dependent on the extracellular calcium concentration (Figure 7.1); (2) agents (verapamil, its analog D600, and La^+) that

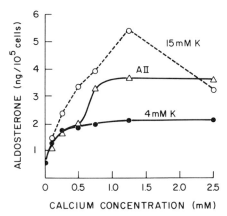

Figure 7.1   Effect of either high (15 mM) or low (4 mM) K^+ or angiotensin (AII) on aldosterone production in dog zona glomerulosa cells as function of the Ca^{2+} concentration of the medium. From Foster et al., (1981), with permission.

block calcium channels in the plasma membrane inhibit both AII- and K+-induced increase in steroid biosynthesis; (3) the ionophore A23187 produces a Ca^{2+}-dependent increase in hormone production; (4) high extracellular Ca^{2+}, *per se,* stimulates aldosterone production; and (5) AII and K+ stimulate calcium uptake (Figure 7.2) and block its efflux from glomerulosa cells. These data not only establish a messenger function of calcium, but indicate that the extracellular calcium pool is a major source for messenger calcium in these responses.

The evidence in support of a major messenger role for cAMP in the action of ACTH on the glomerulosa cell is not quite as unambiguous as that supporting the messenger role of Ca^{2+} in K+ and AII action. The reason is that changes in extracellular Ca^{2+} concentration and various calcium channel blockers inhibit the action of ACTH on glomerulosa cells (Fakunding and Catt, 1980). This effect of calcium lack is a dual one. In the absence of Ca^{2+}, ACTH does not invoke a rise in cAMP concentration, and the action of cAMP is calcium-dependent as shown by the fact that the effect of exogenous cAMP on aldosterone production is less marked in cells incubated in a calcium-free medium. Furthermore, as shown in Figure 7.3, in the glomerulosa cell, just as in the fasiculata cell, there is a discrepancy between the concentrations of ACTH needed to stimulate aldosterone production and those needed to induce a rise in the cAMP content of these same cells (Fujita et al., 1979). These results raise the possibility that an agent other than cAMP (possibly Ca^{2+}) acts as the important second messenger in ACTH action and that cAMP plays some less immediate messenger function. Two experiments by Fakunding and Catt (1980) address this question. In the first, they examined the effect of increasing extracellular lanthanum concentration

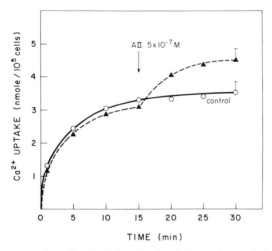

Figure 7.2 Time course of uptake of calcium into beef glomerulosa cells in the presence and absence of AII ($10^{x8}M$). The hormone was added 16 minutes after the addition of $^{45}Ca^{2+}$. From Foster et al. (1981), with permission).

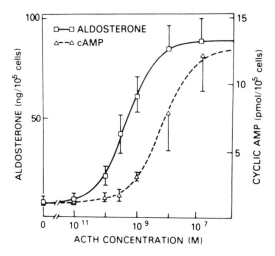

Figure 7.3 Aldosterone production and cAMP content in adrenal glomerulosa cells as function of ACTH concentration. From Fujita et al. (1971), with permission.

on the action of 1 nm AII and 10 nm ACTH. They found (Figure 7.4) that 10^{-6} M lanthanum blocked, nearly totally, the effect of AII but had practically no effect on the ACTH-mediated increase in aldosterone production. However, higher concentration of lanthanum blocked ACTH action. A second experiment was performed to examine the effect of increasing lanthanum concentration upon both the ACTH-mediated increase in cAMP con-

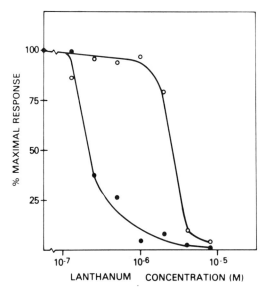

Figure 7.4 Rate of aldosterone production, plotted as percentage of maximal, as function of the lanthanum concentration in the medium when either 1 nM AII (●) or 10 nM ACTH (○) was present. From Fakunding and Catt (1980), with permission.

centration and in aldosterone production rate. The results showed a close correlation between the La^{3+}-induced decrease in cAMP content and in aldosterone production. These results show that cAMP does have a major messenger function in ACTH action on adrenal glomerulosa cell even though it remains possible that at low ACTH concentrations some other messenger also plays a role.

The conclusion from the available data is that AII and K^+ on the one hand and ACTH on the other regulate aldosterone biosynthesis in adrenal glomerulosa cells by activating respectively the calcium and cAMP limbs of the synarchic system, and that the two synarchic messengers act redundantly to modify the behavior of the same ultimate response element within these cells. The molecular basis by which they control the behavior of these response elements is not known.

HEPATIC GLUCOSE PRODUCTION

Introduction

Sutherland and Rall (1958, 1960) discovered the second messenger role of cAMP during their studies of the hormonal control of hepatic phosphorylase. Their finding led, in turn, to the discovery that most, if not all, β-adrenergic effects are mediated by the cAMP messenger system (Robison et al., 1971). The liver system served as a benchmark against which to compare a variety of other adrenergic systems and against which to compare other tissues employing the cAMP messenger system. Recent analyses of the hormonal control of hepatic glycogenolysis and gluconeogenesis indicate that these processes are not controlled solely by this messenger system. Rather, there are two more or less separate messenger systems regulating hepatic glucose production: glucagon and β-adrenergic agonists operating via the cAMP messenger system and vasopressin, angiotensin II, and α-adrenergic agonists operating via the calcium messenger system (Van de Werve et al., 1977; Assimacopoulos-Jeannet et al., 1977; Keppens et al., 1977).

Since the initial discoveries of Sutherland and Rall, the mechanism of action of glucagon has been studied repeatedly. There is general agreement that the major glucagon receptor is coupled to the adenylate cyclase of the cAMP messenger system. The system has met all the criteria established by Sutherland to prove the second messenger role of cAMP: (1) after glucagon administration there is an increase in cellular cAMP; (2) similarly glucagon addition leads to an increase in labeling with phosphate of total and specific phosphoprotein substrates of cAMP-dependent protein kinases; (3) phosphodiesterase inhibitors enhance the metabolic effects of glucagon; (4) exogenous cAMP mimics the metabolic effects of glucagon; and (5) plasma membrane fractions of liver possess a glucagon-stimulatable adenylate cyclase (Exton and Harper, 1975). Major support for the concept that cAMP is the messenger in glucagon action stems from the fact that exogenous cAMP mimics many of these effects of glucagon, including the changes in ion fluxes and plasma membrane potential.

In keeping with the concept of an integrative action of a hormone on a cell function, glucagon regulates a variety of metabolic processes in the liver cell. These include (1) activation of glycogenolysis and inhibition of glycogen synthesis; (2) stimulation of gluconeogenesis, which includes changes in the activity of both mitochondrial and cytosolic enzymes; (3) inhibition of triglyceride synthesis; (4) alteration in the fluxes of K^+ and Ca^{2+} and a change in the Mg^{2+} content of mitochondria; (5) enhanced urea biosynthesis; (6) enhanced lipolysis; (7) enhanced amino acid uptake; (8) enhanced calcium accumulation by a microsomal fraction (Bygrave and Tranter, 1978; Moore et al., 1974; Waltenbaugh and Friedmann, 1978); and (9) hyperpolarization of the cell membrane (Friedmann et al., 1971; Waltenbaugh et al., 1978; Friedmann and Dambach, 1973, 1980). Whether all of these diverse effects are controlled by changes in cAMP content is not known.

Calcium as Messenger

The messenger role of calcium in the hormonal control of hepatic metabolism will be discussed in terms of the evidence pointing to a calcium-dependent, cAMP-independent activation of glycogenolysis and/or gluconeogenesis by vasopressin, angiotensin, and α-adrenergic agonists. The first issue to be addressed is that of defining the calcium pool which serves as source of messenger in these systems and the related question of how changes in calcium flux are brought about. This discussion is followed by a consideration of how the calcium message exerts its effects.

As noted above, the hepatic response to epinephrine was the original system in which cAMP was found to serve a messenger function. It was not until 1972 that Sherline, Lynch, and Glinsman raised the first serious doubts about the role of cAMP as the adrenergic messenger by noting that α-adrenergic agents may also stimulate hepatic glucose production. In the succeeding year, Tolbert, Butcher, and Fain (1973) demonstrated that when the α-agonist phenylephrine and the β-agonist isoproterenol were employed to stimulate hepatic glucose production, there was no correlation between cAMP content and glucose production in the rat liver. Later work (Cherrington et al., 1976) showed a similar difference between the effects of glucagon and phenylephrine. Phenylephrine stimulated glucose production without causing a rise in either cAMP or in the phosphorylated form of phosphorylase kinase, whereas glucagon in a dose sufficient to produce a comparable rise in glucose production caused an increase in both (Figure 7.5). Furthermore, the α-blocker phentolamine suppressed the effect of phenylephrine upon glucose production, but the β-blocker propranolol did not. These workers concluded that in the rat liver, catecholamines activate hepatic glucose production by an α-adrenergic, cAMP-independent mechanism. More recent work has amply confirmed this conclusion and shown, in addition, that either vasopressin or angiotensin II stimulates hepatic glucose

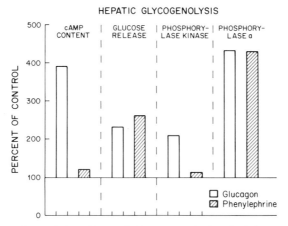

Figure 7.5 Comparison of the effects of glucagon and phenylephrine on cAMP content, glucose release, phosphorylase kinase activity, and phosphorylase a content in liver. Note that in spite of the fact that the two agents cause similar increases in phosphorylase a content and glucose release, they have quite different effects on cAMP content and phosphorylase kinase (the phosphorylated form) content. Replotted from Cherrington et al. (1976).

production by a cAMP-independent mechanism (Birnbaum and Fain, 1977; Van de Werve et al., 1977; Assimacopoulos-Jeannet et al., 1977; Keppens et al., 1977; Exton, 1979; Hutson et al., 1976; Kneer, N. M. et al., 1979; Chan and Exton, 1978; Garrison and Borland, 1979; Jakob and Deem, 1976; Parisa et al., 1977; LeCann and Freychet, 1978; Chen et al., 1978; Shimazu and Amakawa, 1975; Keppens and de Wulf, 1979; Keppens and de Wulf, 1976, 1979; Garrison et al., 1979; Garrison, 1978).

Either angiotensin II, vasopressin, or α-adrenergic agonists increase the rate of hepatic glycogenolysis and gluconeogenesis. Their effects depend upon the calcium concentration in the external medium. In the absence of external calcium, they do not stimulate glucose production (Chan and Exton, 1977; Van de Werve et al., 1977; Keppens et al., 1977). Each of these hormones increases the uptake of calcium into hepatic cells (Figure 7.6) (Keppens et al., 1977; Foden and Randle, 1978; Assimacopoulos-Jeannet, 1977; Chen et al., 1978). These facts would suggest that the hormones cause a rise in the cytosolic Ca^{2+} concentration primarily by increasing the rate of entry of calcium into the cell across the plasma membrane. Consistent with this view are the facts that angiotensin, vasopressin, and adrenaline all stimulate phosphoinositide turnover in liver cells (Billah and Michell, 1979), but glucagon and A23187 do not. Also, A23187, a divalent cation ionophore, produces a calcium-dependent stimulation of glycogenolysis. However, there are other data showing that these same hormones also increase calcium efflux from a subcellular pool (Blackmore et al., 1979a,b; Exton, 1979; Chen et al., 1978; Babcock et al., 1979; Pogglioli et al., 1980), so it is possible that their effects on hepatic cell calcium metabolism are more complex than simply increasing a calcium entry step.

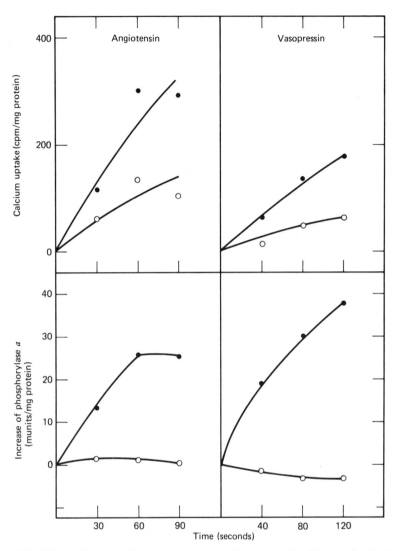

Figure 7.6 Effect of angiotensin or vasopressin on the uptake of calcium and activation of phosphorylase in hepatic cells: (○) control; (●) hormone-stimulated cells. From Keppens et al. (1977), with permission.

The studies of Chen et al. (1978) and Blackmore et al. (1979) have shown that the hormone causes a net release of cellular calcium when the cells are incubated in a calcium-free medium and that the intracellular calcium pool being mobilized is the mitochondrial pool. In contrast, Foden and Randle (1978) reported that phenylephrine caused an increase in cellular and mitochondrial calcium in cells incubated in the presence of calcium. Also, Pogglioli et al. (1980) have shown that, when studying the time course of the α-agonist effect on cellular calcium metabolism, the hormones caused an initial rise in cytosolic calcium and an increase in calcium uptake into mitochondria, and an increase in the efflux of calcium from the cell as well as an increased calcium influx into the cell. These authors concluded that the endoplasmic reticulum was the possible source of the intracellular calcium mobilized by phenylephrine. Complicating any simple interpretation is the finding of Chan and Exton (1977) that when hepatocytes are incubated in calcium-free media and then exposed to phenylephrine, there is a rise in the cAMP content of the cells, indicating that α-agonists can activate the adenylate cyclase under these conditions. It is thus possible that under some experimental conditions the calcium efflux seen is a consequence of the cAMP message. For the present, it appears safe to conclude that phenylephrine increases calcium uptake across the plasma membrane and that it also probably causes the mobilization of calcium from the endoplasmic reticulum. In contrast, the present evidence favors the view that glucagon causes the mobilization of calcium from the mitochondrial pool, an effect mediated by cAMP (see also Randle et al., 1979).

Another line of evidence that supports a coupling between hormone action and the calcium messenger system is the demonstration that phenylephrine, vasopressin, and angiotensin stimulate phosphatidylinositol (PI) breakdown (see Chapter 3 for a discussion of the relationship of this metabolic event to the calcium system) in rat hepatocytes, but glucagon does not (DeTorrentigiu and Berthet, 1977; Billah and Michell, 1979; Michell, 1975; Tolbert et al., 1980; Kirk et al., 1977). Three lines of evidence suggest that this change is receptor mediated and not a consequence of a rise in cytosolic calcium ion concentration: (1) A23187 does not stimulate PI turnover even though it enhances hepatic glycogenolysis; (2) vasopressin, angiotensin, and phenylephrine stimulate PI turnover even in cells incubated in calcium-free media; and (3) α-adrenergic antagonists block the effect of phenylephrine but not that of either vasopressin or angiotensin on PI turnover.

As noted previously, it is still not clear how this change in PI turnover is involved in the calcium messenger system. The most attractive hypothesis (Michell, 1975) is that changes in membrane PI structure are responsible for the gating in the calcium channel. This remains to be established. Recently, Nishizuka and coworkers (Kishimoto et al., 1977; Nishizuka et al., 1978, 1979; Takai et al., 1980) have suggested an alternative function. They discovered a calcium-dependent protein kinase in the cell cytosol which is activated by diacylglycerol. Reference to Figure 3.10 shows that diacylglycerol is the major product of PI hydrolysis, hence it is generated following a receptor-mediated stimulation of PI turnover. Nishizuka suggests that diacylglycerol may serve a messenger function and may specifically increase the sensitivity of a specific protein kinase to activation by calcium (another possible example of sensitivity modulation, see Chapter 3).

A different way of assessing the messenger role of Ca^{2+} is that of searching for cellular events normally thought to be mediated by a rise in the cytosolic Ca^{2+} concentration. One such event is an efflux of K^+. A hormonally mediated increase in K$^+$ efflux is seen in liver cells after treatment with either vasopressin, angiotensin, phenylephrine, *or glucagon* (Weiss and Putney, 1978) and causes an increase in membrane potential (Hayslett and Jenkinson, 1969; Friedmann and Dambach, 1978). The change in K$^+$ permeability induced by either angiotensin or phenylephrine has been found to be calcium dependent. Weiss and Putney (1978) propose that these agents have two effects on the calcium metabolism of the plasma membrane: they cause an immediate release of Ca^{2+} from binding sites on the membrane, and they alter the permeability of (open a gate in) a calcium channel. These calcium-mediated changes in K$^+$ efflux have been taken as further evidence that each of these three hormones causes a rise in the Ca^{2+} content of the cell cytosol, a conclusion consistent with the proposed second messenger role of calcium in their action.

A different approach to defining the messenger role of calcium in hormone action has recently been developed by Murphy et al. (1980). They exposed isolated hepatic cells to low concentrations of digitonin that were sufficient to increase the calcium permeability of the plasma membrane. These cells were then incubated in media containing a calcium buffering system which fixed the free calcium concentration at different values. They then determined the change in Ca^{2+} concentration in the medium using the calcium-sensitive indicator Arsenazo III. The calcium concentration at which free calcium concentration did not change upon addition of cells (exposed to digitonin) was taken as a measure of the cytosolic Ca^{2+} concentration. This value was reported to be approximately 0.2 μM in resting cells, to rise to approximately 0.5 μM upon treatment of the cells with phenylephrine, but not to change when the cells were treated with glucagon. These results are consistent with the conclusion that phenylephrine activates the calcium messenger system and that glucagon does not.

This conclusion leaves unexplained the fact that glucagon also causes an increased K$^+$ efflux and a hyperpolarization of the plasma membrane (Friedmann and Park, 1968; Friedmann and Rasmussen, 1970; Friedmann and Dambach, 1973, 1980) even though it does not stimulate calcium influx or PI turnover. There is no question that on the basis of the available data, one must conclude that cAMP is the major intracellular messenger in the action of glucagon. Nonetheless, glucagon alters cellular calcium metabolism (Friedmann and Park, 1968; Friedmann and Rasmussen, 1970; Foden and Randle, 1978; Chen et al., 1978; Waltenbaugh et al., 1978; Bygrave and Tranter, 1978; Waltenbaugh and Friedmann, 1978; Randle et al., 1979). Most of the evidence indicates that glucagon does not stimulate calcium uptake into liver cells nor that extracellular calcium is required for its action (but see Keppens et al., 1977; Assimacopoulos-Jeannet, 1977), but that it may stimulate the release of calcium from mitochondria and its uptake by microsomes. The current consensus is that the glucagon-induced alterations in hepatic cell calcium metabolism are a consequence of the action of intracellular cAMP. This conclusion is based in large part on the fact that exogenous cAMP mimics the effect of glucagon on cellular calcium metabolism. The question that remains a matter of debate is whether the postulated mobilization of calcium from mitochondria to cytosol and/or the stimulation of calcium uptake by the microsomes play a significant messenger role in the action of glucagon.

Reinhart et al. (1980) showed that trifluoperazine, a drug thought to act by blocking calcium–calmodulin-mediated intracellular events, blocked the effects of phenylephrine on hepatic glucose production but did not influence the action of glucagon. It appears likely that a rise in cytosolic Ca^{2+} concentration, if it does occur after glucagon action, does not play a significant immediate role in coupling stimulus to response. Conversely, the results of Reinhart et al. (1980) lend further support to the conclusion that calcium plays a major messenger role in the action of phenylephrine.

Redox Control and Membrane Potential

The preceding discussion leaves unresolved an intriguing aspect of the control of hepatic cell metabolism—that of the relationship between changes in membrane potential and in metabolism. Since changes in membrane potential are the result of changes in ion fluxes across the plasma membrane, the question really is how or if changes in ion fluxes across the plasma membrane participate in metabolic regulation. The question arises largely as a result of the work of Friedmann and her associates (Friedmann and Park, 1968; Friedmann and Rasmussen, 1970; Friedmann et al., 1971; Friedmann and Dambach, 1973, 1980). They found that following the administration of either glucagon or exogenous cAMP to the isolated, perfused liver, an efflux of K^+ and Ca^{2+} from and an influx of Na^+ into the cell occurred (Figure 7.7) as well as a change in perfusate pH. These changes were associated with a hyperpolarization of the plasma membrane (see also Haylett and Jenkinson, 1969). The question of interest is whether the change in membrane potential is coupled in any way to the change in metabolic events or is merely a reflection of a change in the metabolic activity of the cell.

Friedmann and Dambach (1980) approached this problem by analyzing the effect of agents known to alter membrane potential on the rate of hepatic glucose production. They found a close correlation between the measured membrane potential and the rate of glucose production. In particular, in confirmation of earlier work by Tolbert and Fain (1974), they showed that perfusion of the liver with low doses of valinomysin stimulated gluconeogenesis and caused a hyperpolarization of the plasma membrane. The only known effect of this agent is that of increasing the K^+ permeability of biological membranes. The mechanism by which valinomycin stimulates hepatic glucose production remains to be determined. However, a possible lead is the discovery by Clark and Jarrett (1978) that the redox potential in the cell regulates the activity of a membrane-bound phosphodiesterase. The rate of cAMP hydrolysis by this enzyme is a function of the NADH concentration (or the NADH/NAD).

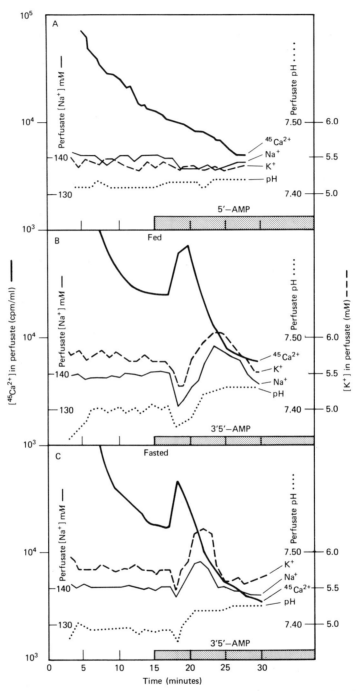

Figure 7.7 Efflux of labeled Ca²⁺, Na⁺, and K⁺ and changes in pH from isolated perfused liver in response to 5'AMP (no significant change) (A) and in response to exogenous cAMP in livers from fed (B) and fasted rats (C). From Friedmann and Dambach 1973, with permission.

The link that is missing at present is that between the redox potential in the cell and the membrane potential across the plasma membrane. However, recent studies by Crane and coworkers (Goldenberg et al., 1978; Low et al., 1978; Low and Crane, 1976; 1978; Crane and Low, 1978) have shown that the plasma membranes of many cells contain a NADH dehydrogenase activity. Also, in the case of the beta cell in the endocrine pancreas (see Chapter 6), it has been found that the redox potential controls the permeability of a K^+ channel in the membrane. Hence, it is quite possible that there is an important dialogue between membrane ion channels and metabolic processes. More work is necessary to understand this dialogue.

The Molecular Basis of Convergence

Accepting for the present that catecholamines, vasopressin, and angiotensin II activate hepatic metabolism via a rise in the calcium ion concentration in the cell cytosol and glucagon via a rise in cAMP concentration, the question that arises is the mechanism by which the increased Ca^{2+} concentration alters cell metabolism and whether this is in any way similar to that observed in the case of glucagon acting via the cAMP messenger system.

Hepatic carbohydrate metabolism appears to be regulated at the same control points whether Ca^{2+} or cAMP is messenger. These control points are (1) phosphorylase b (Sherline et al., 1972; Van de Werve, 1977; Hutson et al., 1976; Keppens and de Wulf, 1976); (2) glycogen synthase (Hutson et al., 1976); (3) pyruvate kinase (Taunton et al., 1974; Chan and Exton, 1978; Stifel et al., 1974; Garrison and Borland, 1979); and (4) mitochondrial pyruvate carboxylation (Foldes and Barrett, 1977; Garrison and Haynes, 1975; Garrison and Borland, 1979; Kneer et al., 1979).

In attempting to define the molecular basis by which these extracellular stimuli control the activities of these enzymes, Garrison (1979) compared the effects of glucagon and catecholamines upon the incorporation of radioactive phosphate into cytosolic proteins (presumed to be the result of hormone-mediated kinase activation) from intact rat hepatocytes treated with different hormones. Treatment of these cells with glucagon or exogenous cyclic AMP increased the extent of phosphorylation of 12 separate protein bands when the cytosolic proteins were separated by slab gel electrophoresis (Figure 7.8). Treatment of similar cells with norepinephrine, in the presence of β-antagonist to block cyclase activation led to an increase in the phosphorylation of 11 of the same 12 proteins phosphorylated after glucagon. The twelfth protein, the one not phosphorylated, was phosphorylase b kinase. The phosphorylation of these 11 proteins in response to catecholamine was abolished by removal of Ca^{2+} from the external medium, but their phosphorylation in response to glucagon was not altered if the calcium content of the medium was decreased. Hence, the same proteins undergo phosphorylation in response to either the calcium or the cAMP message.

It is not yet known if the same protein kinase is regulated by either Ca^{2+} or

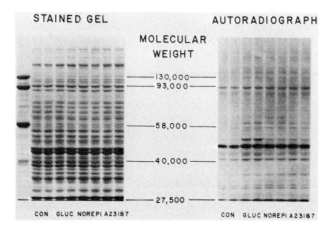

STAINED GEL   AUTORADIOGRAPH

MOLECULAR
WEIGHT

————130,000————
————93,000————

————58,000————

————40,000————

————27,500————

CON GLUC NOREPI A23187   CON GLUC NOREPI A23187

Figure 7.8 Pattern of phosphate incorporation into cytosolic proteins of liver after control (ion), glucagon (gluc), norepinephrine (norepi), or ionophore (A23187) treatment. On the left, the pattern of proteins separated by slab-gel electrophoresis; on the right, an autoradiograph indicating regions (brands) of incorporation of ^{32}P into protein. From Garrison (1978), with permission.

cAMP or whether there are separate cAMP- and Ca^{2+}-dependent kinases. However, in view of the report by Schulman and Greengard (1978a,b) that a distinct calmodulin–calcium-activated protein kinase is present in many tissues and that in other systems it has been found that the same protein can serve as substrate for either a cAMP-dependent or calcium-dependent protein kinase, it is quite likely that Ca^{2+} and cAMP act via separate protein kinases which utilize the same cytosolic proteins as substrates. This conclusion is consistent with the evidence obtained by Cohen (1978) and Roach et al. (1978) showing that the same protein, glycogen synthase, can serve as substrate for three different protein kinases and that when it does so, it is phosphorylated at different sites (see Chapter 4). Furthermore, phosphorylation at each site has a different effect upon phosphoprotein function.

A likely explanation for the greater inhibition of pyruvate kinase by glucagon as compared to phenylephrine is that cAMP-dependent protein kinase leads to phosphorylation of a site on the enzyme that has a more marked effect upon its function then does the phosphorylation of a different site by a calcium-dependent protein kinase.

Conclusion

The model (Figure 7.9) that emerges from this discussion of the hormonal control of hepatic glucose metabolism is one in which *redundant control* is exerted by separate messengers activating, respectively, the calcium and cAMP limbs of the synarchic system. An increase in concentration of either messenger within the cell leads to a stimulation of glycogenolysis and gluconeogenesis by controlling virtually the same metabolic steps by the same mechanism—phosphorylation of the regulated proteins.

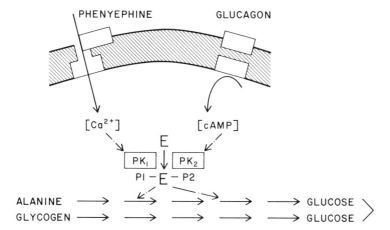

Figure 7.9 Model of redundant control of hepatic glucose metabolism by phenylephrine and glucagon. When phenylephrine interacts with its specific surface receptor, the immediate consequence is a rise in Ca^{2+} concentration, $[Ca^{2+}]$, of the cell cytosol. This rise in $[Ca^{2+}]$ leads to an activation of a calcium-dependent protein kinase PK_1, which in turn catalyzes the phosphorylation (Pl-E) of several different enzymes in both the gluconeogenic (alanine → glucose) and glycogenolytic (glucogen → glucose) pathways. As a result of these phosphorylations, the activities of these enzymes are modified so that glucose production in each pathway is enhanced. When glucagon interacts with its surface receptor, the immediate consequence is a rise in the cyclic AMP concentration, [cAMP], of the cell cytosol. This rise in [cAMP] leads to an activation of a cAMP-dependent protein kinase PK_2, which in turn catalyzes the phosphorylation (E-P2) of the same enzymes (but at different sites E-P2 vs Pl-E). As a result, glucose production in each pathway is enhanced.

FLUID ABSORPTION AND SECRETION IN THE SMALL INTESTINE

One of the most characteristic properties of epithelia, ranging from frog skin and rabbit cornea to seminal vesicles and the various segments of the gastrointestinal tract, is that of the absorption and/or secretion of fluids and electrolytes. This net transfer of fluid and electrolytes is possible because of the polar nature of the cells lining these tissues. As in many other tissues, regulation of these highly specialized functions is under neural and hormonal control and, as is so often the case, these controls involve cAMP and Ca^{2+} as second messengers.

Two aspects of epithelia transport need consideration before discussing the control of absorptive and secretory activities. The first is the categorization of epithelia as either loose or tight. The second aspect is the question of whether the same or different cell types are responsible for the absorptive and secretory activities of an intact tissue, such as the small intestine, possessing both attributes.

In general, epithelia have been classified as tight or loose on the basis of their electrical and absorptive properties. The basis of this distinction rests upon a difference in the rate of paracellular fluid and electrolyte transport. In tight epithelia, there is practically no fluid or electrolyte transport between cells, hence any net transport of fluid and/or electrolyte takes place via a transcellular pathway. An example of this type of epithelium is the toad bladder. A model of the mechanisms of ion and H_2O movement and their hormonal controls in this tissue has been discussed (see Chapter 4). In contrast, in loose epithelia, even though the driving force for net fluid and electrolyte absorption depends upon the transport properties of the membrane, a significant part of the fluid and electrolyte that moves across the tissue does so by moving between the cells via the so-called paracellular pathway.

Normally, cells in both types of epithelia are bound one to another by specific sites, tight junctions, on their lateral surfaces. Hence, the determinant of the looseness of the particular epithelium is the permeability properties of these tight junctions between the cells. In the toad bladder, these junctions are essentially impermeable to either Na^+ or H_2O; but in the mammalian small intestine, they are quite permeable to H_2O, somewhat permeable to Na^+, and relatively impermeable to Cl^-.

One of the most dramatic changes in cell behavior is that exhibited by the mammalian small intestine. Under basal conditions, there is a net flow of fluids and electrolytes from mucosa to serosa, that is, fluid and electrolyte absorption takes place. However, after treatment with a variety of gastrointestinal hormones, neurotransmitters, drugs, or cholera toxin, the net flux of fluid and electrolytes is reversed and secretion is observed. Two schools of thought exist regarding the means by which this reversal of flow is achieved. Field (1974) proposes that absorption and secretion are respective properties of the cell on the villus tips and those in the villus crypts. In this case, secretagogues are thought to act upon both types of cells, inhibiting absorption in the first type and stimulating secretion in the second cell type. Others (Holman and Naflatin, 1979) believe that there is no anatomical separation of these processes and that secretagogues induce absorptive cells to become secretory cells. On the basis of recent evidence (Naflatin and Simmons, 1979), the latter hypothesis appears the more likely.

Largely from the work of Frizzel, Schultz, and their associates (Frizzel and Schultz, 1972; Nellans et al., 1973, 1974; Frizzel et al., 1975a, 1976, 1979; Schultz and Zalusky, 1964a,b), Naflatin, Holman, and Simmons (Holman and Naflatin, 1975a,b, 1976, 1979; Naflatin and Simmons, 1979; Simmons and Naflatin, 1976a,b; Holman et al., 1979), Powell (Powell, 1974; Powell et al., 1972, 1973), and Field (Bolton, 1971, 1974; Field et al., 1972, 1978), the basic aspects of intestinal fluid and electrolyte transport have been defined. Under nonstimulated conditions, there is net absorption of H_2O, Na^+, and Cl^-. Based upon earlier studies of fluid and electrolyte absorption in the gall bladder (Diamond, 1962, 1964; Wheeler, 1963; Dietschy, 1965; Os and Sleegers, 1971; Frizzel et al., 1975b), it has been shown that there is a coupled entry of Na^+ and Cl^- across the luminal cell membrane in both tissues. This conclusion is based upon the facts that (a) replacement of mucosal Na^+ with a nonabsorbed cation blocks active Cl^- absorption; (b) replacement of mucosal Cl^- with a nonabsorbed anion reduces active Na^+ transport without a change in transepithelial potential difference; (c) active absorption of both Cl^- and Na^+ is inhibited in a tissue treated with ouabain; (d) measurements of the unidirectional flux of either Na^+ or Cl^- across the luminal membrane indicate their obligatory one-for-one coupling; and (e) replacement of Cl^- with a nonabsorbed anion does not alter the potential across the mucosal membrane. Thus, the Na^+ gradient existing across the mucosal membrane serves as the driving force for the active uptake of Cl^- into the cell against its electrochemical gradient. This type of Na^+ gradient-dependent transport is called secondary active transport, to distinguish it from primary active transport in which ATP serves as the immediate source of energy for the movement of the transported species against an electrochemical gradient. Direct support for this concept comes from the recent studies of Duffey et al. (1978) in which they demonstrated that the intracellular activity of Cl^- was two to three times higher than that predicted from the Nernst equation for a passively distributed anion when Na^+ was present but was the predicted value when Na^+ was absent from the incubation media.

Having entered the cell by secondary active transport, Cl^- leaves the cell across the basolateral membrane by passive processes driven by the electrochemical potential across the membrane. In contrast, Na^+ leaves the cell by a ouabain-sensitive Na^+ pump. The activity of this pump is essential for maintaining a low intracellular Na^+ and thereby the electrochemical gradient across the mucosal membrane. When the serosal pump is blocked, this mucosal gradient is dissipated and Cl^- entry as well as active Na^+ transport are abolished. Hence, the NaCl present in the lateral intercellular spaces exerts an osmotic pressure across the tight junction which serves as the driving force for fluid movement across the tissue.

The model one can construct to account for fluid and electrolyte movement during the absorption of fluid and electrolyte across the small intestine (Figure 7.10) has four critical components: (1) coupled Na^- and Cl^- entry across the luminal membrane; (2) a very low Cl^- permeability of the luminal membrane so that Cl^- which enters across the mucosal cell face does not exist passively back into the mucosal fluid; (3) a Na^+ pump on the basolateral membrane; and (4) a permselective tight junction which in conjunction with a local increase in Na^+ concentration within the lateral intercellular space determines the magnitude of fluid flow via the paracellular pathway.

An increasing number of agents have been shown to stimulate electrolyte and fluid secretion in the small intestine (Bolton and Field, 1977; Field et al., 1972, 1978; Sheerin and Field, 1975; Desjeux et al., 1976; Hendrix and Paulk, 1977; Powell et al., 1972, 1973; Nellans et al., 1973, 1974; Simmons and Naflatin, 1976a,b) as well as in the mammalian colon (Phillips and Schmalz, 1970; Turnberg, 1970; Edmonds and Marroth, 1968; Schultz et al., 1977; Frizzel et al., 1976; Binder and Rawlins, 1973a,b; Frizzel, 1977; Kimberg et al., 1971; Schwartz et al., 1974). This latter tissue responds with a secretory

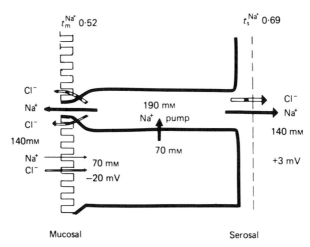

Figure 7.10 Model of the cellular and paracellular pathways of fluid movement in the intestinal mucosa with the Na$^+$ concentration in the respective compartments.

response similar to that seen in the small intestine in that the basic process stimulated is an electronic chloride secretion. The agents include cholinergic neural stimulation, gastrointestinal hormones, enterotoxins, prostaglandins, cholera toxin, serotonin, bile acids, theophylline, calcium ionophore, cAMP, and vasoactive intestinal peptide. Addition of these agents to the small intestine converts this epithelium from an absorptive to a secretory organ. There is an increased electrogenic chloride secretion. This electrogenic chloride secretion is Na$^+$ dependent, ouabain inhibitable, and furosemide inhibitable. It is also inhibited by triaminopyrimidine, an agent thought to convert leaky intercellular junctions into tight ones (Moreno, 1975). The effects of the secretagogues upon transcellular fluxes of Na$^+$ and Cl$^-$ depend upon a number of circumstances; but under short circuit conditions, a decrease in mucosal to serosal flux of both ions and a increase in the serosal to mucosal flux of Cl$^-$ is seen.

Some of the agents that regulate intestinal secretion, for example, cholera toxin and theophylline, are thought to act primarily via the cAMP messenger system, and others, for example, serotonin and prostaglandins, via the calcium system. Studies with agents that act via the cAMP system or with exogenous cAMP, itself, have been more extensive than those with agents acting via the calcium messenger system. For this reason, the mechanism of cAMP action in this tissue will be considered first and in more detail than the mechanism of calcium action.

The change in electrogenic chloride secretion seen after either administration of cholera toxin, theophylline, or exogenous cAMP has been attributed to a change in the Cl$^-$ permeability of the luminal membrane. This conclusion is based upon the following facts: (1) These agents increase electrogenic Cl$^-$ secretion. (2) These agents increase the rate of Cl$^-$ exchange across the luminal membrane even when Cl$^-$ secretion is inhibited by ouabain (Candia et al., 1977; Cuthbert et al., 1969; Hendrix and Paulk, 1977). (3) When theophylline is added to the isolated tissue incubated with ouabain in the serosal medium to inhibit the basolateral Na^+ pump, and hypertonic saline is added to the mucosal medium, an increase in fluid absorption is seen presumably because under these conditions Cl^- enters the cell down its concentration gradient. (4) Triaminopyrimidine, an agent that blocks paracellular Na^+ and H_2O fluxes, inhibits the secretory effect of theophylline.

As noted above, there is a difference of opinion as to whether this change is induced in all mucosal cells lining the intestinal villus or only in a selected population in the clefts of the villi (Field, 1971; Hendrix and Paulk, 1977; Holman and Naflatin, 1979; Naflatin and Simmons, 1979; Holman et al., 1979). Regardless of this controversy, all authors agree that a single change in the Cl^- conductance of the luminal membrane can account for (a) active NaCl secretion; (b) electrogenic Cl^- secretion; (c) an increase in the short circuit current after cAMP action; and (d) an initial increase in the transepithelial conductance of the tissue. In this model, a primary increase in Cl^- permeability leads to a leak of Cl^- out of the cell. This generates a negative transepithelial potential (serosal side positive) that acts as a driving force for the movement of Na^+ from the serosal to the mucosal solution via the paracellular pathway (Figure 7.10).

Although less thoroughly studied, a role of Ca^{2+} in the control of intestinal secretion is also evident. The calcium ionophore A23187 produces a calcium-dependent increase in fluid and electrolyte secretion in the intestine qualitatively similar to that seen after cAMP (Bolton and Field, 1977). These changes are observed even though the ionophore does not cause an increase in the tissue cAMP content. A similar ionophore-induced secretory response is seen in the rabbit colon (Frizzel, 1977). Bolton and Field (1977) have also observed that both carbamylcholine and serotonin (neurotransmitters) stimulate Cl^- secretion in the ileum without causing a change in tissue cAMP content. On the other hand, their effects are dependent upon the presence of extracellular calcium.

These results are consistent with one of several models. It is possible that in this tissue, as in the liver, the final event which mediates the change in mucosal Cl^- permeability is the phosphorylation of a membrane protein and that this protein is a substrate for both a cAMP- and a Ca^{2+}-dependent protein kinase. Alternatively, it is possible that either cAMP or Ca^{2+} is the final mediator and that the other messenger alters its content or the sensitivity of its receptor elements within the cell.

Some data suggest that calcium may be the final mediator and that it acts via calmodulin. First, although as noted above, calcium does not appear to alter cAMP content of the mucosal cell, cAMP stimulates the efflux of calcium from prelabeled cells (Frizzel, 1977); and by analogy with the situation in other tissues, this may reflect the mobilization of an intracellular pool of calcium and a consequent increase in the calcium ion content of the cell cytosol. Second, Holmgren et al. (1978) and Hamilton and Hamilton

(1978) showed that phenothiazines, known to bind to calmodulin and to inhibit its action (Levin and Weiss, 1976), block the increase in intestinal fluid secretion caused by the calcium ionophore A23187. Third, Ilundain and Naflatin (1979) have shown that trifluoperazine (Stelazine) also blocks the effects of theophylline and choleratoxin on Cl⁻ permeability but does not block their effect upon tissue cAMP content. Based on the previous observations of Levin and Weiss (1976) and Fretel and Weiss (1976) that the binding of calcium to calmodulin leads to an increase in the affinity of calmodulin for Stelazine, Ilundain and Naflatin (1979) examined the effect of ionophore, choleragen, and theophylline on the uptake of [³H]Stelazine into intestinal mucosal cells and correlated this uptake with changes in secretory rate. They found that Stelazine blocked the action of both ionophore and cholera toxin, and that under these conditions both extracellular stimuli induced an increase in the uptake of Stelazine. They interpreted this result to mean that an increase in the content of the Ca²⁺–calmodulin complex was an event common to the action of both classes of secretagogues.

A model consistent with the available data is presented in Figure 7.11. Just as in adrenal glomerulosa and hepatocyte, so in the intestinal mucosal cell there is evidence for redundant control of specialized cell function by separate activation of the two limbs of the synarchic system by distinctly different extracellular stimuli. In contrast to the other two systems, in which both limbs are controlled by hormones, in the intestine the cAMP limb is con-

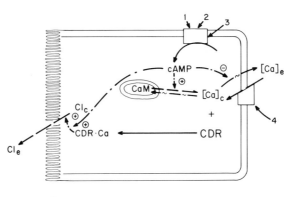

(1) INTESTINAL PEPTIDES
(2) OTHER MESSENGERS
(3) CHOLERA TOXIN
(4) CALCIUM IONOPHORE

Figure 7.11   Model of the interrelated roles of cAMP and calcium in the regulation of intestinal fluid secretion. In this model, the major change in the intestinal mucosal cell is an increase in the permeability of the luminal membrane of the cell (left). This change can be induced either by agents (1–3) that activate adenylate cyclase, or those that increase calcium entry into the cell (4). The final common mediator of the Cl- permeability change may be Ca·CDR (the calcium–calmodulin complex). The action of cAMP may involve a change in the sensitivity of the system to CDR·Ca and/or a mobilization of calcium from in intracellular pool.

trolled hormonally and the Ca^{2+} limb, neurally. Also, in terms of the site of convergence of information flow of the two limbs, there also appears to be a difference. In the case of the liver, convergence is at the level of protein phosphorylation; in the case of the intestinal cell, it may well be at the level of the Ca^{2+}–calmodulin complex. However, considerably more data are needed before this conclusion is accepted. Nonetheless, two conclusions of general significance arise from this discussion. The first is that redundant control can involve the nervous as well as the endocrine system, and the second is that the molecular site of convergence of information flow within the cell may be different in different tissues exhibiting redundant control.

CONCLUSION

Redundancy of control obviously confers considerable physiological regulatory plasticity at the organismal level. We might, therefore, expect that the types of cellular responses controlled in this way would be of great survival value to the organism. In the case of the adrenal glomerulosa, the essence of survival can be related to the critical role of its product, aldosterone, in regulating bodily Na^+ content. Maintenance of total body Na^+ and K^+ is one of the most necessary requirements for the survival of the terrestrial animal. Any number of changes—hemorrhage, diarrhea, lack of Na^+ uptake—can threaten the organism with Na^+ depletion. Survival depends on a prompt increase in Na^+ retention by kidney and intestine. Given the diversity of changes that lead to the same potential consequence, a complex system of extracellular controls has evolved to ensure that regardless of the nature of the pathophysiological change—for example, a decrease in Na^+ concentration, a decrease in blood volume without a change in Na^+ concentration, an increase in K^+ concentration—the organism can respond appropriately. Hence, the plasticity in this control system is at the supracellular level, with the cellular response being stereotyped and redundant.

Another example of a metabolic response critical to the survival of the organism is that of hepatic glucose production. A sufficient supply of glucose is essential to the normal functioning of the brain. Under conditions of fasting, one can anticipate that any number of events, in addition to a fall in blood glucose concentration—for example, a decrease in cerebral blood flow—would lead to an enhanced output of glucose from the liver. This being likely, it is equally likely that different events are communicated to the liver by different extracellular signals. This is the case. Redundant control of hepatic glucose production by glucagon and a group of other hormones operates by controlling separate limbs of the synarchic pathway.

A similar type of redundant control appears to function in the regulation of intestinal fluid secretion, but the interactions of the two limbs are less clearly defined than in the first two systems, and the survival value of this particular response is equally unclear.

Antagonistic Control

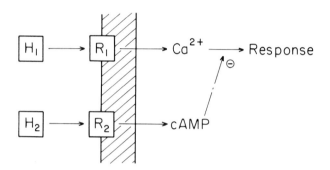

INTRODUCTION

Up to this point in nearly all the systems discussed, cAMP and calcium have acted in either a coordinate or supplementary fashion in mediating the responses of specific cells to one or more extracellular messengers. However, given the number of components in each messenger system and the varied interrelationships between the two systems, it is not surprising that during evolution these interactions have in some tissues led to antagonistic or opposing effects. One can anticipate that, just as in extracellular control systems in which antagonistic controls operate, there is no direct antagonism between the opposing hormones; so in the case of the intracellular effects of calcium and cAMP, it is unlikely that cAMP directly antagonizes the action of calcium. More likely, cAMP acts to alter either the domain of the calcium message or the sensitivity of various response elements to calcium, just as it does in the previously discussed coordinate control systems. Equally, calcium acts to alter either the domain of this cAMP message or the sensitivity of various response elements to cAMP.

Four systems in which antagonistic controls by the messenger systems are observed are (1) smooth muscle contraction, (2) platelet release reaction; (3) histamine release from mast cells; and (4) enzyme release from neutrophils. Each is discussed. In addition, the hormonal control of bone resorption by parathyroid hormone (PTH) and calcitonin (CT) is discussed as an example of a unique kind of antagonistic control in which two hormones with

256

opposing cellular effects both activate the cAMP messenger system. Finally, the role of cAMP in regulating postsynaptic events in the nervous system is discussed as another type of antagonistic control which is in some ways more complex and less well understood than the other examples but which is important in demonstrating again the essential organizational unity between the stimulus–response coupling in neural and endocrine systems.

SMOOTH MUSCLE CONTRACTION

It is now generally accepted that calcium is the coupling factor between excitation and contraction in all forms of muscle (Sandow, 1952; Ebashi, 1976; Bolton, 1979). However, in the case of smooth muscle, a controversy remains concerning the nature of the mechanism by which calcium exerts its effect (Ebashi et al., 1978; Ebashi, 1979; Aksoy et al., 1976; Bremel, 1974; Chacko et al., 1977; Carsten, 1971; Ebashi et al., 1975; Gorecka et al., 1976; Ito and Holta, 1976; Kendricks-Jones et al., 1970; Sobieszek, 1977; Szent-Gyorgyi et al., 1973). Ebashi and coworkers have presented evidence in isolated actomyosin preparation that a new calcium receptor protein, leiotonin, mediates a thin filament control of actomyosin ATPase and presumably, therefore, muscle contraction. On the other hand, work from several different laboratories has presented convincing evidence in favor of a thick filament (i.e., myosin) control of contraction (Szent-Gyorgyi, 1976; Collins, 1976a,b; Hitchcock and Kendrick-Jones, 1975; Horl et al., 1975). In particular, the specific phosphorylation of myosin light chains (MLC), a calcium–calmodulin-dependent myosin light chain kinase, has been correlated with changes in the strength of smooth muscle contraction. There is considerable evidence showing a correlation between the extent of phosphorylation of the light chain, its ATPase activity, and the strength of contraction (Sobieszek, 1977; Dabrowski et al., 1978a,b; Yagi et al., 1978; Waisman et al., 1975, 1978; Kerrick et al., 1980; Conti and Adelstein, 1980).

Studies employing ATPγS have provided additional evidence for thick filament control. The ATP analog ATPγS can serve as a substrate for myosin light chain kinase reaction (Sherry et al., 1978) and results in the thiophosphorylation of myosin light chain. This thiophosphorylated derivative shows ATPase activity but is resistant to dephosphorylation by phosphoprotein phosphatase (Figure 8.1). Using this tool, Hoar et al. (1979) and Cassidy et al. (1979) have examined the effect of calcium-dependent thiophosphorylation of myosin light chain in skinned smooth muscle fibers (avian gizzard, rabbit ileum). Incubation of the strips in the presence of ATPγS and calcium led to a calcium-mediated rise in tension which persisted upon removal of calcium (Figure 8.2). In contrast, when ATP was employed a similar calcium-mediated rise in tension was rapidly reversed upon removal of calcium. Correlated with this sustained tension was the persistent ^{35}S-labeling of the 20,000 M.W. myosin light chain LC_{20}. These results strongly support the concept that LC_{20} phosphorylation is a significant aspect of calcium-mediated tension development in smooth muscle.

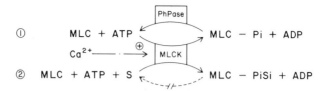

Figure 8.1 A comparison of the events relating to the phosphorylation of myosin light chain kinase (MLC) when ATP and ATPγS are employed as substrate. When either compound is substrate, myosin light chain kinase (MLCK) catalyzes the phosphorylation (MLCpPi) or thiophosphorylation (MLC-PiSi) of myosin light chain. However, the phosphoprotein phosphatase (PhPase) can catalyze the dephosphorylation of only MLC-Pi and not MLC-PiSi.

Barron et al. (1979) have examined the phosphorylation of pig aortic myosin under physiological conditions. They found a correlation between the increase in light chain phosphorylation and strength of contraction in aortic smooth muscle. This norepinephrine-induced contraction is not associated with an action potential (Shibata and Briggs, 1966) and is thought to result from a release of Ca^{2+} from the sarcoplasmic reticulum (SR) (Van Breeman et al., 1972, 1973). Both histamine and angiotensin also induce similar types of contraction, and Deth and Van Breeman (1977) have presented evidence that all three agonists activate the contractile system by a

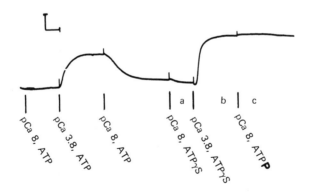

Figure 8.2 The contractile response of skinned smooth muscle to the sequential addition of solutions containing varying concentrations of calcium and ATP or ATPγS. Upon addition of ATP and 10^{-8} M calcium (pCa8), there is no contractile response. Addition of ATP plus $10^{-38}M$ calcium causes contraction, which is reversed by switching to a solution containing 10^{-8} M calcium. The addition of ATPγS caused no contraction in the presence of 10^{-8} M calcium (a) but a prompt contraction in the presence of $10^{-3.8}$ M calcium (b). This contraction was not reversed by exposure to 10^{-8} M calcium. From Kerrick et al. (1980), with permission.

calcium–calmodulin-mediated activation of myosin light chain kinase. Also, Hidaka et al. (1979) have found that psychotropic agents such as chlor- promazine produce relaxation of aortic smooth muscle presumably by inac- tivating a calmodulin-regulated process, because the one known biochemical action of these drugs is that of binding to calmodulin and blocking its action (Levin and Weiss, 1977).

In considering these contrasting hypotheses, a fact of considerable impor- tance is that many smooth muscles maintain some degree of tonus, that is, they are partially contracted, and agents that act on this tissue alter its state of tonus. In addition, oscillations in the extent of contraction can be superimposed upon this basal tonic state. Hence, the regulatory require- ments for smooth muscle are quite different than those for skeletal muscle. In light of these facts, it is possible that both types of calcium-mediated events, that is, thin and thick filament regulation, are components of the mechanism controlling the contractile process: one, leiotonin–calcium, to modulate the oscillatory cycles; the other, calmodulin–calcium–MLCK, to determine the level of tonus or basal contractile state.

From the point of view of our present discussion, the aspect of smooth muscle physiology of most immediate interest is the role of cAMP in regulat- ing these calcium-mediated processes. Before discussing this question, how- ever, it is essential to consider the messenger role of calcium and particularly the question of which pool of cellular and/or extracellular calcium contrib- uted to the messenger pool of calcium when smooth muscles contract. As reviewed by Somlyo and Somlyo (1968), and by Bolton (1979), there is no universal mechanism by which smooth muscle is activated. Receptor type varies, coupling of membrane potential to contraction varies, the source of calcium for contraction varies, and the responses to a host of drugs that alter either cellular calcium or cAMP metabolism differ. Given this complexity, it is not possible to develop a model universally applicable to all situations. However, there are a few rather general effects. For example, acetylcholine or α-adrenergic agonists usually cause muscle contraction (van Breeman et al., 1972), and β-agonists always cause relaxation.

In causing contraction, Ach or α-agonist may or may not produce mem- brane depolarization and an increase in the frequency of action potentials. In the case of aortic smooth muscle, for example, there is no significant change in action potential when norepinephrine induces contraction (Shibata and Briggs, 1966). The altered ion fluxes and ion permeabilities underlying these membrane phenomena cause an increased entry of calcium into the cell and/or an increased release of calcium from sarcoplasmic reticular stores (Figure 8.3) (van Breeman et al., 1973; Bolton, 1979). In different muscles, the relative importance of these two pools varies; and in the same muscle, the importance depends upon the concentration of agonist. As shown by Farley and Miles (1978), acetylcholine-induced contractions of dog tracheal smooth muscle depend upon different calcium pools as the dose of the agonist is increased. At low concentrations of Ach, extracellular calcium is

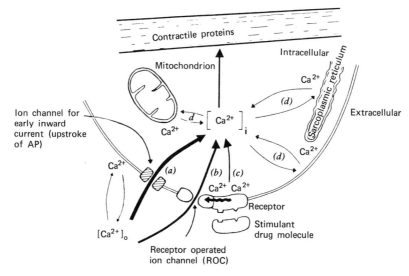

Figure 8.3 Pathways by which the intracellular calcium concentration, $[Ca^{2+}]i$, is raised in smooth muscle cells. Calcium may enter the cell by ion channels related to an action potential (a) or by receptor-operated channels (b or c). It may also arise from either (d) the plasma membrane, the sarcoplasmic reticulum, or the mitochondria. From Bolton (1979), with permission.

required, and the response is blocked by verapamil. At high concentrations, extracellular calcium is not required, and Ach induces a net efflux of calcium from the release of calcium from a tightly bound intracellular pool. The mechanism by which Ach effects this release is not known. These data imply that under physiological circumstances, small changes in Ach concentration alter the contractile state of the muscle primarily by altering the net influx of calcium across the plasma membrane of the cell, and large changes in Ach concentration lead to both altered plasma membrane flux and the motilization of an intracellular calcium pool, that is, the two pools of calcium serve complementary functions.

One of the more universal aspects of smooth muscle behavior is that β-adrenergic agonists nearly always cause muscle relaxation. In doing so, these agonists invariably cause an increase in the cAMP concentration within the cell. The presumption, based on considerable experimental information, is that cAMP is the relaxation messenger under these circumstances. From the foregoing discussion, it is clear that this relaxation must involve either an efflux of calcium from the cell, a redistribution of calcium within the cell, and/or a change in the sensitivity of one or more calcium response elements to calcium. There is evidence showing that each of these changes is produced by a rise in the cAMP content of the cell in some type of smooth muscle cell, but that they may not all occur in each type.

One way in which cAMP may function is that suggested by Scheid et al. (1979). They have shown in isolated smooth muscle cells from toad stomach that addition of isoproterenol leads to an inhibition of contraction associated with a rise in intracellular cAMP content, PK activity, and Phos a activity. A major additional effect is an increase in Na^+ efflux and K^+ influx brought about by activation of the Na^+/K^+ ATPase in the plasma membrane. On the basis of these findings, they proposed that relaxation is brought about by a change in the Na^+ gradient across the plasma membrane leading to an increase in Na^+–Ca^{2+} exchange (Brading, 1978) with a resultant fall in $[Ca^{2+}]_c$ and thus a decrease in the contractile state (Figure 8.4).

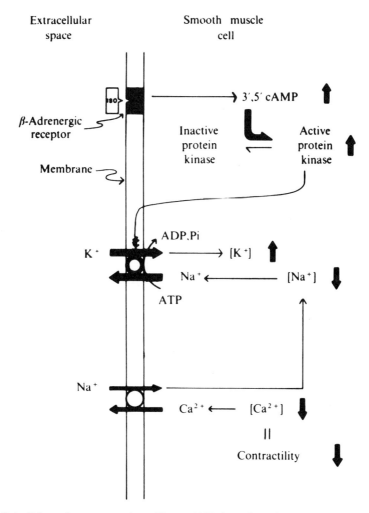

Figure 8.4 Schematic representation of how cAMP-dependent phosphorylation of a component of the Na^+/K^+ ATPase of the smooth muscle cell membrane induces an increase in intracellular Na^+, thereby increasing the exchange of intracellular Ca^{2+} for extracellular Na^+ and causing relaxation. From Scheid et al. (1979), with permission.

A second way in which cAMP may function is to alter intracellular calcium distribution. Support for this mechanism comes from the finding that addition of cAMP and protein kinase to isolated microsomal fractions (containing elements of the sarcoplasmic reticulum) from several different types of smooth muscle (Nishikori and Maeno, 1979; Webb and Bholla, 1976; Andersonn and Nilsson, 1972) leads to a phosphorylation of the membranes and a stimulation of calcium uptake by them (Figure 8.5). By this mechanism, β-agonists act to cause relaxation by inducing the reaccumulation of calcium previously released by this organelle. In this regard, Mueller and van Breeman (1979) have shown that in the smooth muscle of the taenia coli, contraction can be reversed by addition of 8-bromo-cAMP, phosphodiesterase inhibitors, or β-adrenergic agents and that this relaxation is not associated with an increase in the rate of calcium efflux from the cell. These results show that an inwardly directed Na^+ gradient (see above) is not absolutely essential for the relaxing effect of cAMP and suggest that either cAMP-dependent accumulation of calcium and/or alteration of the calcium sensitivity of myosin light chain kinase occur under these circumstances. Work by Casteelo and Raeymaekers (1979) supports this conclusion and indicates that β-agonist pretreatment increases the size of an intracellular calcium pool that participates in stimulus–response coupling.

The third and in some ways the most interesting way in which cAMP can alter smooth muscle contraction is by altering the sensitivity of a calcium response element to calcium. Adelstein et al. (1978, 1979) have shown that the cAMP-dependent protein kinase can use myosin light chain kinase (MLCK) as substrate, and that the phosphorylated MLCK catalyzes the phosphorylation of MLC at only half its normal rate. Following this lead, Silver et al. (1979) showed that the calcium-dependent phosphorylation of MLC in native bovine aortic actomyosin (DiSalvo et al., 1978) is decreased in the presence of cAMP and cAMP-dependent PK and that this decrease correlates with the cAMP-dependent phosphorylation of a 100,000 M.W. protein, the MLCK. Conti and Adelstein (1980) have shown that the phosphorylated MLCK is activated to a lesser extent by calmodulin than is the nonphosphorylated enzyme (Figure 8.6). These results indicate that by inducing the phosphorylation of MLCK, the cAMP-dependent protein kinase decreases the sensitivity of this enzyme to activation by calcium–calmodulin (Figure 8.7).

What emerges from these different lines of investigation is a composite picture of the mediator of relaxation, cAMP, acting at several sites within the cell to coordinate changes in calcium exchange across the plasma membrane with changes in intracellular calcium binding, and in the sensitivity of the cellular response elements to calcium—one more example of the integrative action of a second messenger within a particular cell type. It is very likely that the relative importance of these three cAMP-dependent processes in regulating the contractile state will vary from one type of smooth muscle to another. In some, all three may operate. In others, only one or two of the three mechanisms may be of importance.

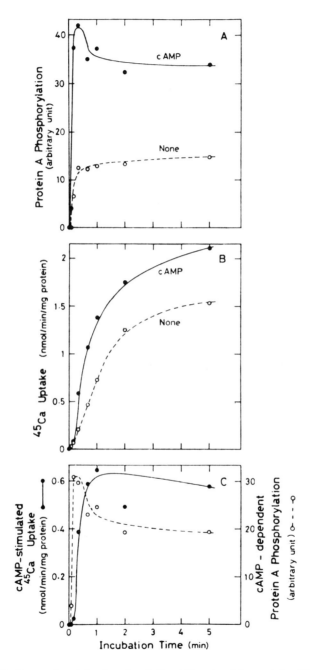

Figure 8.5 Time course of protein phosphorylation (A) and calcium uptake (B) in uterine muscle microsomes in the presence and absence of cAMP (10 μM). In C, plot of cAMP-dependent component of calcium uptake. From Nishikori and Maeno (1979), with permission.

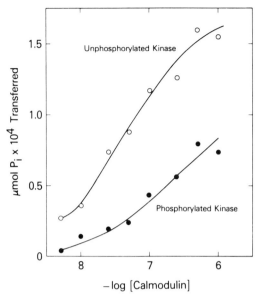

Figure 8.6 Titration curves of the myosin light chain kinase activity of unphosphorylated enzyme (○) and phosphorylated enzyme (●) agonist-log of calmodulin content (calcium ion was present). Note that phosphorylated MLCK is activated much less readily than the unphosphorylated enzyme. From Conti and Adelstein (1980), with permission.

This system of opposing controls of cell function mediated by the two separate messenger systems is of considerable interest because it seems to be at variance with the other systems in which calcium and cAMP act in complementary or coordinating fashion. The system most closely analogous, and seemingly therefore of greatest contrast, is the situation in the heart (see Chapter 9), in which cAMP appears to augment the physiological response induced by the calcium messenger system. However, closer comparison

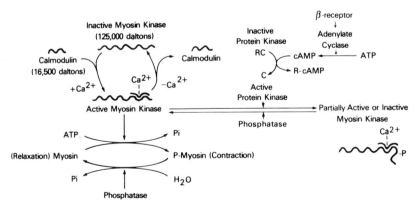

Figure 8.7 Schematic representation of the mechanisms by which cAMP and calcium regulate smooth muscle contraction. From Adelstein and Hathaway (1979), with permission.

reveals that three of the four effects seen in the smooth muscle are also seen in the heart: (1) a cAMP-dependent protein kinase phosphorylates a component of a calcium-regulatory protein complex; (2) cAMP enhances the activity of the Na^+/K^+ ATPase; and (3) cAMP enhances the uptake of calcium by the sarcoplasmic reticulum. The only additional effect of cAMP in the heart is that cAMP enhances calcium entry through the voltage-dependent calcium channel, and this apparently does not occur in most smooth muscles. In fact, in most smooth muscles, activation of the muscle cell by agonists leads to the opening of a receptor-operated rather than a voltage-dependent calcium channel. Voltage-dependent calcium entry is, therefore, not a component of the plasma membrane events when many smooth muscles are stimulated to contract. Thus, a minor variation in the nature of the components of the membrane response, plus a difference in organization of the response elements within the tissue, is sufficient to account for the quite striking difference in physiological behavior of these two types of muscle.

The most illustrative example of how the same biochemical effect can lead to quite different consequences is the cAMP-dependent stimulation of calcium uptake by the SR. This occurs in both organs, heart and smooth muscle, and in both it has the consequence of increasing the rate of relaxation. However, in the heart, because of its periodic behavior, the increase in calcium accumulation is essential in increasing the pool of calcium released at the next systole, and therefore in increasing the force of contraction of the organ in successive systoles.

The situation in smooth muscle, though standing in contrast to heart in terms of physiological consequence, affirms the major thesis we are discussing. The regulation of the specialized function of most cells by extracellular messengers depends on the interaction of the synarchic messengers, calcium and cAMP. It is the particular variations in these universal relationships that define the operational system that regulates function in specific cell types.

REGULATION OF PLATELET FUNCTION

The platelet plays a critical role in hemostasis (Baumgartner, 1972; Reimers et al., 1973; Walsh, 1974). After an injury to a blood vessel, there are a number of events which are integrated into a complex process responsible for the cessation of hemorrhage. These include contraction of the blood vessel, the formation of a platelet plug at the site of injury, initiation at this site of the coagulation cascade with the formation of a clot, and finally the retraction of this clot. The platelet obviously serves in the second of these steps but is also involved in both the third and fourth as well. The most immediate response of the platelets is that of adherence to the damaged vascular wall and to each other. This response involves both a change in cell surface properties and a change in cell shape.

Simultaneous with this response is a secretory response in which a variety of substances stored in secretory granules within the platelet are released from it by an exocytotic process similar to that seen in other secretory tissues. These released substances include ADP and serotonin, which facilitates platelet aggregation (a positive feed-forward control step), and a variety of substances, for example, fibrinogen and platelet factor 4, which promote clot formation and/or vasoconstriction. In addition, activated platelets are induced to synthesize prostaglandins, which act both as positive and negative feedback regulators of platelet function; and the platelet surface membrane change includes the appearance of platelet factor 3 on the platelet surface. This factor catalyzes the formation of thrombin, the critical initial step in the clotting cascade.

These various responses do not occur sequentially but in parallel (Holmsen, 1975; and Holmsen et al., 1969) and together are known as the "release reaction." This release reaction can be initiated by a large number of different agents: thrombin, ADP, collagen, serotonin, epinephrine, arachidonic acid, and the calcium ionophore A23187 (Mustard and Pachham, 1970; Feinstein and Fraser, 1975; Massini and Luscher, 1972, 1974; White et al., 1974; Feinstein, 1978). Regardless of which of these factors initiates the release reaction, all of the components of the release reaction are calcium-mediated events (Feinstein, 1978), that is, a rise in cytosolic Ca^{2+} content appears to activate all the different components of the release reaction. It also stimulates glycogenolysis by an activation of phosphorylase b kinase (Detwiler, 1972; Gear and Schneider, 1975).

The situation in the platelet appears to be similar to that in smooth muscle in the sense that either extracellular calcium or one or more pools of intracellular calcium can serve as the source for the signal calcium (Murer, 1972; Sneddon, 1972; Hovig, 1963; Feinstein et al., 1976; Miller et al., 1975; Wolfe and Shulman, 1970; Morse et al., 1965; Feinstein and Fraser, 1975; Massini and Luscher, 1972, 1974; LeBreton et al., 1976; Steiner and Tateishi, 1974; Salganecoff et al., 1975; Detwiler and Feinman, 1973). With different agents, there is a difference in the requirement for extracellular calcium. The problem is complicated by the fact that platelet aggregation (the membrane-to-membrane fusion) requires extracellular calcium, but the secretory response may or may not. For example, extracellular calcium is essential for collagen-induced release and enhanced secretion induced by low concentration of thrombin, but it is not required for the release reaction initiated by high concentrations of thrombin. These responses are similar to those seen in certain smooth muscles wherein low and high agonist concentration appear to employ different calcium pools as the source of messenger calcium.

What is clear is that in many circumstances extracellular calcium is not required. This means that one or more pools of calcium exist within the platelet and serve as a source of messenger calcium. At least four possible pools have been identified. These are secretory granules, the plasma membrane, microsomes or the so-called dense tubular system, and the open canalicular system which represents infolding of the plasma membrane. On the basis of present evidence, it seems unlikely that the calcium in the secretory granules of the platelets plays a coupling function. Also, the available evidence does not support plasma membrane depolarization as the initiator of calcium release. The two most attractive possibilities are either the open canalicular system and/or the microsomes.

In either case, the unresolved issue is how the initial interaction of, for example, thrombin or ADP with a surface membrane receptor induces the release of internal calcium. The one study of interest is that of LeBreton et al. (1976) in which chlortetracycline was used as a fluorescent probe to monitor "membrane-bound" calcium. They found a decrease in fluorescence which they interpreted as indicating a release of plasma membrane calcium. In a later study (LeBreton and Dinerstein, 1977), these investigators showed that the same change in fluorescence and a change in shape was seen even when the platelets were treated with TMP-8 [8-(N,N-diethylamino)octyl 3,45-trimethoxybenzoate HCl). TMP-8 has the properties of a local anesthetic, and it blocked secretions. The fact that it blocked secretion but not shape change led to the suggestion that a second pool of calcium is required for coupling stimulus to secretion than the pool controlling shape change.

Support for this possibility has been reported by Charo et al. (1976) and Feinstein et al. (1976). They showed that TMB-8 and other local anesthetics block the secretory response induced by thrombin or A23187. The inhibition of the ionophore-induced response could be overcome by addition of extracellular calcium. They suggest that this second pool of calcium may be the microsomal pool, and the mechanism involved might be a calcium-induced calcium release similar to that in cardiac muscle (see Chapter 9). As an alternative, they suggest that an initial release of calcium from the plasma membrane causes an activation of phospholipase A_2 leading to release of arachidonic acid and the subsequent synthesis of thromboxane A_2 and/or PG endoperoxides (Pachham et al., 1973; Pickett et al., 1977), one of which could serve a messenger function. The possibility that prostaglandins, thromboxanes, or their metabolites may play such a messenger function in the calcium messenger system has also been raised by Rubin and Laycock (1978) from studies of the calcium-dependent activation of phospholipase A_2 by ACTH in the adrenal cortex.

Within the context of the major thesis of this chapter, the question of most interest is that of the relationship of the cAMP to the calcium messenger system in the control of platelet function. As in smooth muscle, so in the platelet, a rise in the cAMP content of the platelet inhibits the activity of the calcium messenger system. For example, PGE_1 inhibits the release reaction induced by agents ranging from ADP to the ionophore A23187 (Salzman, 1972; Feinstein, 1978). The actions of PGE_1 are potentiated by phosphodiesterase inhibitors, and this agent has been shown to stimulate platelet adenylate cyclase (Steer and Wood, 1979). A variety of other prostaglandins activate adenylate cyclase (Best et al., 1971; Gorman et al., 1977; Tateson et al., 1977), and there is a good correlation between their ability to activate the cyclase and to inhibit platelet aggregation (Gryglewski et al., 1976; Smith et al., 1976). Furthermore, dibutyryl cAMP will also inhibit the release reaction.

In analogy with the situation in smooth muscle, the mechanism by which cAMP alters platelet function could involve either an effect of cAMP upon intracellular calcium metabolism and/or an effect upon the sensitivity of various response elements to calcium. Kaser-Glanzman et al. (1977) have reported that cAMP and protein kinase cause a threefold stimulation of calcium uptake in a "microsomal" fraction from platelets (Robblee et al., 1973), so one modality of cAMP control may well be the control of intracellular calcium distribution. However, this cannot be the only mechanism because PGE_1, or dibutyryl cAMP, inhibit the aggregation of platelets induced by A23187 (Feinstein and Fraser, 1975; White et al., 1974). In this circumstance, one would predict that all the calcium entering the cell as a consequence of ionophore action could not be accumulated rapidly enough to prevent a rise in cytosolic calcium. If so, the data suggest that cAMP must also alter the sensitivity of the calcium response elements to calcium ion. Although this is not yet established, it is noteworthy that control of the contractile system in platelets involves thick filament regulation via calmodulin-regulated myosin light chain kinase just as seen in smooth muscle. As discussed above, in smooth muscle the sensitivity of this calmodulin-regulated system is altered by a cAMP-dependent phosphorylation of the myosin kinase. It seems quite likely that the control of the sensitivity of the platelet enzyme will also be mediated in this way.

HISTAMINE RELEASE BY MAST CELLS

Anaphylactic allergic reactions are due to the release of histamine (and other mediators) from tissue mast cells and circulating basophils. This release is normally triggered by the reaction of an allergen with an immunoglobulin E (IgE) bound via its F_c locus to specific receptors on the surface of the cell. The system is operationally similar to a hormone–receptor system with the allergen serving the role of hormone and the bound IgE serving the role of receptor. Allergen–IgE interaction initiates a secretory response with exocytotic release of the substances normally stored within secretory vesicles inside the cell (Figure 8.8). A variety of other agents such as 48/80, ATP, dextran, and A23187 will initiate release even in nonsensitized cells, and concanavalin A will initiate release in sensitized cells (Kazimierczak and Diamant, 1978; Foreman and Mongar, 1975; Foreman et al., 1973, 1974, 1976, 1977; Johnson and Moran, 1969, 1970; Kanno et al., 1973; Cochrane and Douglas, 1975; Lawson et al., 1978; Cockcroft and Gompertz, 1979).

Under most circumstances, histamine release requires the presence of extracellular Ca^{2+}. Antigen–antibody-induced release is associated with a rapid but brief (1 minute) uptake of calcium into the cell. Under a variety of

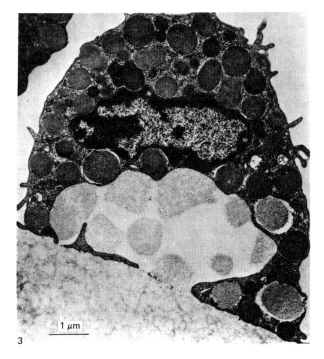

1 μm

3

Figure 8.8 A mast cell adhering to a Con A–Sepharose bead (bottom) in the presence of 1.7 m*M* calcium. Note degranulation has occurred and is confined to region of contact between bead and cell. From Lawson and Raff (1979), with permission.

circumstances there is a good correlation between the magnitude of the calcium uptake and of the release of histamine (Figure 8.9). Both processes are pH dependent, being maximal at a medium pH of 7.5. Addition of either dibutyryl cAMP or theophylline inhibits the antigen–antibody-mediated increases in both calcium uptake and histamine release. Catecholamines, with β-agonist activity, block secretion (Lichtenstein and Margolis, 1968; Ishizaka et al., 1970; Johnson and Moran, 1970; Johnson et al., Sullivan et al., 1975; Kaliner and Austin, 1974), presumably by stimulating an adenylate cyclase system in the membrane. When the calcium ionophore A23187 is added to these cells, calcium uptake and histamine secretion are both stimulated. In this case, neither dibutyryl cAMP nor theophylline alter the response (Figure 8.10).

Finally, preincubation of cells with phosphatidyl serine increases the extent of calcium uptake and the magnitude of histamine release induced by an antigen–antibody reaction, by dextran, or by concanavalin A. Phosphatidyl serine does not by itself increase calcium uptake or histamine release in unstimulated cells, but only enhances these responses of the stimulated cell (Goth et al., 1971; Foreman et al., 1977), probably by pro-

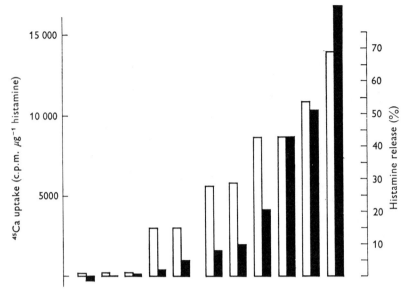

Figure 8.9 Relationship between antigen-induced histamine release (□) and calcium uptake (■) in 11 separate experiments. From Foreman et al. (1976), with permission.

longing the period of time during which the Ca^{2+} channel in the plasma membrane is open.

Taken *in toto,* these data indicate that Ca^{2+} is the factor that couples stimulus to response in the mast cell and that antigen–antibody interaction leads to the opening of a calcium gate or channel in the plasma membrane analogous to receptor-operated channels in smooth muscle. In keeping with this concept are the data of Cockcroft and Gompertz (1979) showing that antigen–antibody interaction or Con A addition leads to an increase in the rate of incorporation of both inositol and phosphate into the phosphatidylinositol pool in these cells. However, as noted previously (see Chapter 3), there is also recent evidence that activation of the phospholipid methylation pathway is involved in the calcium gating phenomenon. Based on the earlier observations of Ishizaka et al. (1978) showing that linking of the IgE receptors on the mast cell surface increases both calcium entry into the cell and histamine release, Ishizaka and coworkers (1980) studied the relationship of these events to phospholipid methylation. They demonstrated that addition of either antibodies against IgE receptors or the F(ab')$_2$ fragments of these antibodies induces histamine release, whereas Fab' monomer fragments do not, even though they bind to the receptor. Those reagents that caused histamine release had the property of bridging IgE receptors on the cell surface. When this occurred, the methylation of phosphatidylethanolamine (PE) to monomethyl PE and phosphatidylcholine took place and preceded in time the increase in calcium uptake and histamine release (see Figure 3.12).

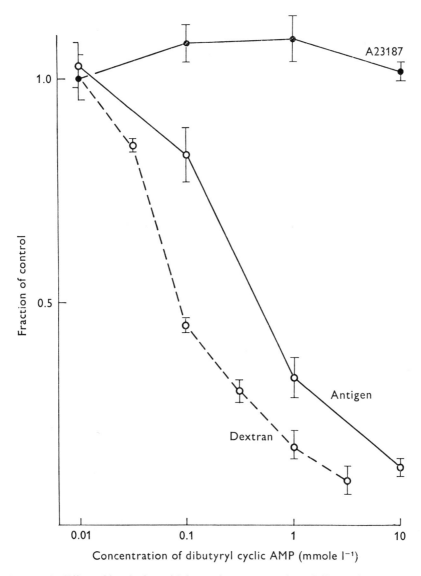

Figure 8.10 Effect of incubation with increasing concentration of dibutyryl cAMP upon the release of histamine (plotted as per cent of control value seen in absence of DB-cAMP). Histamine release was initiated by addition of either dextran (O—O), antigen (O—O), or A23187 (●—●). Note that DB-CAMP blocked responses to dextran and antigen but not to A23187. From Foreman et al. (1976), with permission.

When an inhibitor of the *S*-adenosyl-L-methionine methylation reaction, *S*-isobutyryl-3-deazaadenosine, was incubated with the cells before addition of the antibody against IgE receptors, methylation, calcium uptake, and histamine release were all inhibited. Varying the concentration of

S-isobutyryl-3-deazaadenosine over a 100-fold concentration range led to a comparable dose dependence in all three processes. From these results, Ishizaka et al. (1980) proposed that phospholipid methylation leads to an opening of a calcium channel in the plasma membrane (see Figure 3.13). Thus, at present there is evidence linking both PI turnover and phospholipid methylation to an opening of the calcium channel in these cells.

The precise role which Ca^{2+} plays in initiating secretion is not yet known, but it is known that the secretory process is dependent on an adequate supply of metabolic energy as well as an entry of calcium into the cell (Peterson, 1974; Foreman et al., 1977; Diamont, 1976). Of note is the fact that spontaneous histamine secretion can be evoked by the addition of strontium ion to calcium-free buffers (Foreman, 1977). Secretion increases as the external Sr^{2+} concentration rises, is enhanced in the presence of phosphatidyl serine, depends on adequate metabolic energy, and is blocked by addition of either theophylline or dibutyryl cAMP. It is proposed that Sr^{2+} enters the calcium channel in the resting cell, that is, in this cell the permeability of the channel is higher for Sr^{2+} than for Ca^{2+} but can be lowered by some cAMP-dependent mechanism.

As already mentioned in a previous section (see Chapter 2) this cell is one of the few systems in which the question of the spatial domain of calcium has been examined. Lawson et al. (1978) and Lawson and Raff (1979) linked concanavalin A (Con A) covalently to beads of Sepharose 4B and then mixed the beads with a population of sensitized rat peritoneal mast cells. Localized degranulation of the mast cells was calcium dependent and was restricted to that sector of the cell in direct contact with the beads (Figure 8.8). Subsequent addition of soluble Con A caused degranulation in the other sectors of the same cells. From these findings, the authors concluded that the opening of Ca^{2+} channels in the plasma membrane of the activated cell is a local event when Con A interacts with IgE molecules on the cell surface, and that the intracellular domain of the calcium that entered the cell was restricted to that portion of the cell just beneath that particular area of surface membrane. It is of interest that even though these cells contain few mitochondria, they appear capable of effectively buffering this local influx of calcium.

The question of most interest to the general thesis under discussion concerns the interaction between the calcium and cAMP messenger systems. The fact that dibutyryl cAMP or agents that cause an increase in cAMP within the cell block antigen–antibody-induced histamine release but do not block A23187-induced release has been taken as evidence that cAMP blocks the secretory process by inhibiting the increase in calcium uptake normally seen in antigen-induced activation. Direct support for this proposal has been provided by Foreman et al. (1977). They found that prior treatment of the cells with either dibutyryl cAMP or theophylline blocked the stimulation of calcium uptake normally caused by antigen–antibody interaction. An attractive hypothesis to account for the effects of catecholamine on antigen–

antibody-mediated histamine release is one in which a hormone-induced rise in cAMP concentration activates a protein kinase that catalyzes the phosphorylation of a membrane component which in some way blocks the opening of the calcium channel that normally occurs after antigen interacts with surface-bound antibody. It is of interest that the drug Cromolyn®, which inhibits histamine release induced by antigen–antibody interaction, is thought to act by inhibiting calcium gating (Foreman and Garland, 1974) and has been found to induce the phosphorylation of a 78,000 M.W. protein in the mast cell (Theoharides et al., 1980). The subcellular location of this protein is not yet known.

The modulatory role of cAMP discussed above relates to the ability of other external agents that influence the cAMP messenger system to alter the response of the cell to a normal primary stimulus, antigen–antibody interaction. In this regard, it is worth contrasting this situation to that seen in the beta cell of the pancreatic islets (see Chapter 6). In the beta cell, changes in the cAMP content of the cell alter the response of the cell to the normal primary stimulus, glucose. The response to the glucose stimulus is greater the greater the cAMP content of the cell, that is, cAMP enhances the temporal and/or spatial domain of the calcium signal. In contrast, in the mast cell, the response to the primary stimulus is an inverse function of the cAMP content of the cell, that is, the cAMP messenger system restricts the temporal and/or spatial domain of the calcium signal. It is noteworthy that in both systems, the cAMP messenger system appears to influence calcium fluxes across the plasma membrane. In the beta cell, low cAMP values are associated with low rates of calcium entry; and in mast cells, high cAMP values are associated with low rates of calcium entry in response to their respective primary stimulators.

There remains the possibility that cAMP also plays an immediate role in the response of the cell to stimulation by antigen—antibody interaction. Early data had suggested that the cAMP content of mast cells fell after antibody activation. However, Sullivan et al. (1976) showed that when either Con A or anti-IgE antibody induced histamine release, there was a transient rise in the cAMP content of mast cells which peaked within 20 seconds and then fell back toward normal values by 1 minute. These authors suggested that this transient rise in cAMP content might play an essential role in initiating the secretory process. However, their data are equally consistent with the concept that this transient rise in cAMP is an integral part of the normal response, but that it functions as the termination signal to inactivate the calcium gating process. If so, it seems likely that the extracellular messenger, that is, antigen–antibody reaction, would function both to open the calcium channel and to activate adenylate cyclase because Foreman and Mongar (1975) have shown that if mast cells are activated by addition of antigen to IgE-coated cells incubated in the absence of calcium and then calcium is added at different times after antigen, there is a rapid decay in the secretory response after calcium addition. This result means that the inactivation of the calcium channel is not dependent on calcium. An attractive possibility is that it is dependent on cAMP. It is of interest that preincubation of these cells with phosphatidyl serine slows the decay in response. The molecular basis of this effect is not known, but this effect could account for the ability of phosphatidyl serine to enhance histamine secretion.

The present proposal, if validated, would mean that cAMP is an essential second messenger both in the modulation of the immediate response as well as in the long-term adaptations of responsiveness occurring in response to catecholamines. However, it remains possible that the rise in cAMP is a calcium–calmodulin-mediated event which serves another role in the cellular response.

REGULATION OF NEUTROPHIL FUNCTION

The circulating polymorphonuclear leucocyte, or neutrophil, is one of the major phagocytic cells in the blood stream (Ignarro, 1977). It can, however, under other conditions secrete lysosomal enzymes or display a chemotactic response to a variety of stimuli. Its activation is also associated with an increase in the activity of intracellular superoxide dismutase. All four of the responses can be induced by appropriately sensitized particles (Ignarro and George, 1974a,b; Weissman et al., 1971). All of these functions, except obviously phagocytosis, can also be activated by addition of small-molecular-weight fragments of the fifth component of complement (Goldstein et al., 1973) or by the synthetic peptide formylmethionylleucyl-phenylalanine (FMLP). In addition, the effect of FMLP is greatly enhanced in the presence of cytochalasin B.

Starting with the initial work of Woodin and Wieneke (1968), all studies (Naccache et al., 1977a,b, 1979a,b; Ignarro and George, 1974a,b; Becker and Showell, 1972) have indicated that Ca^{2+} serves to couple stimulus to response in this system. Under most circumstances, external Ca^{2+} is necessary in order for a response to be seen. Addition of any of a variety of stimuli leads to a significant increase in rate of uptake of both labeled calcium and sodium into the cell. There is usually a close correlation between the extent of calcium uptake and the measured response. Addition of the calcium ionophore A23187 induces a similar calcium uptake and all of the cellular responses produced by FMLP (Naccache et al., 1977). If cells are prelabeled with $^{45}Ca^{2+}$ and then stimulated with FMLP, there is a transient decrease in $^{45}Ca^{2+}$ content followed by a marked increase in the steady state level of $^{45}Ca^{2+}$ within the cell. If a similar experiment is done in cells incubated in a medium containing a low concentration of extracellular calcium (> 0.1 mM), then there is a fall in the ^{45}Ca content of the cell (Petroski et al., 1979). The addition of FMLP causes a decrease in the fluorescence of chlor-tetracycline-labeled neutrophil (Naccache et al., 1979) and the inhibitor nordehydroguaerelic acid selectively inhibits the FMLP-induced increase in calcium influx without altering the FMLP-induced initial release of ^{45}Ca from the cell (Naccache et al., 1979).

These results have led to the conclusion that chemotactic and other stimuli induce an initial increase in the release of calcium from a plasma membrane-bound pool followed by an increase in the influx of calcium into these cells across the plasma membrane. This situation is comparable to that in other tissue such as the adrenal medulla (see Chapter 9). In fact, just as in the adrenal medulla, the extracellular messenger causes a depolarization of the plasma membrane. Using phorbol myristate to activate the neutrophil and superoxide production as an index of its response, Whitin et al. (1980) measured the membrane potential using the fluorescent probe di-S-C$_3$-(5) (3,3'-dipropylthiocarbocyanine). They found that phorbol myristate causes a depolarization of the membrane potential which correlated in onset and magnitude with the change in superoxide production. These data are consistent with the presence of a voltage-dependent calcium channel in the plasma membrane of these cells which is activated when the membrane is depolarized by any of a variety of extracellular agents.

Ignarro (1977) has recently reviewed the possible role of cAMP in modulating neutrophilic function. As early as 1970, Scott (1970) showed that homogenates of human leucocytes possessed catecholamine- and PGI-sensitive adenylate cyclase. Work by several different groups (May et al., 1970; Weissman et al., 1971, 1975; Ignarro and George, 1974a,b; Ignarro et al., 1974) demonstrated that cAMP or dibutyryl cAMP inhibited lysosomal enzyme secretion. Similarly, PGE, theophylline, and β-adrenergic agonists, all of which caused a rise in cellular cAMP content, blocked enzyme release induced by serum-coated particles or by soluble components derived from the complement system. Furthermore, cAMP or agents which increase its concentration block the other responses of these cells such as chemotaxis, intracellular killing of bacteria, and phagocytosis.

In spite of the clear evidence that the effect of cAMP is antagonistic to the action of calcium in this cell type, there has been very little work aimed at defining the mechanism of action of cAMP. The most attractive possibility is that this nucleotide acts in the neutrophil much as it does in the mast cell, and that it acts by altering the entry of calcium into the cell.

The other feature of this cellular response which has received considerable attention is that an accompaniment of cell activation is a calcium-dependent rise in cGMP content. Addition of cGMP alone does not cause cell activation, so it seems unlikely the cGMP is the direct messenger causing the various cellular responses. On the other hand, cGMP enhances the response to a standard immune reactant and is caused to increase in concentration by such a reactant. This suggests that cGMP serves as a feed-forward amplifier of the calcium message in the cell either by enhancing the sensitivity of the calcium response element or by altering the temporal and/or spatial domains of calcium within the cell. What emerges from the analysis of the control properties of neutrophils is that they are operationally similar to those found in the mast cell. Secretory processes and contractile processes are both quite common, and both contain a common attribute— calcium is the primary factor that couples stimulus to response.

In previous chapters, both contractile and secretory systems were described in which cAMP functions to augment the calcium-mediated contractile or secretory response. The systems reviewed in this chapter illustrate that an equally common relationship is one in which cAMP functions to minimize or negate the calcium- mediated contractile or secretory response. What also emerges is that cAMP can modulate the transport of calcium across the plasma membrane by altering the properties of the calcium channels in this membrane. In some cells, cAMP causes inactivation of these channels; but in others, it prolongs the duration of the period of activation. In addition, there is evidence that cAMP stimulates the microsomal accumulation of calcium and indirect evidence that it enhances the efflux of calcium from mitochondria. Viewed from the perspective of cellular function, this means that one of the major physiological functions of cAMP is that of modulating cellular calcium metabolism and the activity of the calcium messenger system.

PARATHYROID HORMONE, CALCITONIN, AND BONE RESORPTION

One of the most complex but nonetheless potentially most interesting instances of antagonistic hormonal control of a physiological process is the regulation of bone resorption by parathyroid hormone (PTH) and calcitonin (CT) (see Barrett and Rasmussen, 1981). The major complexity is that in bone, these two peptides hormones have opposing effects. PTH increases and CT decreases osteoclastic bone resorption, even though both cause an increase in the tissue content of cAMP. This system points up a number of the difficulties one has in relating physiological response to biochemical events in a complex tissue. The problem in bone is that there are at least three functional cell types—osteoclasts, osteoblasts, and osteocytes—plus at least two types of precursor cells—those giving rise to osteoclasts, preosteoclasts, and those giving rise to osteoblasts, preosteoblasts. The issue is further complicated by the fact that there is a constant turnover of osteoclasts and osteoblasts and a coupling between the turnover of these two cell populations. Because of this feature of a constant turnover of cell populations, the hormones have both immediate and long-term effects on bone function. Failure to distinguish between long-term physiological responses and immediate biochemical effects has led to a considerable confusion concerning the relationships between biochemical events and cellular response.

In order to restrict this discussion to a point of considerable theoretical import, attention will be confined to a consideration of the control of osteoclast function by PTH and CT. The specific question to be considered is whether these two hormones produce opposite cellular responses even though they both cause an increase in the cAMP content of these cells.

Abundant physiological and histological data suggest that PTH increases the bone resorptive activity of osteoclasts and that CT decreases their activity. The most convincing evidence that these hormones have opposing actions on osteoclast function is that of Mears (1971). He showed that PTH induced a stable 8 mV depolarization of the membrane potential and calcitonin induced a 7 mV hyperpolarization of this potential. These data argue that the two hormones have opposing effects upon the same cell. However, analysis of the situation is complicated by the fact that PTH increases the size of the osteoclast cell population and CT decreases it. These effects on cell pool size take hours to develop, but in many cases changes in bone resorption are also only detectable after several hours. Hence, effects on cell turnover may be misinterpreted in terms of changes in cell response.

Some facts support the hypothesis that PHT causes an increase in cAMP in osteoclasts. Infusion of dibutyryl cAMP or cAMP causes an increase in release of calcium from the bone of a parathyroidectomized rat (Rasmussen et al., 1968). This response develops slowly and is not of the same magnitude as that seen after PTH infusion. In particular, there is very little associated increase in hydroxyproline excretion (an index of bone matrix removal). It is quite possible that the source of urinary calcium in these studies was that mobilized from soft tissue cells in response to cAMP (see Chapter 2) or that mobilized from a labile calcium pool in osteocytic lacunae (Talmage et al., 1980) and did not represent an increase in osteoclast bone resorption.

This conclusion is consistent with the facts that effects of PTH upon bone cell metabolism are produced by concentrations of hormone 10- to 100-fold lower than those necessary to increase cAMP content (Herman-Erlee et al., 1978); that phosphodiesterase inhibitors do not enhance the resorptive action of PTH (Rasmussen et al., 1968); and that cholera toxin, an agent which causes a marked rise in bone cAMP content, does not mimic but actually inhibits this action of PTH (Nagata et al., 1977). Furthermore, structural analogs of PTH modified at the N-terminal region of the molecule (desamino PTH, 1-34; PTH, 2-34; and PTH, 3-34) stimulate bone resorption even though they are incapable of activating adenylate cyclase (Herman-Erlee et al., 1978). On the other hand, pretreatment of rats with CT blocks the calcium-mobilizing effect of DB-cAMP as well as that of PTH (Munson and Hirsch, 1968). So if CT activates adenylate cyclase as its primary effect, one still faces the paradox of a hormone acting via a cyclase-coupled system inhibiting the effect of exogenous cAMP. It is noteworthy that CT blocks the bone resorbing-action of PTH but does not inhibit the ability of PTH to increase the cAMP content of bone (Rodan and Rodan, 1974).

Attempts have been made to approach this problem by separating the different types of bone cells (Luben et al., 1974, 1976, 1977; Chen and Feldman, 1978; Peck et al., 1977; Puzas et al., 1979; Smith and Johnson, 1973, 1974). These separations methods have not yet been developed to the point where completely homogeneous populations of cells are obtained. In general, it has been found that populations rich in "osteoblasts" respond to PTH but not to CT with a marked increase in cAMP content. Cells identified as "osteoclasts" respond to both CT and PTH with an increase in cAMP content.

On balance, one way to interpret the data is to conclude that PTH and CT activate the adenylate cyclases in different cell populations. The difficulty with this conclusion is that the two hormones clearly have opposing effects upon the activities of both osteoclasts and osteocytes. If, for example, we conclude that osteoblasts but not osteoclasts have a PTH-responsive cyclase, and conversely that osteoclasts but not osteoblasts have a CT-responsive cyclase system, then the osteocyte is a problem. These cells are derived from osteoblasts, not from osteoclasts. Yet in terms of their behavior, they appear to increase calcium mobilization in response to PTH and calcium storage in response to CT (Talmage et al., 1980). One would logically expect them to possess a PTH-responsive cyclase. If so, then CT inhibits calcium mobilization in these cells by a mechanism different than the one by which it inhibits the calcium mobilization caused by PTH activation of osteoclast function.

Studies of the correlation between PTH-mediated metabolic effects and cAMP production have also been carried out. PTH causes a marked increase in aerobic lactate production (Cohn and Forscher, 1962). Structural analogs of PTH which have little effect on cAMP content have little effect of lactate production (Herman-Erlee et al., 1978). Conversely, CT and Verapamil inhibit PTH-induced bone resorption without blocking the effects of PTH on lactate metabolism (Nisbet et al., 1970; Hermann-Erlee, 1977). These results imply that the effect of PTH upon lactate production is cAMP linked. Furthermore, because PTH inhibits bone collagen synthesis, an osteoblast function, by a cAMP-dependent mechanism (Cohn and Wong, 1978), the metabolic evidence is consistent with the data derived from separated cells. It leads to the conclusion that PTH activates the adenylate cyclase in osteoblasts and the subsequent rise in cAMP is responsible for a stimulation of lactate production and an inhibition of collagen synthesis. In addition, the data suggest that CT does not inhibit these actions of PTH.

In contrast to these data are the observations that osteoblast-like cells respond to PTH with a decrease in citrate decarboxylation (Luben et al., 1976, 1977; Cohn and Wong, 1978). Addition of 10^{-4} M DB-cAMP produces a similar effect. Nonetheless, in the absence of extracellular calcium, neither agent produces any effect. Furthermore, simply raising the medium calcium concentration to 5 mM inhibits citrate decarboxylation without altering cellular cAMP content. Likewise, the hormone 1,25-dihydroxy vitamin D_3 induces a similar calcium-dependent inhibition of citrate metabolism without altering cAMP content. These data lead to the conclusion that in the osteoblast both cAMP and Ca^{2+} serve second messenger functions in the actions of PTH.

Another metabolic effect thought to be related to osteoclast function is that of hyaluronate synthesis. PTH induces a rapid increase in the incorporation of [^{3}H] glucosamine into hyaluronate (Luben et al., 1974). This effect is antagonized by CT when measured in osteoclast-like cells. These cells respond to both hormones with an equal threefold increase in cellular cAMP content (Luben et al., 1977). One might dismiss the effect of PTH upon cAMP as being unimportant and representing the fact that this bone cell population is heterogeneous except for the fact that $10^{-4}M$ DBcAMP also stimulates hyaluronate synthesis. Its effect is also blocked by CT (Wong et al., 1977). Neither DBcAMP nor PTH is effective if calcium is removed from the medium, and simply raising the Ca^{2+} content of the medium will enhance the production of hyaluronate without causing an increase in cellular cAMP content.

These results bring our discussion full circle. There is biochemical evidence that PTH and CT each cause a rise in cAMP content of a separated bone cell population capable of hyaluronate synthesis, but that the two hormones produce different effects: PTH stimulates and CT inhibits hyaluronate synthesis. In addition, in both osteoblast-like and osteoclast-like cells, there is evidence that calcium ions may serve a messenger function in the action of PTH, just as they do in the action of PTH upon kidney cells (see Chapter 5).

Support for this messenger function of calcium in PTH actions comes from several experimental findings. First, PTH administration leads to an increase in calcium uptake by bone cells (Parsons and Robinson, 1971); Rasmussen and Feinblatt, 1971; Boelkins et al., 1976). Second, the magnitude of the calcium-mobilizing effect of PTH is enhanced if calcium is infused into a parathyroidectomized animal at the time of PTH administration (Parsons and Robinson, 1971). Third, the steroid hormone 1,25(OH)$_2$D$_3$, when added to bone in organ culture, stimulates calcium release, citrate production, and hyaluronate synthesis just as PTH does without, however, altering cAMP concentrations (Raisz et al., 1972; Stern et al., 1975; Herman-Erlee and Gaillard, 1978; Gebauer and Fleisch, 1978; Wong et al., 1977). Fourth, PTH added to bone in culture increases calcium influx into cells within 1 minute after its addition (Dziak and Stern, 1974). Neither exogenous cAMP nor DB-cAMP produce this effect: also, addition of methylisobutylxanthine has no effect, even though it causes a twofold increase in cAMP content. Fifth, addition of Verapamil, a calcium channel blocker in heart and other tissues, markedly inhibits the action of PTH upon bone resorption in organ culture, even though it has no effect on the PTH-induced increase in cAMP content (Herman-Erlee, et al., 1977). The inhibition by Verapamil can be partially overcome by raising the ambient calcium concentration. Sixth, as noted above, structural analogs of PTH modified in the N-terminal region enhance bone resorption, though they do not stimulate bone cell adenylate cyclase.

These observations provide considerable support for a messenger role of calcium in PTH action on bone resorption. Taken together with the previously discussed data on the role of cAMP in the action of this hormone, they lead to the conclusion that PTH regulates osteoclast function via a dual, possibly coordinate, messenger system (Figure 8.11).

If this conclusion is accepted, and it is also concluded that cAMP serves a second messenger function in CT action on osteoclasts, then CT must have an effect on cellular calcium metabolism which differs from that of PTH. Support for this assumption has been provided by the studies of Rasmussen and Feinblatt (1971). They showed that CT causes an initial efflux of calcium from bone, presumably from bone cells, in contrast to the PTH-mediated uptake of calcium into bone. Whether this is a direct effect on the plasma membrane calcium pump or is mediated indirectly is not known. It is possible that it is indirect and is brought about by a primary effect upon cellular phosphate metabolism (Talmage et al., 1972). For example, if CT increases phosphate uptake into osteoclast, this would cause an increase in calcium uptake into mitochondria with a resultant fall in cytosolic Ca^{2+} content and a decrease in calcium efflux from the cell. This model is supported by the studies of Borle (1969) who showed that in the isolated kidney cell exposed to CT for some time, the steady state rate of calcium efflux from the cell was decreased. Also, work in the intact kidney has shown that PTH and CT have opposite effects upon pyridine nucleotide oxidation which are thought to be reflections of differences in their effects on cytosolic calcium (see pp. 169 and 348 in Rasmussen and Bordier, 1974).

The emerging model (Figure 8.11) is one in which the two hormones increase cAMP in the same cell but have different effects upon the calcium messenger system, leading to different cellular responses. This model is of considerable interest because it represents a possible instance in which the calcium and cAMP messenger systems can be regulated in opposite direc-

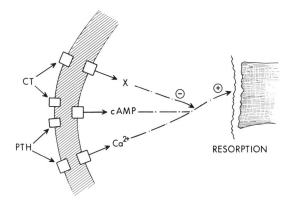

Figure 8.11   Interrelated messenger functions in actions of PTH and CT on osteoclasts. When PTH acts, both calcium uptake and cAMP-synthesis increase, and these increases are associated with the cellular response of increased bone resorption. When CT acts it blocks the cellular effect of PTH even though it, too, activates adenylate cyclase. It appears that CT calls forth an unidentified second messenger (X) which alters the properties of the calcium messenger system.

tions by the same primary stimulus, CT. Unfortunately, the evidence concerning the effects of CT upon cellular calcium metabolism is not conclusive.

This model is also of interest from the point of view of two hormones with opposite physiological effects, both activating the cAMP messenger system. However, before the model is accepted, additional studies are needed in order to rule out the alternative, but no less interesting possibility that PTH exerts its effects upon one class of bone cells, the osteoclasts, by activating the calcium messenger system and upon another, the osteoblasts, by activating the cAMP messenger system. As reviewed, the available data are more consistent with a dual messenger control of the activities of both cell types by PTH and, hence, with the activity of the osteoclast being controlled by PTH and CT in opposite directions, even though both activate the cyclase system in these cells. The opposing cellular responses to these two extracellular messengers may depend upon different effects on the calcium messenger system.

MODULATION OF POSTSYNAPTIC EVENTS

The most widely studied systems in which cAMP has been implicated as a modulator of postsynaptic events are the mammalian nervous system, particularly sympathetic ganglia, and specific neurons in the locus coeruleus, which send axons to cerebellar Purkinje, hippocampal, and cerebrocortical pyramidal neurons. In all these areas, there is evidence that norepinephrine can stimulate cAMP production (Bloom, 1979 There is also evidence that dopamine receptors coupled to adenylate cyclase constitute the site of action of this neurotransmitter, dopamine, at several central synapses (Greengard, 1978). Evidence is also available indicating that histamine, serotonin, and octopamine are associated with the cAMP messenger system in the nervous system (Greengard, 1978; Bloom, 1979).

Much of this work has not progressed beyond the demonstration of appropriate cyclase activation occurring upon addition of the neurotransmitter or beyond showing that specific antagonists which block the physiological response also block the neurotransmitter-induced increase in cAMP concentration. However, in the case of dopamine-activated adenylate cyclase in the brain, there is evidence showing that phenothiazines inhibit this response. In view of the evidence that these drugs block calcium-dependent calmodulin-induced responses, it seems likely that activation of adenylate cyclase by central dopamine receptors involves the participation of calcium—calmodulin.

The fact of most significance to emerge from the study of central neuron function is that neurotransmitter activation of postsynaptic adenylate cyclase is associated with changes in membrane potential of the postsynaptic neuron but not with initiation of action potentials. Thus, in the postsynaptic as well as presynaptic responses, cAMP serves as a modulator of the response of the postsynaptic membrane to primary excitatory neurotransmitters.

Although in several cases the suggestion has been made that in modulating postsynaptic events, cAMP regulates the Ca^{2+} conductance of the membrane, this is by no means established. In fact, in some systems it is clearly not the case (Bloom 1979). Nonetheless, if considered in the context of our previous discussion, the data are consistent with the hypothesis that cAMP, directly or indirectly, alters the functioning of the calcium messenger system in the postsynaptic neuron, as it does at presynaptic termini. Our previous discussion (see Chapter 3) focused on the fact that even though acetylcholine–nicotinic receptor interaction did not lead to a direct change in membrane calcium permeability, it did so indirectly by altering membrane potential which was in turn responsible for the eventual influx of calcium into the cell via a voltage-dependent channel. This calcium influx is responsible for the eventual response of the cell, namely, neurosecretion. If we accept as a valid thesis that in the nerve cell the primary intracellular messenger in stimulus–response coupling is Ca^{2+} and that the primary mechanism by which the cytosolic Ca^{2+} concentration is changed in the stimulated cell is via a voltage-dependent calcium channel, then it is immediately obvious that an alternative messenger system, such as the cAMP system which acts to modify the resting membrane potential, ultimately acts to alter the properties of the calcium messenger system.

Mammalian Sympathetic Ganglion

Because of the complexity of the mammalian central nervous system, it is difficult to isolate specific nerve cells and study their response in isolation. In an effort to elucidate the possible postsynaptic role of cAMP, the superior cervical ganglion of the sympathetic nervous system has been studied in some detail by Greengard and associates because of its relative structural simplicity. Within this ganglion, preganglionic fibers terminate upon two groups of nerve cells (Greengard (1974, 1976, 1978; Greengard and Kebabian, 1976). In the first, acetylcholine released from the presynaptic termini initiate either fast- or slow-excitation potentials in the postsynaptic neurons. In the second, acetylcholine activates a cell of a particular type, the SIF cell, which in turn secretes a catecholamine, probably dopamine, from termini innervating the same postsynaptic neurons as innervated by cholinergic fibers. The release of catecholamine from the presynaptic termini of these interneurons leads to a hyperpolarization of the postsynaptic neuron, a so-called slow inhibitory postsynaptic potential (Eccles and Libet, 1961; Libet, 1970).

The likelihood that this slow inhibitory postsynaptic potential is the consequence of a rise in cAMP concentration within the postsynaptic neuron is supported by the following observations (McAfee et al., 1971; Kebabian and Greengard, 1971; Kalix et al., 1974; Greengard and Kebabian, 1974; McAffee and Greengard, 1972; Kebabian et al., 1975; Study and Greengard, 1978): (1) Stimulation of presynaptic fibers leads to a rapid fivefold rise in the cAMP content of the ganglion. (2) This rise is blocked by atropine, suggesting that if the muscarinic receptors for acetylcholine are blocked, then, even though neurosecretion takes place, the interneuron is not stimulated and hence does not release dopamine. (3) Exogenously applied dopamine induces a hyperpolarization of postganglionic neurons and a rise in the cAMP content of the isolated ganglion. (4) Dopamine increases the cAMP concentration within postganglionic neurons as measured cytochemically. (5) Phosphodiesterase inhibitors potentiate the effects of dopamine on the membrane potential and on cAMP content. (6) Cyclic AMP, monobutyryl cAMP, and dibutyryl cAMP are each able to cause a hyperpolarization of postganglionic neurons. However, there is no universal agreement on this point (Busis et al., 1978; Gallagher and Shinnick-Gallagher, 1977; Lindl, 1979). No effect on a membrane depolarization has been described in response to cAMP in these other studies, leading their authors to suggest that cAMP has a function other than altering the ionic conductance of the membrane.

Central Noradrenergic Projections

Detailed anatomical and electrophysiological studies in mammalian brain have shown that there is a connection between neurons of the locus coeruleus (LC) and four sets of target neurons: cerebellar Purkinje neurons, hippocampal and cerebrocortical pyramidal neurons, and unidentified neurons in the septum (Bloom, 1979; Hoffer et al., 1971, 1973; Moore and Bloom, 1979; Siggins et al., 1969, 1971a,b,c). Of particular interest are the findings that norepinephrine (NE) is found in these four regions and that within them NE stimulates the synthesis of cAMP. Stimulation of these presumptive NE-secreting neurons produces a hyperpolarization of the membranes of the postsynaptic neuron in either the cerebellum or hippocampus. These effects of LC stimulation are blocked by prior inhibition of NE synthesis and storage.

These effects of NE on membrane potential are mediated via the cAMP messenger system. The evidence in support of this view is the following: (1) Iontophorectic application of NE to these neurons causes a hyperpolarization. (2) The hyperpolarizing effects of NE are enhanced by either parenteral or iontophorectic application of phosphodiesterase inhibitors. (3) Iontophorectic application of cAMP produces a similar change in membrane potential. (4) The effect of cAMP is enhanced by the application of PDE inhibitors. (5) Either topically applied NE or stimulation of LC neurons leads to a marked increase in the number of cerebellar Purkinje neurons which react positively to an immunocytochemical assay for intracellularly bound cAMP. (6) NE and cAMP alter membrane potential in cultured Purkinje neurons. (7) NE activates an adenylate cyclase in membranes prepared from this region of the cerebellum.

These data are similar to those discussed above concerning the action of dopamine in the superior cervical ganglion. They demonstrate that the cAMP messenger system can modulate postsynaptic as well as presynaptic events and that cAMP may influence nerve cell function by altering either the local neurosecretory events at the synapse or by altering the responsiveness of the nerve body to other neurotransmitters. Both effects lead ultimately to a change in the functioning of the calcium messenger system, although they appear to achieve this end by modifying different properties of the nerve cell membrane. Equally important, it is already evident that activation of the cAMP messenger system within specific neurons can have either a facilitatory or inhibitory effect upon the response of a particular neuron. The point to be made is that the ultimate manner in which a nerve cell responds is by neurosecretion, a calcium-dependent process. The efficiency of synaptic transmission can be modified by the activity of the cAMP messenger system. Modification can occur either at the secretory step or at the response step in the process of synaptic transmission, and modification can lead either to an enhancement and/or prolongation of information flow or to inhibition and/or shortening of information flow.

Associative Learning in *Hermissenda Crassicornis*

In the elegant studies of Alkon and associates, the nudibranch *Hermissenda crassicornis* has been employed to analyze the neurophysiological correlates of associative learning (Alkon, 1974, 1975, 1976a,b, 1979; Alkon and Grossman, 1978). This organism is positively phototactic, that is, it moves toward light. It also responds to rotation by moving in a direction opposite to a gravitational force. If a light step is paired with rotation, the animals's movement toward a light source is greatly reduced. This behavioral change requires that the light and rotational stimuli be paired and not presented sequentially. Associative training of *Hermissenda* behavior has many of the features of associative learning seen in vertebrates.

A major site of change in cell behavior within the nervous system of this primitive organism has been identified as the membrane of the type B photoreceptor cell. Exposure of the organism to a light step causes a depolarization and increased firing of type B cells. Rotation is also followed by a depolarization of the membrane of the type B cell. However, no impulse activity is produced. Of particular interest is the observation that a 30-second light step leads to a long-lasting depolarization (LLD) of 1 to 2 minutes in duration. When rotation is paired with light, a light stimulus is always followed by a greater and longer-lasting membrane depolarization and increased firing of the type B cell. The striking feature of this altered behavior of the type B cell is that the sensitivity to the light is not changed in response to rotation, only the magnitude and duration of the LLD of the type B cell to a particular light step change.

Studies of type B cell membrane responses under voltage or current clamp conditions have shown that the sustained depolarization results from calcium influx across the membrane via a voltage-dependent calcium channel and from an inhibition of resting K^+ efflux probably regulated by intracellular calcium.

   The intracellular iontophoretic injection of cAMP into the anatomically isolated type B cell leads to an inhibition of the calcium current seen under voltage clamp conditions and a decrease in the magnitude and duration of the membrane depolarization when no voltage clamp is applied (Figure 8.12). These data indicate that an increase in intracellular cAMP decreases the rate of flow of Ca^{2+} via the voltage-dependent channel in this neuron and raises the possibility that the effect of rotation is mediated by a reduction in the cAMP content of these neurons.

   These data are of particular interest in that the effect of cAMP in this cell, that of inhibiting calcium flux via a voltage-dependent channel, is the exact opposite to that of cAMP in the heart (see Chapter 9) and the abdominal ganglion of *Aplysia* (see Chapter 6), where cAMP leads to an enhancement of calcium flux via a similar voltage-dependent channel. Within the nervous system, the cAMP messenger system can modify the properties of the

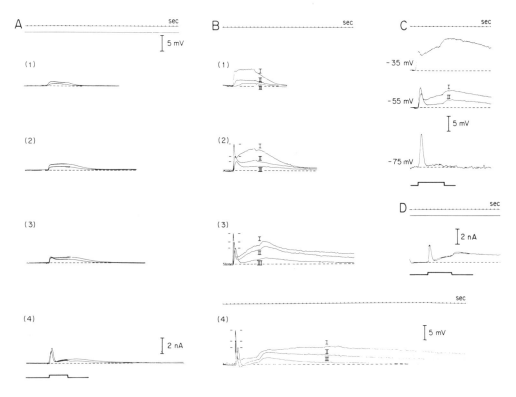

Figure 8.12   Effect of intracellular cAMP on membrane potential across the plasma membrane of a photoreceptor cell (B cell) in *Hermissenda crassicornis*. In experiment B, light steps are indicated by the bottom trace. With light steps of increasing intensity (1 through 4) there is an increase in membrane depolarization. At each light intensity (1 through 4) intracellular injection of cAMP causes a reduction in magnitude of depolarization (Control—I; after intracellular cAMP—II), and a second injection of cAMP reduced the voltage response even further (III). From Alkon (1979), with permission.

calcium messenger system in such fashion as to either expand or restrict the temporal and/or spacial domain of the calcium message and thereby influence the flow of information from one cell to the next.

CONCLUSION

All the clearly defined examples of antagonistic synarchic regulation discussed in this chapter have been examples in which cAMP serves in some way to either block the generation or shorten the duration of the calcium signal and/or to decrease the sensitivity of response elements to activation by Ca^{2+}. No well-defined cases of the opposite circumstance has been described in which Ca^{2+} serves to antagonize a primary cAMP messenger. However, one can predict that systems of this type exist and will eventually be discovered.

9

Sequential Control

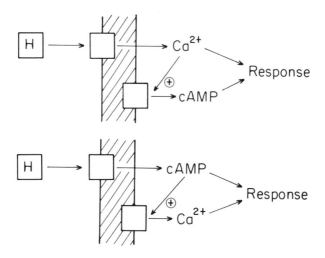

INTRODUCTION

One of the most interesting types of synarchy is one in which messenger generation is brought about sequentially. An extracellular messenger interacting with its surface receptor gives rise to either of the two messengers which in turn is responsible for the generation of the second. For example, in the mammalian heart and the brain, a primary cAMP messenger initiates a secondary calcium message, and the two together control cellular response. Conversely, in the adrenal medulla, a primary calcium message initiates a secondary cAMP message, and together they determine cellular response.

The earliest examples, phytogenetically, of sequential messenger function can be found in stimulus–response coupling in certain unicellular organisms. Of particular interest is the process of aggregation in the cellular slime mold *Dictyostelium discordeum,* in which cAMP serves as an extracellular messenger of communication between two or more cells in the aggregating population and by its action gives rise to a calcium message that initiates, in turn, directed movement of the cells toward one another. Furthermore, this calcium message gives rise, in turn, to a new cAMP message, so that sequential communication obtains throughout the entire population.

CARDIAC MUSCLE

Since the early recognition of the relationship between β-receptors and adenylate cyclase (Sutherland and Rall, 1958), a subject of considerable interest has been the role of cAMP in the positive inotropic response of the heart to epinephrine. Our knowledge concerning this question has grown as our knowledge of the molecular events underlying the cyclic contractions in the heart has developed. This subject has been reviewed in depth recently by Chapman (1979) and so will not be presented in detail.

An oversimplified summary of the sequence of events in each contractile cycle is necessary in order to fully comprehend the ensuing discussion. With the initiation of the electrical systole, an action potential is propagated across the surface of the cardiac muscle cell. As a consequence of this event, the calcium conductance of the membrane increases, leading to the entry of calcium into the cytosol. Careful estimates of the amount of the calcium indicate that it represents only 25% of that required to induce the contractile response. Hence, in addition to calcium entering the cell across the sarcolemma (plasma membrane), there is a release of calcium from an internal store. This store has been identified as the sarcoplasmic reticulum (SR). Debate continues as to how the message of the action potential leads to the release of calcium from the SR. One school holds that it is triggered by the influx of calcium across the plasma membrane. Calcium-induced calcium efflux from isolated cardiac SR has been demonstrated by Fabiato and Fabiato (1978). However, Chapman (1979) points out that this would seem to be an all-or-none type of response which is inconsistent with the known capability of the heart to show a graded response. He, on the other hand, suggests that in the heart, as in skeletal muscle, there is a coupling between the invaginations of the sarcolemma, the so-called dyads, and the SR that involves some type of electrotonic coupling between the two membrane systems. In either case, there is general agreement that a significant portion of the calcium involved in initiating the contractile response comes from the SR (Tsien, 1977; Chapman, 1979).

The calcium from the two sources interacts with troponin C and initiates contraction by a mechanism thought to be similar to that seen in skeletal muscle (see Chapter 4). With repolarization of the plasma (and possibly endoplasmic reticular) membrane, calcium is pumped out of the cell and into the SR. As the Ca^{2+} concentration in the cytosol falls, calcium dissociates from TNC, and the muscle relaxes.

The effects of catecholamines on two of the properties of this system are shown in Figure 9.1. Isoproterenol causes an increase in the amplitude of the contractile twitch while it simultaneously shortens the time-to-peak tension (Nathan and Beeler, 1975; Tsien, 1977). Thus, both an increase in rate and magnitude of tension development and in rate of subsequent relaxation occur in response to the drug. Also, as shown in Figure 9.1, drug addition leads to a change in the profile of the action potential involving an elevation of the plateau phase and acceleration of the repolarization phase. These

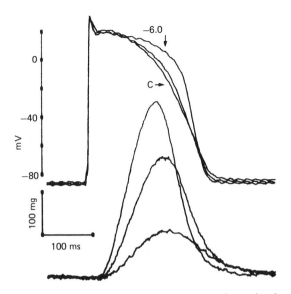

Figure 9.1   Effect of catecholamines on the heart. Upper trace shows the change in membrane potential with time following electrical systole. Catecholamines prolong the duration of the plateau after the initial depolarization. Lower trace shows the change in mechanical force. Catecholamines increase both the rate of rise and the peak strength of contraction as well as the subsequent rate of relaxation. From Nathan and Beeler (1975), with permission.

changes are associated with or preceded by a rise in the cAMP content of the tissue. Hence, it is thought that they are mediated by this messenger. In support of this view is the fact that pharmacological manipulation of the cAMP messenger system leads to many of the expected changes. However, as discussed thoroughly by Tsien (1977), many of these experiments are difficult to interpret because many of the agents employed have effects on the plasma membrane which are dissimilar from those seen after β-agonist addition. On the basis of his own detailed investigations, Tsien (1977) concludes that cAMP or its analogs can reproduce the same alterations in cardiac function as seen after β-agonist treatment (Tsien, 1973).

The mode of action of cAMP has been studied by a number of different investigators using a variety of tools. This work has been reviewed by Tsien (1977), Krause and Wollenberger (1977), Mayer et al. (1978), and Katz (1979) and so is not extensively reviewed here. The essential facts established to date are that cAMP may and probably does act on at least three sites: the sarcolemma, the sarcoplasmic reticulum, and the troponin system in the contractile apparatus.

In the case of the sarcolemma, Reuter (1973) and Tsien (1977) have shown that the increase in the height of the plateau phase is due to enhanced calcium entry into the cell after epinephrine addition (Reuter and Scholz, 1976). Reuter (1973) proposed that cAMP alters calcium influx by increasing the number of voltage-sensitive calcium channels in the membrane, and

Krause and Wollenberger (1977) have demonstrated cAMP-dependent phosphorylation of sarcolemmal proteins. As yet, it has not been possible to relate the one finding directly to the other. The situation is of considerable interest in the sense that gating of the same ion channel is regulated both by electrical (voltage-dependent) and chemical (cAMP) mechanisms.

There is also an increase in the Na^+/K^+ ATPase activity of this membrane after addition of catecholamines, but the functional significance of this change is not known. Finally, there is an increase in rate of calcium efflux and an increase in the activity of sarcolemmal Ca^{2+}/Mg^{2+} ATPase activity after catecholamine action (Krause and Wollenberger, 1977), but this may be a consequence of the rise in cytosolic calcium ion content. On the other hand, Fine et al. (1975) have shown that cAMP will stimulate an intrinsic protein kinase in plasma membrane-enriched preparations of myocardium. These phosphorylated membranes accumulate calcium at twice the rate of the nontreated membranes. Even so, this enhanced efflux rate is not sufficient to compensate completely for the increase in calcium entry induced by catecholamine treatment, so that the total calcium content of the heart increases.

Studies of the effect of cAMP on the phosphorylation of proteins in the cardiac SR and their relationship to calcium transport have been described by several investigators (Kirchberger et al. 1974; LaRaia and Morkin, 1974; Wollenberger, 1972; Kirchberger and Tada, 1976; Katz et al., 1975; Katz, 1979). There is a substrate for cAMP-dependent protein kinase, now called phospholamban, which is associated with the calcium transport system of the SR membrane. Phosphorylation of the protein increases the rate of calcium accumulation and the extent of calcium accumulation and decreases the final steady state calcium ion concentration outside (cytosolic side) the membrane. These findings, associated with observations that catecholamines increase the calcium content of the SR in the intact heart, have led to the proposal (Katz, 1979) that phosphorylation of the protein increases the rate and extent of calcium accumulation by the SR in the catecholamine-treated heart. As a consequence, both the rate of relaxation, and the magnitude of the calcium pulse released at the time of the next cystole increase thereby accounting for a major part of both the increase in contractile strength and the increased rate of muscle relaxation.

However, the situation is more complex and more interesting than this simple model implies. Studies by LePeuch et al. (1979), Horl and Heilmeyer (1968) and Horl et al. (1978) have shown that the rate of calcium uptake by canine cardiac sarcoplasmic reticulum (SR) is regulated by either a calcium-calmodulin-dependent on a cAMP-dependent phosphorylation of the regulatory protein phospholamban, and by a phosphoprotein phosphatase reaction. Previous work (Wray and Gray, 1977; Will et al., 1976; Kirchberger and Tada, 1976; Horl et al., 1975; Kirchberger et al., 1979; Cohen et al., 1978) had shown that either cAMP-dependent protein kinase or the calcium-dependent phosphorylase kinase, could cause the phosphorylation of cardiac SR and thereby stimulate the rate of calcium transport. LePeuch et al. (1979) developed a method for preparing a more highly purified cardiac SR fraction. They showed that the isolated catalytic subunit of cAMP-dependent protein kinase could stimulate the phosphorylation of phospholamban. However, this phosphorylation did not alter the rate of calcium transport. They also found that addition of calcium and calmodulin (without an associated protein kinase) led to an increase in the extent of phospholamban phosphorylation. This calcium–calmodulin-mediated phosphorylation caused an increase in the rate of calcium transport. If the catalytic subunit of cAMP-dependent protein kinase was added to SR incubated with calcium–calmodulin, it caused a further increase in the extent of phospholamban phosphorylation and a further increase in the rate of calcium transport. Finally, the cAMP-dependent and calcium-dependent protein kinase activities catalyzed the phosphorylation of different serine residues in the phospholamban molecule.

The model that emerges is one in which the activity of a protein kinase intrinsic to the SR membrane is controlled by the calcium–calmodulin complex in the cytosolic compartment of the cell. When this rises, the protein kinase is activated and catalyzes the phosphorylation of phospholamban, and this in turn leads to an increase in the rate of calcium uptake into the SR. Hence, the primary and most immediate regulator of calcium uptake by the SR is the calcium–calmodulin content of the cell cytosol (Figure 9.2). This situation is operationally similar to that seen in the calcium–calmodulin activation of the calcium pump in the plasma membrane (see Chapter 3), but functionally it differs from this situation in that calmodulin activation of the plasma membrane pump does not appear to involve phosphorylation of a regulatory protein similar to phospholamban. In any case, as regards the SR system, the soluble cAMP-dependent protein kinase represents a supplementary means of regulating calcium transport in the SR. A rise in cAMP

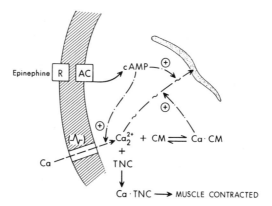

Figure 9.2 Model of the actions of cAMP in cardiac muscle in which cAMP enhances calcium entry into the cell (left) via a voltage-dependent channel and enhances the calcium–calmodulin ($Ca^{2+} \cdot CM$)-mediated increase in rate of calcium accumulation by the SR (right).

within the cell leads to an increase in the content of the free catalytic subunit of cAMP-dependent protein kinase. This enzyme catalyzes the further phosphorylation of phospholamban at a distinct site, and this phosphorylation causes a further activation of calcium transport. Operationally, cAMP operates as a sequential messenger in regulating this transport process, and thereby directly modifies the temporal domain of the cytosolic calcium messenger (Figure 9.2).

The other site at which cAMP functions is at the calcium-binding site on the contractile apparatus. This possibility has been actively explored ever since Bailey and Villar-Pilasi (1971) reported that cAMP could stimulate the phosphorylation of TN-I via a protein kinase reaction. Work in the laboratories of Krebs (Stull et al., 1972; England et al., 1972, 1973), Heilmeyer (Pratje and Heilmeyer, 1972, 1973), and Perry (Perry and Cole, 1974) extended this work. In addition, Perry and Cole (1974) showed that phosphorylase kinase could catalyze the phosphorylation of the TN-I subunit of the troponin complex. Furthermore, England (1975) and Solaro et al. (1976) have shown that the phosphate content of TN-I is increased in TN-I subunits extracted from muscle previously treated with catecholamines. They also showed a correlation between the dose–response curve for adrenaline-induced increase in contractile force and in the phosphorous content of TN-I. In spite of this evidence, the relationship between TN-I phosphorylation and the inotropic effect of catecholamines remains an unresolved question because in isolated systems phosphorylation of TN-I leads to a shift to the right in the binding curve of calcium to TN-I and to calcium activation of myosin ATPase. However, Holroyde et al. (1979) in restudying this problem found no significant effect of phosphorylation on calcium binding and concluded that this phosphorylation was not of significance in the beat-to-beat control of myocardial contractibility.

On the basis of the above results, a strong case can be made for a cAMP-mediated sequence of events (Figure 9.3) which alter primarily myocardial calcium metabolism and thereby are responsible for the inotropic action of catecholamines. However, there are other data which still cloud the issue. Foremost among these are the results by Ventener et al. (1975) and Mayer et al. (1978) who have shown that if the catecholamine agonist is attached to glass beads and these beads applied to the heart, a significant inotropic response occurs even though there is no change in the cAMP content of the tissue.

These results are in sharp contrast to the situation in the mast cell, where application of immobilized agonist leads to a secretory response confined to its site of contact with the cell (see Chapter 8). However, the heart operates as a syncytium, and a *sine qua non* for its proper function must be an intrinsic ability to produce a coordinated response. Viewed in this light, and taking the proposal of Mayer et al. (1978) that the initiating event in the glass bead experiment is the activation of adenylate cyclase and a rise in cAMP in the local region leading to an increased influx of calcium into the cell, it is

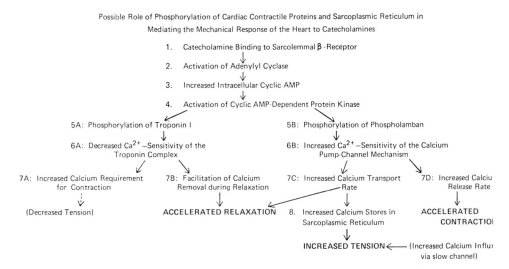

Possible Role of Phosphorylation of Cardiac Contractile Proteins and Sarcoplasmic Reticulum in
Mediating the Mechanical Response of the Heart to Catecholamines

1. Catecholamine Binding to Sarcolemmal β -Receptor
2. Activation of Adenylyl Cyclase
3. Increased Intracellular Cyclic AMP
4. Activation of Cyclic AMP-Dependent Protein Kinase

5A: Phosphorylation of Troponin I   5B: Phosphorylation of Phospholamban

6A: Decreased Ca^{2+} −Sensitivity of the   6B: Increased Ca^{2+} −Sensitivity of the Calcium
    Troponin Complex   Pump-Channel Mechanism

7A: Increased Calcium Requirement   7B: Facilitation of Calcium   7C: Increased Calcium Transport   7D: Increased Calciu
    for Contraction   Removal during Relaxation   Rate   Release Rate

(Decreased Tension)   ACCELERATED RELAXATION   8. Increased Calcium Stores in   ACCELERATED
                                                                  Sarcoplasmic Reticulum   CONTRACTIOI

                                                               INCREASED TENSION ◄── (Increased Calcium Influ›
                                                                                        via slow channel)

Figure 9.3 Schematic representation of the sequence of events by which catecholamines alter myocardial contractility. Not represented is an effect of cAMP-dependent phosphorylation of the sarcolemma leading to a prolongation of the calcium current across this membrane. From Katz (1979), with permission.

then possible to propose that this calcium influx is the trigger for the propagated response. This could involve activation of calcium-dependent protein kinases which catalyze the phosphorylation of sites on plasma membrane, SR, and the contractile system, hence sharing with cAMP the role of mediating the inotropic response. Evidence for such a calcium-dependent reaction has already been discussed.

The data in the mammalian heart lead to a model in which sequential control appears to operate at several levels. The first is that the rise in cAMP concentration induced by epinephrine appears to be responsible for the subsequent increase in the calcium conductance of the plasma membrane and thereby for an increase in the strength of the calcium signal. The second is at the level of the control of glycogenolysis where cAMP activates the first enzyme and calcium the second in the phosphorylase cascade. The third is at the level of the sarcoplasmic reticulum where calcium-dependent phosphorylation of a membrane protein allows for a subsequent cAMP-dependent phosphorylation to cause a further increase in the rate of energy-dependent calcium accumulation (Figure 9.2).

DOPAMINERGIC NEURONS

The fact that a number of central dopaminergic neurons exhibit a rise in their cAMP content in response to activation has already been discussed (see Chapter 6). However, studies of the mechanism by which dopamine regulates cAMP metabolism in this tissue has revealed a complex system involving calcium–calmodulin in the sequential regulation of both membrane-bound adenylate cyclase and soluble phosphodiesterase (Gnegy et al., 1981; Hanbauer et al., 1981). The sequential pattern is the opposite of that found in the erythrocyte.

The finding of prime importance is that if a plasma membrane fraction from a dopaminergic-rich region of the brain, the striatum, is used as an *in vitro* system to study dopamine-regulated adenylate cyclase, an association of calmodulin with this membrane is an essential component of the cyclase complex. Various *in vivo* and *in vitro* manipulations lead to an alteration in membrane calmodulin content and thereby change the sensitivity of the cyclase system to activation by dopamine (DA).

Before discussing these data, it is useful to review the fact that in the central nervous system, the calmodulin–calcium complex has been shown to activate both phosphodiesterase and adenylate cyclase. At first glance, one might consider this a wasteful kind of simultaneous control of both cAMP synthesis and degradation. However, if one views cellular response either in a temporal or a spatial domain, a number of control possibilities exist. If the activation of the two enzymes are not synchronous in time, then a sequential activation of adenylate cyclase and then phosphodiesterase could lead to a transient rise in cAMP content within the cell. A difference in the sensitivity of the two calmodulin-regulated enzymes to Ca^{2+} could represent a second type of sequential control. Such a situation has been shown to exist in the guinea pig brain (Piascik et al., 1980). As shown in Figure 9.4, the activation of adenylate cyclase by calcium occurs at a lower calcium concentration ($10^{-7} M$) than does activation of PDE ($6\text{-}7 \times 10^{-7} M$). Another possibility is that if both enzymes are activated simultaneously, they could nevertheless, because of their spatial arrangement—cyclase in the membrane and PDE in the cytosol—restrict the subcellular domain in which a rise in cAMP concentration occurred. A fourth possibility, as already discussed in the case of the red cell, is that the calcium receptor protein, calmodulin, is translocated from one subcellular compartment to another so that, depending upon its distribution the particular component of the cyclase—PDE system, one or the other of the components will dominate.

The following data have been obtained in the case of dopaminergic neurons: (1) Removal of calmodulin from membrane *in vitro* causes a decrease in dopamine (DA) activation of cyclase, and an increase in calmodulin increases the DA responsiveness both by increasing the V_{max} and lowering the K_a of activation by DA. (2) Chronic stimulation of cells with DA leads to a decrease in membrane-bound calmodulin and an increase in soluble calmodulin. (3) This increase in soluble calmodulin is associated with an increase in PDE activity in cytosol. (4) Under circumstances where supersensitivity to DA develops, there is an increase in calmodulin content of isolated membranes. (5) A cAMP-dependent phosphorylation of the membrane decrease calmodulin binding. (6) Phenothiazines block the binding of calmodulin to membranes and thereby inhibit cyclase. (7) The effect of

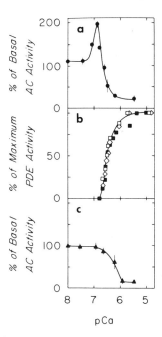

Figure 9.4 Basal activity of adenylate cyclase as function of Ca^{2+} concentration (plotted apCa) in the presence (*a*) and absence (*c*) of calmodulin. Also plotted is the activity of the soluble PDE from the same tissue as a function of pCa (*b*). From Piascik et al. (1980), with permission.

calmodulin requires the guanine nucleotide-regulating subunit of the cyclase molecule. (8) Calcium increases the binding of calmodulin to the membrane.

At low calcium and calmodulin concentrations, an activation of the cyclase is seen; at high concentrations, an inhibition occurs. These data are consistent with a model in which both cAMP and Ca^{2+} regulate the binding of calmodulin to the cyclase complex and thereby determine the responsiveness of the cell to the neurotransmitter dopamine. Continued exposure of the cell to excess dopamine leads to a desensitization of the cell to further stimulation. This involves, in part at least, a sequence in which the dopamine-induced rise in cAMP leads to a phosphorylation of the membrane and a dissociation of calmodulin from the cyclase system. This alone would lead to a decrease in rate of cAMP synthesis. In addition, the calmodulin released by the membrane would activate the soluble PDE and cause an increase in the rate of cAMP hydrolysis. If, as is likely, other synapses impinging on these same neurons regulate the calcium messenger system in these neurons, a very complex interaction between the two messenger systems would exist in these cells.

These observations in dopaminergic neurons illustrate yet another means of altering the flow of information in the cell. As discussed previously, one way in which information is transmitted in the calcium messenger system is by an increase in the Ca^{2+} concentration of the cell cytosol, so-called amplitude modulation. A second way, also discussed, is one in which the affinity of the calcium receptor protein, for example, calmodulin, for calcium is changed due to the interaction of this protein with another protein, so-called sensitivity modulation. The situation in both the red cell (see Chapter 4) and dopaminergic neuron is an extension of one possible consequence of sensitivity modulation in the spatial domain. If, for example, the Ca^{2+} concentration in the cell cytosol were fixed and a dopaminergic neuron were stimulated chronically with DA, then a shift of calmodulin from membrane to cytosol without a change in cytosolic Ca^{2+} concentration would lead to the activation of the calcium-sensitive enzyme phosphodiesterase, a situation one might call *translocational modulation,* to distinguish it from the other types of modulation previously described.

ADRENAL MEDULA

Althouugh an emphasis on the role of the cAMP and calcium messenger systems in the nervous system has been alluded to in general terms throughout this discussion, few specific examples have been presented. The reason is rather obvious. In contrast to liver or salivary gland, it is not possible to identify, isolate, and study messenger events in a homogeneous population of nerve cells all having more or less the same function. However, there is an exception to this general rule, the adrenal medulla. This is a neuroendocrine organ composed primarily of a single cell type (90% chromaffin cells), carrying out a single function (secretion of catecholamines), and innervated exclusively by cholinergic nerves which regulate cell function by activating a population of surface receptors, predominantly of the nicotinic type (Coupland, 1965; Douglas, 1966, 1968; Rubin, 1970). The properties of the chromaffin cell membrane are similar to those of nerve membranes in general. Activation of the nicotinic receptors leads to a sharp increase in Na^+ conductance, which leads in turn to a fall in membrane potential thus activating a voltage-dependent calcium channel. As first shown by Douglas (Douglas and Rubin, 1961; Douglas, 1966), Ach induces an increase in calcium uptake into the gland and a calcium-dependent secretion of catecholamines (Figure 1.9). A variety of other agents which can depolarize the membrane lead to catecholamine secretion as long as calcium is available in the medium, but not in its absence (Douglas, 1966, 1968). Furthermore, A23187, a divalent cation ionophore, which does not cause membrane depolarization but does increase calcium entry into the cell, evokes calcium-dependent catecholamine secretion (Garcia et al., 1975). Lastly, it is possible to evoke release (Gutman et al., 1979) by addition of calcium–containing liposomes to adrenal medullary tissue incubated in calcium-free Locke's solution. Presumably this occurs because fusion of the liposomes with the cell membrane delivers calcium to the cell cytosol.

In addition to triggering the release process, the rise in cytosolic calcium leads to an activation of the rate-limiting enzyme in catecholamine biosynthesis, tyrosine hydroxylase (TH) (Figure 9.5). Calmodulin is present in the adrenal medulla (Kuo and Coffee, 1976a,b) and it plays a role in the calcium-dependent activation of tyrosine hydroxylase (Morgenroth et al., 1975; Yamauchi and Fujisawa, 1979). There is also evidence that tyrosine hydroxylase is a substrate for cAMP-dependent protein kinase, and phosphorylation by this kinase causes an activation of the enzyme (Vulliet et al., 1980). Activation of this single enzyme both by calcium and cAMP represents another instance in which both messenger systems activate the same cellular response element.

One of the most interesting aspects of the control system in this tissue relates to its long-term adaptive response to stress. For example, exposure of the rat to a cold environment, 4°C for 30 minutes or more, leads to hyperplasia and hypertrophy of the tissue. One of the biochemical events occurring in this adaptive response is the induction of tyrosine hydroxylase (Figure 9.5). The striking aspect of this response as deduced by Guidotti et al. (1975) is that tyrosine hydroxylase induction is always preceded by a rise in the tissue cAMP content occurring in the first 2 hours of the stressful response. Tissue levels of cAMP then decline, even if the stress is continued, and some 12 to 24 hours later the tyrosine hydroxylase content of the tissues rises. Any situation which blocks the initial increase in cAMP content blocks the subsequent rise in tyrosine hydroxylase content. In a previous discussion of this problem, we erroneously concluded that the mechanism of the cAMP increase was an activation of a β-receptor–cyclase system on the chromaffin cell surface by the secreted catecholamine (Rasmussen and Goodman, 1977). However, on the basis of the data of Guidotti et al. (1975), such a mechanism is unlikely in view of the fact that the rise is

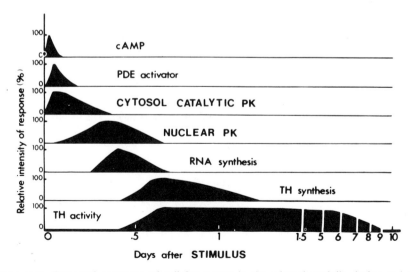

Figure 9.5 Temporal sequence of cellular events in the adrenal medulla during and after exposure to cold. TH = Tyrosine hydroxylase. From Guidotti et al. (1978), with permission.

mediated directly by Ach or its analogs, is not blocked by propranolol, and is blocked by agents which block nicotinic receptor activation.

However, in particulate preparations of medullary tissue, it is not possible to demonstrate a direct activation of adenylate cyclase by carbamylcholine even though the drug is highly effective in inducing a rise in the cAMP content of the tissue when added to intact tissue *in vitro* (Guidotti et al., 1975). In view of the finding that a calcium–calmodulin activation of adenylate cyclase is frequently observed in nervous tissue (Brostrom et al., 1976), it is quite possible that the sequence of events in the adrenal medulla is, as proposed by Guidotti et al. (1978) (Figure 9.6), an Ach-induced increase in plasma membrane calcium conductance followed by a rise in intracellular Ca^{2+} content which initially leads to synthesis of catecholamine by directly altering the activity of tyrosine hydroxylase. An activation of adenylate cyclase by calcium–calmodulin leads to a rise in cAMP concentration which in turn enhances the calmodulin-mediated secretory response and which causes the activation of tyrosine hydroxylase. The catalytic subunit (C) of this enzyme translocates into the nucleus where it initiates the synthesis of

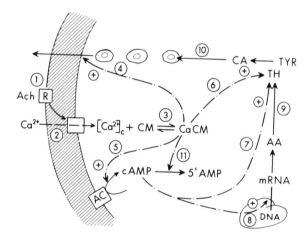

Figure 9.6 Sequential model of Ca^{2+} and cAMP-dependent control of adrenal medullary catecholamine secretion and biosynthesis. Interaction of acetylcholine with its surface receptor (1) leads to an increase in the Na^+ permeability of the membrane which in turn leads to membrane depolarization and the activation of a voltage-dependent calcium channel (2) in the membrane. The subsequent rise in cytosolic calcium ion concentration, $[Ca^{2+}]_c$, increases the concentration (3) of the calcium–calmodulin complex ($CM \cdot Ca^{2+}$). This complex mediates an immediate secretory response (4), an activation of adenylate cyclase (5), and an activation of the enzyme tyrosine hydroxylase (TH) (6). The activation of cyclase leads to a rise in cAMP concentration which interacts with protein kinase to liberate the free catalytic subunit. This subunit activates TH (7) and is translated to the nucleus where it stimulates the synthesis of the TH-mRNA (8) and eventually the synthesis of more TH (9). The combination of increased amount of TH and increased activity of TH leads to an increase in catecholamine (CH) synthesis (10). With continued acetylcholine exposure, the $CM \cdot Ca^{2+}$ concentration increases to the point where cAMP hydrolysis is activated (11) and cAMP concentration falls back to basal levels.

the mRNA for tyrosine hydroxylase (and other proteins). The reason for the subsequent fall in cAMP content even in the face of continued stress is thought to be a rise in the content of calcium–calmodulin in the cytosol leading to an activation of the cytosolic phosphodiesterase. This rise in calcium–calmodulin concentration could result from a cAMP-dependent release of calmodulin from the membrane; Gnegy et al. (1977) have shown that cAMP-dependent phosphorylation of a membrane fraction from brain caused the release of membrane-bound calmodulin.

These data are of considerable interest in focusing attention on the obvious question of why calcium–calmodulin would activate both adenylate cyclase, the cAMP source, and phosphodiesterase, the cAMP sink, in the same tissue. Obviously, if the purpose is to regulate cAMP content, simultaneous activation of both enzymes might well lead to no change in cAMP content and only a futile cycling of ATP. However, in the case of the adrenal medulla, the available evidence raises the distinct possibility that following hormonal (or neurotransmitter) activation of a tissue, there is a temporal and/or spatial separation of the two effects with an initial binding of calcium to the membrane-bound calmodulin which causes an activation of adenylate cyclase. The subsequent rise in cellular cAMP content (an increase in the amplitude of the cAMP signal) would have a number of the consequences, as described by Guidotti et al. (1978), but would also initiate the sequence of events leading to the termination of this cAMP signal. This sequence would be as follows: a rise in cAMP concentration, activation of cAMP-dependent protein kinase, phosphorylation of a membrane protein, dissociation of calmodulin from the membrane, a calmodulin-dependent activation of phosphodiesterase, a fall in cellular cAMP content. Thus, by a sequential activation of adenylate cyclase and phosphodiesterase involving the interplay of the two messenger systems, both the initial rise and the subsequent fall in cAMP concentration result from control of the activities of the respective enzymes by calcium–calmodulin.

UNICELLULAR ORGANISMS

Having considered the possible relationships between calcium and cAMP in the most complex of tissues, the central nervous system, it is worth considering the simplest and most primitive systems, various unicellular organisms.

One characteristic feature of these unicellular organisms is motility, and a nearly universal feature of motile animal cells is the control of the motile systems by calcium ion. It is, therefore, not unexpected that recent work has (1) identified both actin and myosin in these cells, (2) shown that calcium regulatory elements are present, (3) indicated that calcium currents across the plasma membrane function to couple stimulus to motile response, and (4) identified cAMP as a modulator of these calcium-regulated systems. Although much has been learned, we still have no complete picture of cAMP–calcium relationships in most of these organisms. Emphasis in the study of certain of them has been on the role of calcium, and in others, on the function of cAMP. In what follows, the description of the control properties of several of these systems will emphasize known aspects and only speculate on their possible general significance.

The unicellular systems in which the role of cAMP has been most thoroughly studied is the cellular slime mold *Dictyostelium discoideum*. The nucleotide is the principal extracellular messenger in the aggregation of this unicellular organism. This aggregation requires directed motility of the amoebae so that a calcium-mediated system is responsive to cAMP control. For these reasons, this system is the first to be discussed. An example of sequential control of a metabolic process in a unicellular organism, *Tetrahymena*, is discussed subsequently.

Aggregation in Slime Mold

The cellular slime molds, in particular *Dictyostelium discoideum*, have been a focus of investigative attention because of their ability to communicate with one another. When these amoebae starve, the isolated cells undergo a biochemical transformation from a population of noncommunicating individuals into a single communicating aggregate. Some of them begin to send out chemical messages to which others respond by both relaying the message and moving toward the source of the original message. This process continues until the individual amoebae have made contact and then joined together to form a slug, a multicellular organism, which undergoes a process of differentiation to form a spore within which a few viable amoebae remain alive and dormant until nutritional conditions are appropriate for population growth.

The part of this sequence from the initiation of signal generation by the lead amoebae to the point of slug formation is known as the process of aggregation. The messenger system underlying this process has been intensively studied and been shown to involve both cAMP and calcium (Gerisch et al., 1975; Konjin et al., 1967; Wurster et al., 1976, 1977; Bonner, 1967, 1977; Newell, 1978; Loomis, 1979; Mason et al., 1971; Wick et al., 1978; Malchow et al., 1972, 1975, 1978; Clarke and Spudich, 1974; Farnham, 1975; Gerisch and Hess, 1974; Gerisch and Wick, 1975; Goldbeter and Segal, 1977; Henderson, 1975; Mockrin and Spudich, 1976; Roos et al., 1977; Rossomando et al., 1973; Sampson, 1977).

When viewed by time lapse cinematography, aggregate dense populations of starved amoebae show a characteristic pattern of movement. The cell movement is periodic. The cells move at a rate of approximately 20 μm/min for 100 seconds, and then stop for approximately 4 minutes before a second period of movement. The initial signal is given off by a cell(s) in the center and is propagated outward. In dense populations of cells, this gives rise to periodic waves of inward movement of cells. As the cells come closer together later in the process of aggregation, movement may be lateral toward their neighbors as well as centrally so that the cells eventually form streaming branches pulsing toward the center.

The sequence of events in this aggregation process is depicted in Figure 9.7. The sequence consists of at least seven steps: (1) pulsatile signal generation, (2) reception of this signal by neighboring amoebae, (3) signal destruction, (4) relay of the message to further cells with entrainment of their motile responses, (5) chemotactic response by the recipient cell, (6) a developmental initiation response, and (7) cell docking. A feature of this signaling sequence is that once a cell has received a message and has responded by both moving and relaying the message, it becomes refractory for several minutes to stimulation by another message. When viewed on agar surface with dark-field optics, concentric light and dark bands are seen to radiate slowly out from the aggregation center. This change in optical behavior is considered to represent moving and stationary amoebae, respectively. A similar periodic change in light scattering (Figure 9.8) can be seen when aggregation-competent cells are suspended in a cuvette and viewed with a spectrophotometer (Gerisch and Hess, 1974). These oscillations have the same periodicity as the waves seen in an aggregating colony and are thought to represent periodic contraction and relaxation of the cells, and thus are apparently the counterpart of the chemotactic phase of the aggregation sequence.

The extracellular signal that is released by the amoebae is cAMP (Konjin, 1972). The pulsatile nature of the release of this signal has been established best by the studies of Gerisch et al. (1977), showing that the cAMP concentration in a cell population rises and falls periodically in synchrony with the alterations in light scattering (Figure 9.8).

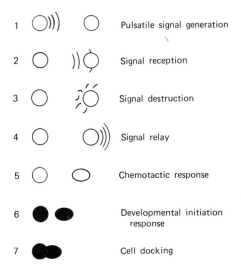

Figure 9.7 Sequence of events in slime mold aggregation. From Newell (1978), with permission.

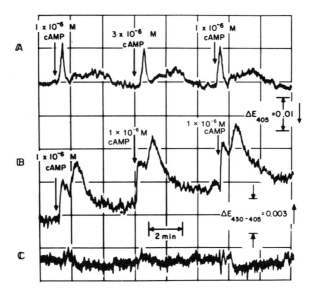

Figure 9.8 Periodic changes in light scattering induced in a culture of *Dictystelium discordeum* are treated with cAMP. From Gerisch and Hess (1974), with permission.

Reception of the cAMP by the recipient cells occurs by binding to a specific receptor on the cell surface (Malchow and Gerisch, 1974; Henderson, 1975; Green and Newell, 1975). These receptors are not present in the fed organism but appear hours after food deprivation. These are highly specific for cAMP and exhibit apparent negative cooperative binding (Mullens and Newell, 1978).

Signal destruction is essential if the system is to display periodicity. This means a system for the rapid destruction of cAMP must exist. Both membrane-bound (Pannbacker and Bravard, 1972; Malchow et al., 1972) and soluble phosphodiesterase has been found (Chassy, 1972; Riedel et al., 1972). However, an inhibitor of the soluble enzyme is also secreted, so it appears that the membrane-bound enzyme is the more important. This enzyme displays kinetics consistent with negative cooperative subunit interactions (Malchow et al., 1975; Green and Newell, 1975).

The relay of the signal is equally important for the propagation of the signal throughout the colony. This is achieved by activation of the adenylate cyclase in the recipient amoebae in response to the cAMP signal. The sequence of biochemical events induced by a pulse of cAMP to a cuvette containing competent amoebae is shown in Figure 9.9. Addition of cAMP induces a nearly immediate increase in the uptake of calcium into the cell, a rise in cGMP concentration, and a decrease in extracellular pH. These changes are followed by a fall in cGMP concentration, a temporary activation of adenylate cyclase leading to a brief rise in cAMP concentration, and a slow efflux of calcium. The change in light scattering is synchronous with the influx of calcium.

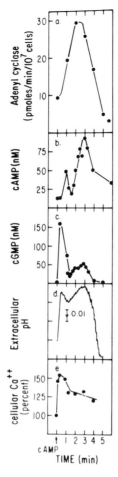

Figure 9.9 Sequence of biochemical events induced by a pulse of cAMP added to a cuvette containing aggregation-competent amoebae. From Loomis (1978), with permission.

The motion of the amoebae toward the aggregating center appears to be a calcium-dependent process (Mason et al., 1971) and probably involves the contraction of an actomyosin system. Taylor and coworkers (Taylor et al., 1973, 1976; Condeelis et al., 1976) have shown that in the amoeba *Chaos carolinensis,* motion involves a calcium-controlled contractile system analogous to that seen in the skeletal muscle of higher organisms. Also, Nuccitelli et al. (1977) have shown that a calcium current across the plasma membrane is related to the direction of movement in this amoeba. Spudich and co-workers (Clarke and Spudich, 1974; Mockrin and Spudich, 1976; Spudich and Cooke, 1975; Spudich and Clarke, 1974) have extracted actin and myosin from *Dictyostelium*. The actin is membrane-bound and may serve as the anchor of the contractile system. Mockrin and Spudich have also found a fraction from *Dictyostelium* which inhibits the myosin ATPase activity of recombined actin and myosin. This inhibited system is reactivated by calcium. This behavior is similar to that described in the case of thin filament control of myosin ATPase in mammalian skeletal muscle. It argues for thin filament (actin) control of the contractile apparatus by calcium. The calcium-binding protein from *Dictyostelium* has not yet been characterized. At present it is not clear whether this protein is similar to the calcium-dependent regulatory protein gelsolin found by Yin and Stossel (1979) to dissolve actin networks and therefore to regulate gel–sol transformations in the cytoplasm of macrophages, or whether it is related to troponin.

The fact that cAMP induces light scattering changes in the presence of 10 m*M* EGTA (Gerisch et al., 1975) has been taken as evidence that calcium is not necessarily involved in signal transduction. However, until it is known how rapidly amoebae lose their calcium under these circumstances, it remains possible that cAMP also increases the release of calcium from these cells. Based on the many observations discussed in preceding sections of this monograph, it seems most likely that the minimal role calcium plays in this system is to couple stimulus (cAMP reception) to chemotactic response (actomyosin contraction). However, given the fact that in many cells from higher organisms, calcium activates guanylate cyclase and adenylate cyclase, it is quite possible that calcium couples stimulus to all three of the major responses of the cell. The point of greatest importance is that a fundamental relationship exists between the calcium and cAMP messenger systems in this very primitive example of intercellular communication.

Metabolism in *Tetrahymena*

The unnicellular eukaryote *Tetrahymena pyriformis* has been found to possess a membrane-bound adenylate cyclase and to employ calcium as a second messenger in several responses. Calcium is utilized to control ciliary motion much as in *Paramecium* (Eckert, 1972). It is also involved in regulating the cell's response to glucose (Nandini-Kishore and Thompson, 1979; Kusamran et al., 1980). In this case, exposure of stationary phase cells to 0.5 to 1% glucose leads to an eightfold increase in the cAMP content of these cells within 1 hour. This rise in cAMP concentration is dependent on extracellular calcium but is blocked by dichloroisoproterenol, a β-catecholamine antagonist. Also, a rise in cAMP content can be induced by epinephrine even in the presence of EGTA, a calcium chelator. These findings have led to the proposal that the sequence of events is as follows: (1) a glucose-induced depolarization of the membrane, (2) the opening of a voltage-dependent calcium channel in the membrane, (3) a calcium-induced secretion of epinephrine, and (4) activation of the membrane-bound adenylate cyclase by epinephrine.

The significance of this rise in cAMP is not known, nor has there been any systematic exploration of other possible cAMP–calcium relationships in this organism. However, Charp and Whitson (1978) have shown that the intracellular concentrations of both cAMP and cGMP fluctuate in relation to the cell cycle in synchronized cultures of *Tetrahymena pyriformis*. The cAMP content is highest before the onset of cell division and is lowest at the end of division. The content of cGMP is lowest before the onset of division and highest at the time of division, and the intracellular calcium fluctuates in relation to the division cycle. There is an influx of calcium preceding division, followed 10 minutes later, at the peak of cytokinesis, by an efflux of calcium. These authors suggest that the alterations in cellular calcium content are responsible for the changes in cyclic nucleotide levels seen during the cell cycle. Although this hypothesis remains to be validated, the results do suggest that the calcium and cAMP messenger systems interact in this unicellular organism as they do in the cells of higher organisms.

The results of Whitson and his collaborators address another important area in which there is considerable evidence for a calcium–cAMP interaction. This area is the control of cell division. Although of great interest and importance, this area is not reviewed in the present monograph.

CONCLUSION

Although apparently less widespread than some of the other variants of synarchic regulation, *sequential control* is clearly evident in several cases of stimulus–response coupling. The fact that this type of control is found in the adrenal medulla, a neuroendocrine tissue, and that the effects of calcium on the two major components of the cAMP system, cyclase and phosphodiesterase, in the adrenal medulla are similar to those found in mammalian brain suggests that this type of control may be common in various types of nerve cells.

In discussing sequential control it is useful to conclude by pointing out that there is experimental evidence showing that each of the synarchic messengers, cAMP and Ca^{2+}, can control the concentration of the other in one of several ways. A rise in cytosolic Ca^{2+} concentration can either activate or inhibit the generation of the cAMP message, that is, activate phosphodiesterase. A rise in cytosolic cAMP concentration can lead either to a more prolonged opening or a more rapid closing of the voltage-dependent calcium channel in the plasma membrane, can enhance the termination of the calcium message by stimulating calcium uptake by the smooth endoplasmic reticulum (SR in muscle), and can delay the termination of the Ca^{2+} message by altering mitochondrial calcium efflux (see Chapter 2). These many different types of control suggest that sequential regulation will be found to be a common mode of operation of the synarchic system.

10

Summary

$$R_1 \quad \longrightarrow Ca^{2+} + CM \longrightarrow Ca_4CM$$

$$R_2 \quad \longrightarrow cAMP \longrightarrow \;\big\downarrow$$

$$R_1 \quad \longrightarrow Ca^{2+} + CM \longrightarrow Ca_4CM$$

GENERAL ASPECTS OF SYNARCHIC REGULATION

Having reviewed a broad spectrum of cellular responses, it is now possible to return to a consideration of the question raised early in our discussion. This question was whether or not in the course of biological evolution, control of stimulus-response coupling was achieved first by primitive mechanisms that were discarded as more complex patterns of cell behavior developed, or whether the early control mechanisms were of such simple elegance and adaptability that they have survived so that a few universal patterns of stimulus-response coupling account for the behavior of nearly all differentiated cells. The answer to that question is clearly that primitive mechanisms of stimulus-response coupling have survived through the millenia. They are as universal as the mechanisms responsible for controlling oxidative phosphorylation, glycogenolysis, and glycolysis. The slime mold and the liver cell share common control elements. The nerve cell and the adrenal cortical cell share cAMP and calcium ion as control elements in their response to stimulation. The amoeba and the brain cell have structurally similar cAMP and calcium receptor proteins. The beta cell and the adrenal medullary cell have the same voltage-dependent calcium channel in their plasma membranes. Yet each of these cells is unique in structure and function, and each, in addition to its heritage of common control elements, possesses some subtle variation upon this universal theme which makes its pattern of response unique. In the end, the discovery of the universality of certain cell control systems should not be surprising. Evolution has been, after all, a conservative process. Nonetheless, it is rather exciting to see a whole complex fabric of intracellular communication woven from such simple cloth. It is useful at this juncture to summarize the key points developed in the preceding chapters.

Synarchic regulation by calcium and cAMP is a universal mechanism by which stimulus–response coupling is achieved in differentiated cells when these are activated by extracellular messengers interacting with surface receptors. The type of cellular response involved is that of a differentiated cell being called upon to perform its specialized function.

The system constitutes a major means by which information flows from cell surface to cell interior. This flow of information can be categorized as a multistep process involving recognition, transduction, transmission, intracellular reception, modulation, response, and termination.

The role of this information transfer system is to alter the function of a number of cellular response elements in a coordinated fashion so that changes in their activities produce an integrated cellular response.

Although a universal system, synarchic regulation exhibits considerable organizational plasticity. Its particular organizational mode in a given cell type is defined by the nature of the interactions between calcium and cAMP. These include coordinate, hierarchical, redundant, sequential, and antagonistic patterns of interaction. However, in any particular cell, elements of more than one of these patterns may operate.

Viewed from this new perspective, there is no difference in stimulus–response coupling between so-called excitable and nonexcitable cells: both employ the same means to couple stimulus to response.

A change in an intracellular response can be achieved either by amplitude, sensitivity, or translocational modulation. The first of these involves changes in the concentration of either calcium or cAMP; the second involves a change in the sensitivity of (affinity for) a particular response element for either calcium or cAMP; and the third involves a translocation of a response element from one subcellular site to another.

The source of the messenger cAMP always is adenylate cyclase in the plasma membrane: the sink can be either cytosolic or membrane-bound phosphodiesterase. The source of calcium varies from one cell type to another. In some instances, cell activation is associated with an increased efflux of cellular calcium reflecting the mobilization of calcium from an internal source. There is circumstantial evidence that the internal source is the endoplasmic reticulum in some cases and the mitochondria in others. In other instances, activation of the surface receptor by hormone or neurotransmitter leads to an increase in Ca^{2+} influx into the cell. In most of these circumstances, the calcium influx is preceded or accompanied by a release of calcium bound to the plasma membrane and/or the endoplasmic reticulum. The exact mechanism by which calcium release from the endoplasmic reticulum is regulated is not known. The major intracellular sink for calcium is the mitochondrial matrix space but the plasma membrane calcium pump also helps terminate the calcium message.

The exact relationship of cGMP to this universal system remains to be defined. Present evidence indicates that the cGMP system modulates the activity of the calcium messenger system, but this evidence is incomplete.

Recent findings indicate that the activity of an electron transport chain in the plasma membrane can modify the properties of both transport systems within the membrane and the activities of membrane-bound enzyme. These findings lead to the obvious suggestion that this membrane redox system may play a role in integrating metabolic events within the cell to transport and metabolic events at the cell surface. Equally likely, this redox system may be a means of coupling ionic fluxes across the plasma membrane to metabolic events within the cell. Clearly, the role of this redox system in cell function and its coupling both to the cell ionic net and the calcium–cAMP messenger systems are areas of great potential interest and should be exciting areas for further exploration. Likewise, the possible roles of other messengers such as phosphoinositides and diacylglycerol have just begun to receive investigative attention. Similarly, the recent discovery of the phospholipid methylation pathway and the associated increase in phospholipase A_2 activity as important aspects of the transduction events in the plasma membrane illustrates the fact that the regulatory events under discussion are considerably more complex than our present working models. That these areas of research are largely unexplored should serve as a reminder that although the development of an understanding of the elegantly simple, yet amazingly complex interrelationships between the calcium and cAMP messenger system has given us a window through which we can begin to explore the regulation of cell function, other equally interesting windows remain to be opened. Nonetheless, the window that has been opened has given us important new insights into the control of cellular metabolism. None more so than the identification of the intracellular receptor proteins for cyclic AMP and calcium, and the characterization of their function in modulating the activity of various response elements. In closing, it is useful to bring this aspect of modulation into the context of overall regulation of cellular calcium metabolism and cell regulation.

INTRACELLULAR MODULATION AND REGULATION OF CELL FUNCTION

One feature of the present discussion is that of depicting the phenomena of cellular regulation in terms of information flow (Chapter 3). This focus has led in turn to an identification and analysis of the discrete steps in the flow of information from cell surface to cell interior. From this analysis a distinction has been made between two means by which intracellular receptor proteins modulate the function of intracellular response elements. These two mechanisms are *amplitude* and *sensitivity* modulation.

This term modulation has been introduced to describe the interaction between intracellular receptor proteins and response elements. These interactions can be characterized in terms of intra- and intermolecular communication. These intra- and intermolecular conversations are the final steps in the information flow process described in Chapter 3. An understanding of the molecular interactions involved in these conversations helps explain many of the most significant features of both amplitude and sensitivity modulation. These will be discussed in relation to the molecular basis of calmodulin action.

Molecular Basis of Calmodulin Action

Calmodulin function can be understood most easily by contrasting the concentration dependence of calcium binding to isolated calmodulin with the calcium dependence of activation of the calcium–calmodulin regulated enzymes, phosphodiesterase (PDE), and the plasma membrane Ca^{2+}/Mg^{2+}-ATPase or calcium pump (Crough and Klee, 1980; Waisman et al., 1981; Huang et al., 1981; Cheung, 1980; Cheung et al., 1981). When these data are plotted (Fig. 10.1), it is readily apparent that the K_D of calcium binding to calmodulin is in the range of 6 to 8 μM, but the K_m of activation of PDE is only 0.6 μM and that of the calcium pump 0.8 μM. This 10-fold difference might be accounted for in one of several ways: (1) the $Ca_1 \cdot CM$ form of calmodulin is the form that activates these enzymes; (2) calmodulin (CM) may be present in large excess of the enzymes hence only a small percentage is in the $Ca_4 \cdot CM$ form and serves as activator; or (3) the binding of CM to a response element like PDE induces a conformational change in CM leading to a marked enhancement in the affinity of CM for calcium.

Recent results indicate that both CM excess, and a PDE-induced conformation change in CM are involved (Blumenthal and Stull, 1980; Huang et al.,

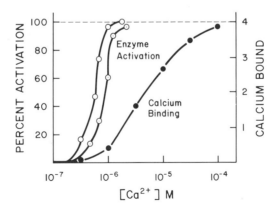

Figure 10.1 The binding of calcium to calmodulin (●—●) and the activity of the enzyme soluble phosphosidesterase (○—○) and membrane-bound Ca^{2+}-Mg^{2+}-ATPase (☉—☉) plotted as a function of the negative log of the calcium ion concentration (pCa). From (Crouch and Klee, 1980; Waisman et al., 1981a; and Huang et al., 1981).

1981). The first has implications to the question of sensitivity modulation, and is discussed subsequently. The second has implications for both amplitude and sensitivity modulation, and is discussed next. Before doing so it is worth summarizing the properties of calcium binding to calmodulin.

When the first calcium binds to isolated CM, a conformational change takes place leading to the enhanced binding of calcium to a second site (Klee, 1977; Crouch and Klee, 1980). The binding of the second calcium causes a further change in CM conformation, but the binding of Ca^{2+} to the third and fourth sites (in isolated calmodulin) causes only a small further change in conformation. From these results, it is reasonable to postulate that the first step in modulation is

$$2Ca^{2+} + CM \underset{k_2}{\overset{k_1}{\rightleftharpoons}} :Ca_2 \cdot CM^* \qquad (1)$$

where CM is calmodulin, and $Ca_2 \cdot CM^*$ is conformed calmodulin to which two calcium atoms are bound, and which is now capable of interacting with a response element. This leads to the next step,

$$Ca_2 \cdot CM^* + RE \underset{k_4}{\overset{k_3}{\rightleftharpoons}} :Ca_2 \cdot \overset{* \ *}{CM} \cdot RE \qquad (2)$$

where RE is a response element, and $Ca_2 \cdot CM \cdot RE$ is a complex of two calciums, a response element, and calmodulin, whose conformation has been further changed so that its two remaining calcium-binding sites have a much higher affinity for calcium than do the same two sites in isolated $Ca_2 \cdot CM^*$. As a consequence of this RE-induced conformational change in CM, the next step is,

$$Ca_2 \cdot \overset{* \ *}{CM} \cdot RE + 2Ca^{2+} \underset{k_6}{\overset{k_5}{\rightleftharpoons}} :Ca_4 \cdot \overset{* \ *}{CM} \cdot RE^* \qquad (3)$$

Where $Ca_4 \cdot CM \cdot RE^*$ is calmodulin with all four calcium-binding sites occupied leading to an activation of RE (RE $\rightarrow$ RE*).

This formulation oversimplifies the true situation, but is convenient because it emphasizes the two types of interacting sites on the calmodulin molecule: those that bind calcium (four in number) and those that bind response elements (one or more in number). Binding to the first calcium site changes the binding of calcium to the second; binding of two calciums changes the binding of RE to the other type of site(s); binding of RE changes the binding of calcium to the two remaining sites; and binding of the two last calciums alters the interaction of substrate with a second type of site on RE (the substrate binding site). Lastly, not shown in this three step model, when substrate, cAMP, binds to PDE (a response element) it enhances the rate of association of (equation 2), and/or the rate of activation of PDE (equation 3) by calmodulin (Teo et al., 1973; Cheung et al., 1981). Thus, all four types of sites, two on CM and two on the RE, influence ligand binding at other sites on both interacting molecules.

The most interesting feature in terms of amplitude modulation is that the association constant for calcium in the reaction 3,

$$Ca_2 \cdot \overset{* \ *}{CM} \cdot RE + 2Ca^{2+} \underset{k_6}{\overset{k_5}{\rightleftharpoons}} Ca_4 \cdot \overset{* \ *}{CM} \cdot RE^*$$

is greater than that for calcium in reaction 1,

$$2Ca^{2+} + CM \underset{k_2}{\overset{k_1}{\rightleftharpoons}} Ca_2 \cdot CM^*$$

$(k_5/k_6 > k_1/k_2)$.

Amplitude Modulation in the Calcium Messenger System

Considered in terms of the sequence of information flow discussed in Chapter 3, the accepted model by which either Ca^{2+} or cAMP serves its messenger function is one of amplitude modulation. In each case, the proposed sequence is the interaction of an extracellular messenger with its cell surface receptor, causing an increase in the concentration (amplitude) of an intracellular messenger (Fig. 10.2). This increase is perceived by a specific receptor protein because this protein has a high affinity for the intracellular messenger, and a narrow concentration range over which it binds to the messenger (Fig. 10.2). When the cell is not activated, the intracellular messenger concentration is below the range of detectability of the receptor protein. When the cell is activated, messenger concentration rises into the range of receptor protein detectability. If the binding affinity of calcium for calmodulin were invariant, then one would predict that all calmodulin-activated response elements would be inactive when the intracellular calcium ion concentration is below 0.1 μM and fully active when the calcium ion concentration is above 10 μM. However, as already noted, this is not the case, the affinity of the various binding sites on calmodulin for calcium is influenced by events at the response element binding sites on calmodulin. This fact has important implications for any discussion of amplitude as well as sensitivity modulation.

One of the most interesting features of sustained cellular responses mediated via activation of the calcium messenger system is that following an initial marked increase in cytosolic calcium ion concentration $[Ca^{2+}]_c$, lasting 3 to 6 minutes, there is a fall in $[Ca^{2+}]_c$ to a steady state concentration only 1.5- to 2.0-fold greater than that found in the nonactivated cell. Yet the cell remains fully activated. This means that the amount of $Ca_4 \cdot \overset{* \ *}{CM} \cdot RE^*$ (see equation 3) remains high if one assumes that there is a direct relationship between the concentration of $Ca_4 \cdot \overset{* \ *}{CM} \cdot RE^*$ and the magnitude of cellular response.

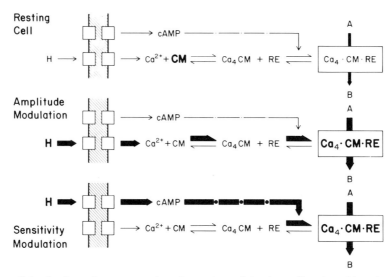

Figure 10.2 A schematic representation of a resting cell (top), a cell activated by a hormone and displaying amplitude modulation in the calcium messenger system (middle), and a cell activated by a hormone and displaying sensitivity modulation in the calcium messenger system secondary to a hormonally induced increase in cAMP. A→B represents the expression of activity of a particular response element (RE); CM represents calmodulin; and $Ca_4 \cdot CM \cdot RE$ represents the calcium-calmodulin–activated form of a particular response element. See text for discussion. Note that this representation is for pictorial purposes and is slightly different from the three step model developed in the text.

Other aspects of calmodulin physiology and cellular calcium metabolism must be discussed in order to understand these different time dependent changes in $[Ca^{2+}]_c$ and $[Ca_4 \cdot \overset{* \; *}{CM} \cdot RE^*]$. First the amount of calmodulin in the cell is large (20 μmol/kg cell H_2O) (Scharff, 1981) compared to the free calcium concentration (0.1 μmol/kg cell H_2O); and second the calmodulin concentration is greater than that of any given response element.

If we assume that to activate an appropriate group of response elements, 25% of the CM must be converted to $Ca_4 \cdot \overset{* \; *}{CM} \cdot RE^*$, then 20 μmoles of Ca^{2+} per kg cell H_2O must be added to the cell cytosol. If we consider that cytosolic (and other) calcium buffer systems continue to operate, a value closer to 50 μmol is probably necessary to achieve this result. The normal rate of calcium entry into a typical cell is 5 μmol/kg cell H_2O/min. This is normally balanced by a similar rate of efflux. During cell activation as much as fourfold increase in calcium influx rate may occur, leading to the influx of 20 μmol/kg cell H_2O/min. At this rate, enough additional calcium to activate CM would enter the cell within 3 minutes.

These calculations lead to the suggestion that the initial bolus of calcium entering the cell after activation is responsible for shifting the calmodulin system rapidly from an inactive (CM) to an active $(Ca_4 \cdot \overset{* \; *}{CM} \cdot RE^*)$ state.

The reason that $[Ca_4 \overset{* \ *}{\cdot} CM \cdot RE^*]$ remains high after this bolus of calcium, even though the steady state $[Ca^{2+}]_c$ falls to values only slightly greater than the concentration seen in the resting cell, is that the K_D for Ca^{2+} in reaction 3 is significantly lower than the K_D for Ca^{2+} in reaction 1 $(k_6/k_5 < k_2/k_1)$. This means that once the system has been shifted to the $Ca_4 \overset{* \ *}{\cdot} CM \cdot RE^*$ configuration, it remains in that configuration even though the $[Ca^{2+}]_c$ is lower than the $[Ca^{2+}]_c$ required to drive it into this configuration initially.

An additional feature of this activated cellular state is that the absolute rate of calcium influx into the cell remains high, and a small but sustained net influx of calcium into the cell is seen. The absolute influx rate is three- to fourfold greater than that seen in the resting cell. Nonetheless, the absolute increase in calcium ion concentration is less than 1.5-fold. This means that the efflux rate of calcium across the plasma membrane is also increased. This increased flux is mediated by activation of the plasma membrane calcium pump $Ca_4 \cdot CM$ (Fig. 10.1). Hence, the $Ca_4 \cdot CM$ (or some other form of $Cx_x \cdot CM$) couples events in the cytosol to those in the plasma membrane. Furthermore, there appears to be some type of coupling between influx and efflux rates across the plasma membrane such that the higher the influx rate, the lower the coupling ratio between influx and efflux, that is, for every incremental increase in influx rate, the incremental increase in efflux rate is slightly less, so that the higher the influx rate the higher the steady state level of ionized calcium in the cell cytosol. Thus, the increased cycling of calcium in the activated cell is not simply a futile metabolic cycle, but part of an elegant cellular control device that couples events at the plasma membrane to those in the cytosol and determines in particular the steady state level of messenger calcium in the cell cytosol, and therefore the concentrations of various $Ca_4 \overset{* \ *}{\cdot} CM \cdot RE^*$ complexes.

A final feature of this system is that in some cells, the change in calcium entry rate after cell activation is not sufficiently great to account for the rapidity of cell activation. In these cases, a transient release of calcium from one or more intracellular calcium pools is evoked by one of several poorly defined mechanisms and accounts for the rapidity of cell activation. However, even in this type of stimulus-response coupling, an increased plasma membrane cycling of calcium is necessary to achieve a sustained response (see discussion of the exocrine pancreas in Chapter 6). Hence, the intracellular pools serve primarily as a source for the initial bolus of calcium needed to trigger the shift of the calmodulin system from an inactive to an active state.

This discussion leads to the conclusion that the process of amplitude modulation is considerably more complex and elegant than previously considered. However, it is its very complexity that allows for the considerable plasticity of cellular response in a system employing a single messenger system. Given this very plasticity one might consider that other means of modulating cellular response are unnecessary. On the other hand, if one accepts the central hypothesis of synarchic regulation, an important validation of this hypothesis is the demonstration of many examples of their interaction at the level of modulation of cellular response. Many such examples do exist. A knowledge of them has led to the recognition of the second type of modulation, *sensitivity modulation* (see Chapters 3, 4, and 8).

Sensitivity Modulation in the Calcium Messenger System

By definition sensitivity modulation is a change in concentration of $Ca_4 \cdot \overset{* \; *}{CM} \cdot RE^*$ (on the simplifying assumption that this represents the only way that a $Ca \cdot CM$-mediated response is triggered, see equations 1 to 3) without a change in the $[Ca^{2+}]_c$. Reference to equations 1 to 3 shows that this could occur either by an increase in $[CM]$, an increase in k_1/k_2, k_3/k_4, or k_5/k_6. The key feature that distinguishes this type of modulation from amplitude modulation is that calcium is the message but in serving as message its concentration in the cytosol does not change (Fig. 10.2).

There are now several well studied examples of this type of modulation in the calcium messenger system. They are all cases in which a rise in $[cAMP]$ leads to a phosphorylation of a component of the response element. In these examples neither the $[CM]$ nor k_1/k_2 are changed. Either k_3/k_4 and/or k_5/k_6 are increased, that is, a covalent modification of the response element alters the apparent affinity of $Ca_2 \cdot CM^*$ for the Re and/or $Ca_2 \cdot \overset{* \; *}{CM} \cdot RE$ for Ca^{2+} leading to an increase in $[Ca_4 \cdot \overset{* \; *}{CM} \cdot RE^*]$.

The first enzyme system in which a cAMP-mediated change in the sensitivity to activation by calcium was described is the phosphorylase system. The key features of this system have already been presented (Figs. 4.9 and 4.10). From the point of view of molecular interactions, the system is of interest because phosphorylation of a subunit of the protein other than either the calcium-binding or catalytic subunits modifies the nature of the interaction between the two. This modification causes an increase in the apparent affinity of the subunit (calmodulin) for calcium. This type of sensitivity modulation can be characterized as *positive* sensitivity modulation. Cases of *negative* sensitivity modulation are also known (see Chapter 8). Both types have as their basis a covalent modification of a response element with a consequent change in the binding affinity of the response element $Ca_2 \cdot CM^*$ and/or Ca^{2+} (see equations 2 and 3).

An example of negative sensitivity modulation is seen in the neurohumoral control of smooth muscle contraction (see Chapter 8). It is instructive to consider this example because in this case the calcium receptor protein is calmodulin, the same calcium receptor protein involved in positive sensitivity modulation in the phosphorylase system. Even though calcium ion is known to couple excitation to contraction in smooth muscle as it does in skeletal and cardiac muscle, its molecular basis of action is quite different. A major calcium dependent change in smooth muscle proteins is a phosphorylation of the light chain of myosin (Dabrowska et al., 1977). There is a more or less direct correlation between the extent of myosin light chain phosphorylation and strength of smooth muscle contraction (Chapter 8). A variety of neural and humoral agents activate contraction by inducing a rise in the cytosolic calcium ion concentration thereby activating the calcium-dependent protein kinase, myosin light chain kinase (MLCK). The calcium binding component of this kinase is calmodulin. When calcium binds to calmodulin, the resulting complex (calcium-calmodulin) activates the enzyme, MLCK. This catalyzes the phosphorylation of the light chain of myosin resulting in a contraction. The K_m for calcium activation of this enzyme is approximately 3 μM, but varies according to the amount of calmodulin (Blumenthal and Stull, 1980).

In most smooth muscles, epinephrine and other β-adrenergic agonists cause a relaxation of the muscle which is mediated by an increase in intracellular cAMP concentration. The rise in cAMP concentration acts in several ways to lower cytosolic calcium ion concentration, but also acts to alter the sensitivity of the myosin light chain kinase to activation by calcium. To achieve this end, cAMP catalyzes the phosphorylation of the enzyme, and thereby shifts the calcium activation curve to a higher range of calcium-calmodulin concentrations (Fig. 8.6). Again, phosphorylation of a protein other than calmodulin alters the interaction of calcium-calmodulin with a response element.

Another form of sensitivity modulation involves regulation of the concentration of the calcium binding protein. In the case of calmodulin, it has been shown that cAMP-dependent phosphorylation of membranes can induce the release of calmodulin from the membrane (Hanbauer, 1980). The net effect of this release is to increase the concentration of CM in the cell cytosol, thereby increasing the concentration of $\overset{**}{Ca_2 \cdot CM}$ and thus $\overset{**}{Ca_4 \cdot CM \cdot RE^*}$ (equations 1 to 3). Likewise, membrane phosphorylation mediated by cAMP-dependent protein kinase can increase the binding of calmodulin to a membrane bound phosphodiesterase (Clayberger et al., 1981), and thereby enhance its activity presumably at a fixed $[Ca^{2+}]_c$.

As already noted, when cAMP binds to PDE it alters the interaction of CM with Ca^{2+} (Teo et al., 1973; Cheung, et al., 1981). This observation has important implications to the whole question of sensitivity modulation. For this reason, it is worth considering it in more detail. When cAMP binds to PDE it causes an increase in the association of $\overset{**}{Ca_2 \cdot CM \cdot RE^*}$ with Ca^{2+} and thus increase the formation of $\overset{**}{Ca_4 \cdot CM \cdot RE^*}$ (or the association of $Ca_2 \cdot$ CM with RE). This means that a rise in cAMP concentration can activate the system (PDE) responsible for terminating the cAMP message.

This situation represents a case where occupation of a substrate binding site on a response element leads to a shift in the equilibrium of either the Ca_2 $\cdot \overset{*}{CM} + RE \rightleftharpoons \overset{**}{Ca_2 \cdot CM} \cdot RE$ and/or the $\overset{**}{Ca_2 \cdot CM} \cdot RE^* \rightleftharpoons \overset{**}{Ca_2 \cdot CM} \cdot RE^*$ reaction. In theory there is every reason to believe that binding of an allosteric modifier to, rather than either substrate binding to or covalent modification of, a response element could bring about a similar change in these equilibria. This being the case there are an infinite number of potential examples of sensitivity modulation in the Ca^{2+}-messenger system.

The fact that any of three structural modifications (allosteric ligand binding, substrate binding, or phosphorylation) can alter the conformation of a given response element, and, thereby, its interaction with CM has implications beyond the concept of sensitivity modulation. If at any given cytosolic $[Ca^{2+}]$, several species of $Ca_4 \cdot \overset{**}{CM} \cdot RE^*$ exist ($Ca_4 \cdot \overset{**}{CM} \cdot \overset{**}{RE}{}^*$, $Ca_4 \cdot \overset{**}{CM} \cdot \overset{*}{RE}_2$, etc.) a change in the structure of one, for example, $Ca_4 \cdot \overset{**}{CM} \cdot \overset{*}{RE}_1$, such that an increase in affinity of CM for RE_1 increases, the concentrations of the other species of $Ca_4 \cdot \overset{**}{CM} \cdot RE_{2,3,...}$ would decrease. How important this particular mechanism would be depends on the ratio of the total concentrations of CM to those of the various response elements. Nonetheless, the ability of the common complex $Ca_2 \cdot \overset{**}{CM}$ to bind to a variety of response elements links these response elements functionally. A change in the binding affinity of one response element induced by an interaction with a drug, a steroid hormone, an ion, a metabolite, a protein, a membrane, or a cyclic nucleotide could influence the activity of several other response elements; the magnitude of this influence being determined both by the amount of the other response elements, and their individual degrees of association with calmodulin. There is, then, a metabolic network of calmodulin response elements all of which respond to some degree to changes not only in $[Ca^{2+}]_c$ but to changes in $[cAMP]_c$ and a host of other factors each of which may interact with only one component (a particular response element) of this nct.

Sensitivity Modulation in the cAMP Messenger System

Sensitivity modulation is not confined to the calcium system; at least one example is known in the cAMP messenger system. The known example is the regulation of glycogen metabolism by insulin (see Chapter 3). When insulin acts on muscle or liver, it causes an increase in glycogen synthesis. If the same cell is also stimulated by epinephrine, a rise in [cAMP] occurs leading to an activation of glycogenolysis. The cAMP controls the activity of a protein kinase which catalyzes the phosphorylation of phosphorylase b kinase (see above). If the two hormones (insulin and epinephrine) are given together, then even though epinephrine causes the same rise in cAMP concentration, there is a markedly reduced activation of the cAMP-dependent protein kinase, and therefore less of a phosphorylation of phosphorylase kinase. The explanation (Walkenbach et al., 1980) for this difference is that a second messenger (probably a glycopeptide), released by the plasma membrane into the cell cytosol as a consequence of insulin-receptor interaction, modifies the cAMP-dependent protein kinase in such a way that its sensitivity to activation by cAMP is altered (Fig. 3.21). As far as is presently known, this second messenger of insulin action does not regulate the state of phosphorylation of the cAMP-dependent protein kinase, but brings about its effect by some other means.

This example is important for two reasons. It illustrates the fact that sensitivity modulation is seen in the cAMP messenger system as well as the calcium messenger system. It also shows that such modulation can be achieved by noncovalent modification of a cellular response element.

The molecular basis of cAMP action is less well defined than that of Ca^{2+}. Nonetheless, recent data show that the classic cAMP receptor consists of the complex R_2C_2 where R is the cAMP receptor protein, and C is the catalytic subunit of protein kinase. Each R is known to possess two cAMP binding sites, hence the basic reaction is $R_2C_2 + 4cAMP \rightleftharpoons 2(cAMP)_2 \cdot R + 2C$. Recent data show that the binding of cAMP to R_2C_2 displays positive cooperative kinetics (Smith et al, 1981). This finding suggests that the control of response element function by cAMP and receptor protein may be operationally equivalent to that mediated by calcium ion and calmodulin.

Other examples of sensitivity modulation in the cAMP messenger system remain to be discovered. It seems quite likely that examples of positive as well as negative modulation will be found in this system as in the calcium messenger system.

Significance in Cell Regulation

This discussion leads to the conclusion that allosterically mediated conformational changes in both intracellular receptor proteins and their response elements lead to a variable rather than a fixed sensitivity of these systems to activation by a given change in intracellular messenger concentration. The present concepts imply that there are potentially an enormous number of discrete cellular processes whose activities are all controlled by the same intracellular messenger-receptor protein complex interacting with a discrete response element that has a distinctive and variable sensitivity to activation by that particular intracellular messenger. Cellular responses, even those that are highly specialized, are not stereotyped but plastic in character. This plasticity underlies the organizational elegance of intracellular control mechanisms.

Conclusion

The characteristics and molecular basis underlying each type of modulation have been considered. The key molecular feature that underlies both types is that the messenger receptor proteins possess two types of ligand-binding sites: one for the particular intracellular messenger, and one for a variety of other protein response elements. Binding of ligand to the messenger-binding site alters protein conformation and thereby ligand binding at the other site. Equally as important, binding of a response element (protein) at the second type of site also alters the conformation of the receptor protein and thereby the characteristics of the binding interaction between messenger and protein at the other type of site. It is these intramolecular and intermolecular conversations that are the ultimate intracellular dialogue in the flow of information from a change in extracellular messenger concentration to an appropriate cellular response. It is this dialogue which is the focal point of synarchic regulation.

References

Abell, C. W., and Monahan, T. M. (1973) *J. Cell. Biol.* 59: 549–558.

Adelstein, R. S., Conti, M. A., Hathaway, D. R., and Klee, C. B. (1978) *J. Biol. Chem.* 253: 8347–8350.

Adelstein, R. S., and Hathaway, D. R. (1979) *Am. J. Cardiol.* 44: 783–786.

Aguilera, G., and Catt, K. J. (1978) *Proc. Natl. Acad. Sci. USA* 75: 4057–4061.

Aguilera, G., and Catt, K. J. (1979) *Endocrinology* 104: 1046–1052.

Aksoy, M. P., Williams, D., Sharkey, E. M., and Hartshorne, D. J. (1976) *Biochem. Biophys. Res. Commun.* 69: 35–41.

Alkon, D. L. (1974) *Fed. Proc.* 33: 1083–1090.

Alkon, D. L. (1975) *J. Gen. Physiol.* 65: 385–397.

Alkon, D. L. (1976a) *J. Gen. Physiol.* 67: 197–211.

Alkon, D. L. (1976b) *J. Gen. Physiol.* 68: 341–358.

Alkon, D. L. (1979) *Science* 205: 810–816.

Alkon, D. L., and Grossman, Y. (1978) *J. Neurophysiol.* 41: 1328–1342.

Allen, J. E., and Rasmussen, H. (1972) *In* Prostaglandins in Cellular Biology. P. W. Ramwell, and B. B. Pharriss, Eds. Plenum, New York, pp. 27–51.

Ammon, H. P. T., and Verspohl, E. (1976) *Endocrinology* 99: 1469–1476.

Anderson, B., Osborn, M., and Weber, K. (1978) *Eur. J. Cell. Biol.* 17: 354–360.

Andersson, R., and Nilsson, K. (1972) *Nature (London) New Biol.* 238: 119–120.

Andersson, R. N., Isson, K., Wikberg, J., Johannson, S., and Lundholm, L. (1975) *Adv. Cyclic Nucl. Res.* 5: 491–518.

Appelman, M. M., and Teraski, W. L. (1975) *Adv. Cyclic Nucl. Res.* 5: 153–162.

Argent, B. E., Smith, R. K., and Case, R. M. (1976) *In* Stimulus Secretion Coupling in the Gastrointestinal Tract. R. M. Case, and H. Goebell, Eds. MPT Press, Lancaster, pp. 237–254.

Arthur, J. R., and Boyd, G. S. (1974) *Eur. J. Biochem.* 49: 117–127.

Ashby, J. P., and Speake, R. N. (1975) *Biochem. J.* 150: 89–96.

Ashcroft, S. J. H., Weerasinghe, L. C. C., and Randle, P. J. (1973) *Biochem. J.* 132: 223–231.

Ashley, C. C. (1978) *Ann. N.Y. Acad. Sci.* 307: 308–329.

Ashley, C. C., and Ridgway, E. B. (1968) *Nature (London)* 219: 1168–1169.

Ashley, C. C., and Ridgway, E. B. (1970) *J. Physiol. (London)* 209: 105–130.

319

Assimacopoulos-Jeannet, F. D., Blackmore, P. F., and Exton, J. H. (1977) *J. Biol. Chem.* 252: 2662–2669.

Atwater, I., Ribalet, B., and Rojas, E. (1978) *J. Physiol.* 278: 117–139.

Babcock, D. F., Chen, J.-L., Yip, B. P., and Lardy, H. A. (1979) *J. Biol. Chem.* 254: 8117–8120.

Bailey, C., and Villar-Palasi, C. (1971) *Fed. Proc.* 30: 1147.

Baker, P. F. (1973) *Fed. Proc.* 32: 1944–1950.

Baker, P. F. (1976) *In* SEB Symposium XXX, Calcium in Biological Systems. Cambridge University Press, New York, pp. 67–88.

Baker, P. F. (1978) *Ann. N.Y. Acad. Sci.* 307: 250–268.

Baker, P. F., and Carruthers, A. (1980) *Nature* 286: 276–279.

Balban, R. S., and Mandel, L. J. (1979) *Biochem. Biophys. Acta* 555: 1–12.

Bär, H. P., Hechter, O., Schwartz, I. L., and Walter, R. (1970) *Proc. Natl. Acad. Sci. USA* 67: 7–12.

Bárány, K., Bárány, M., Gillis, M. J., and Kushmerick, M. J. (1979) *J. Biol. Chem.* 254: 3617–3623.

Bárány, K., Bárány, M., Gillis, J. M., and Kushmerick, M. J. (1980) *Fed. Proc.* 39: 1547–1551.

Barker, W. C., Ketcham, L. K., and Dayhoff, M. O. (1977) *In* Ca^{2+} Binding Proteins and Ca^{2+} Function. R. H. Wasserman, R. A. Corradino, E. Carofoli, R. H. Kretsinger, D. H. MacLennan, and F. L. Seigel, Eds., Elsevier, New York, p. 110.

Baron, G., Demaille, J., and Dutruge, E. (1975) *FEBS Lett.* 56: 156–160.

Barrantes, F. J., Changeux, J. P., Lunt, G. G., and Sobel, A. (1975) *Nature* 256: 325–327.

Barrett, P., and Rasmussen, H. (1981) *In* Physiology of Cyclic Nucleotides. J. A. Nathanson, and J. W. Kebabian, Eds. Springer-Verlag, New York, In Press.

Barron, J. T., Bárány, M., and Bárány, K. (1979) *J. Biol. Chem.* 254: 4954–4956.

Batzri, S., Amsterdam, A., Selinger, Z., Ohad, I., and Schramm, M. (1971) *Proc. Natl. Acad. USA* 68: 121–123.

Batzri, S., and Selinger, Z. (1973) *J. Biol. Chem.* 248: 356–360.

Batzri, S., Selinger, Z., Schramm, M., and Rabinovitch, M. R. (1973) *J. Biol. Chem.* 248: 361–368.

Baumgartner, H. R. (1972) *Thromb. Diath. Haemorrh. Suppl.* 51: 161–198.

Bdolah, A., and Schramm, M. (1962) *Biochem. Biophys. Res. Commun.* 8: 266–270.

Bdolah, A., and Schramm, M. (1965) *Biochem. Biophys. Res. Commun.* 18: 452–454.

Beall, R. J., and Sayers, G. (1972) *Arch. Biochem. Biophys.* 148: 70–76.

Beaudoin, A. R., Marois, G., Dunnigan, J., and Morisset, J. (1974) *Can. J. Phys. Biochem.* 52: 174–182.

Beavo, J. A., Bechtel, P. J., and Krebs, E. C. (1975) *Adv. Cyclic Nucl. Res.* 5: 241–251.

Becker, E. L., and Showell, H. J. (1972) *J. Immunitaets forsch.* 1435: 466–476.

Becker, G. L., Fiskum, G., and Lehninger, A. L. (1980) *J. Biol. Chem.* 255: 9009–9012.

Bell, J. J., and Harding, B. W. (1974) *Biochim. Biophys. Acta* 348: 227–233.

Bell, R. L., Kennerly, D. A., Stanford, N., and Majerus, P. W. (1979) *Proc. Natl. Acad. Sci. USA* 76: 3238–3241.

Bentley, P. J. (1958) *J. Endocrinol.* 17: 201–209.

Bentley, P. J. (1960) *J. Endocrinol.* 21: 161–170.

Bentley, P. J. (1966) *Biol. Rev.* 41: 275–316.

Benzoana, G., Capony, J.-P., and Pechère, J.-F. (1972) *Biochim. Biophys. Acta* 278: 110–116.

Berridge, M. J. (1970) *J. Exp. Biol.* 53: 171–186.

Berridge, M. J. (1973) *Calliphora J. Exp. Biol.* 59: 595–606.

Berridge, M. J. (1975) *Adv. Cyclic Nucl. Res.* 6: 1–98.

Berridge, M. J. (1976a) *Adv. Cyclic Nucl. Res.* 6: 1–96.

Berridge, M. J. (1976b) *In* SEB Symposium XXX, Calcium in Biological Systems. Cambridge University Press, New York, pp. 219–231.

Berridge, M. J. (1980) *Cell Calcium* 1: 217–227.

Berridge, M. J., and Fain, J. N. (1979) *Biochem. J.* 178: 59–69.

Berridge, M. J., Lindley, B. D., and Prince, W. T. (1975) *J. Physiol. (London)* 244: 549–567.

Berridge, M. J., and Lipke, H. (1979) *J. Exp. Biol.* 78: 137–148.

Berridge, M. J., Oschman, J. L., and Wall, B. J. (1975) *In* Ca^{2+} Transport in Contraction and Secretion. E. Carafoli, F. Clementi, W. Drabikowski, and A. Margreth, Eds., North-Holland, Amsterdam. pp. 133–138.

Berridge, M. J., and Patel, N. G. (1968) *Science* 162: 462–463.

Berridge, M. J., and Prince, W. T. (1972a) *Adv. Insect Physiol.* 9: 1–18.

Berridge, M. J., and Prince, W. T. (1972b) *J. Exp. Biol.* 56: 139–153.

Berrie, C. P., Birdsall, N. J., Burgen, A. S. V., and Hulme, S. (1979) *Biochem. Biophys. Res. Commun.* 87: 1000–1005.

Berzins, K., Cohen, R. S., Blomberg, H., Siekevitz, P., Veda, T., and Greengard, P. (1978). *J. Cell. Biol.* 79: 92a.

Best, L. C., Martin, J. T., Russel, R. G. G., and Preston, F. E. (1977) *Nature* 267: 850–852.

Bihler, I. (1972) *In* The Role of Membranes in Metabolic Regulation. M. A. Hamlman, and R. W. Hanson, Eds. Academic, New York, pp. 411–422.

Bikle, D. D., Murphy, E. W., and Rasmussen, H. (1975) *J. Clin. Invest.* 55: 299–304.

Bikle, D. D., Murphy, E. W., and Rasmussen, H. (1976) *Biochim. Biophys. Acta* 437: 394–402.

Bikle, D. D., and Rasmussen, H. (1974a) *Biochem. Biophys. Acta* 362: 439–447.

Bikle, D. D., and Rasmussen, H. (1974b) *Biochem. Biophys. Acta* 362: 425–438.

Bikle, D. D., and Rasmussen, H. (1978a) *Biochem. Biophys. Acta* 538: 127–138.

Bikle, D. D., and Rasmussen, H. (1978b) *J. Biol. Chem.* 53: 3042–3048.

Billah, M. M., and Mitchell, R. H. (1979) *Biochem. J.* 182: 661–668.

Binder, H. J., and Rawlins, C. L. (1973a) *J. Clin. Invest.* 52: 1460–1466.

Binder, H. J., and Rawlins, C. L. (1973b) *Am. J. Physiol.* 225: 1232–1239.

Birks, R. I., and MacIntosh, F. C. (1957) *Br. Med. Bull.* 13: 146–161.

Birmingham, M. K., Elliot, F. H., and Valere, P. H. C. (1953) *Endocrinology* 53: 687–689.

Birmingham, M. K., Kurlents, E., Lane, R., Muhlstock, B., and Traikov, H. (1960) *Can. J. Biochem. Physiol.* 38: 1077–1085.

Birnbaum, M. J., and Fain, J. N. (1977) *J. Biol. Chem.* 252: 528–535.

Birnbaumer, L. (1973) *Biochim. Biophys. Acta* 300: 129–158.

Birnbaumer, L. (1977) *In* Cyclic 3′,5′-Nucleotides: Mechanisms of Action. H. Cramer, and J. Schultz, Eds. Wiley, New York, pp. 13–36.

Blackmore, P. F., Assimacopoulos-Jeannet, F., Chan, T. M., and Exton, J. H. (1979) *J. Biol. Chem.* 254: 2828–2834.

Blackmore, P. F., Brumley, F. T., Marks, J. L., and Exton, J. H. (1978) *J. Biol. Chem.* 253: 3851–3858.

Blackmore, P. F., Dehaye, J.-P., and Exton, J. H. (1979) *J. Biol. Chem.* 254: 6945–6950.

Blair, E. L., Brown, J. C., Harper, A. A., and Scratcherd, T. (1966) *J. Physiol. (London)* 184: 812–824.

Blaustein, M. P. (1974) *Rev. Physiol. Biochem. Pharmacol.* 70: 33–82.

Blaustein, M., Ratzstaff, R. W., and Kendrick, N. K. (1978) *Ann. N.Y. Acad. Sci.* 307: 195–212.

Blinks, J. R., Prendergast, F. G., and Allen, D. G. (1976) *Pharmacol. Rev.* 28: 1–93.

Blomberg, H., Cohen, R. S., and Siekevitz, P. (1977) *J. Cell. Biol.* 74: 204–225.

Bloom, H. E. (1979) *Fed. Proc.* 38: 2203–2207.

Blume, A. I., Lichtenstein, D., and Boone, G. (1979) *Proc. Natl. Acad. Sci USA* 76: 5626–2630.

Blumenthal, D. K., and Stull, J. T. (1980) *Biochemistry* 19: 5608–5614.

Boelkins, J. N., Mazurkiewiez, M., Mazar, P. E., and Mueller, W. J. (1976) *Endocrinology* 98: 403–412.

Bolton, J. E., and Field, M. (1977) *J. Membr. Biol.* 35: 159–173.

Bolton, T. B. (1979) *Physiol. Rev.* 59: 607–718.

Bond, G. H., and Clough, D. L. (1973) *Biochim. Biophys. Acta* 323: 592–599.

Bonner, J. T. (1967) The Cellular Slime Molds, 2nd ed. Princeton University Press, Princeton.

Bonner, J. T. (1977) *Mycologia* 69: 443–459.

Borle, A. (1970) *J. Gen. Physiol.* 55: 163–171.

Borle, A. B. (1972) *J. Membr. Biol.* 10: 45–66.

Borle, A. (1973) *Fed. Proc.* 32: 1944–1950.

Borle, A. (1974) *J. Membr. Biol.* 16: 221–228.

Borle, A. B., and Anderson, J. H. (1976) *In* SEB Symposium XXX, Calcium in Biological Systems. Cambridge University Press, New York, pp. 141–160.

Borle, A. B., and Uchikawa, T. (1978) *Endocrinology* 102: 1725–1732.

Borle, A. B., and Uchikawa, T. (1979) *Endocrinology* 104: 122–129.

Bougeois, J. P., Popot, J. L., Ryter, A., and Changeux, J.-P. (1973) *Brain Res.* 62: 557–563.

Bowman, R. H. (1970) *J. Biol. Chem.* 245: 1604–1612.

Bowman, W. C., and Nott, M. W. (1969) *Pharmacol. Rev.* 21: 27–72.

Bowyer, F., and Kitabchi, A. E. (1974) *Biochem. Biophys. Res. Commun.* 57: 100–105.

Boyd, G. S., Arthur, J. R., Beckett, G. J., Mason, J. I., and Trzeciak, W. H. (1975) *Steroid Biochem.* 6: 427–436.

Boynton, A. L., Whitfield, J. F., Issaics, R. J., and Morton, H. J. (1974) *In Vitro* 10: 12–17.

Brading, A. F. (1978) *Proc. Physiol. Soc.* 12P–14P.

Bremel, R. D. (1974) *Nature (London)* 252: 405–407.

Brinley, F. J., Jr. (1978) *Ann. Rev. Biophys. Bioeng.* 7: 363–392.

Brinley, F. J., Jr., Tiffert, T., and Scarpa, A. (1978) *FEBS Lett.* 91: 25–29.

Brisson, G. R., and Malaisse, W. J. (1973) *Metabolism* 22: 455–465.

Brisson, G. R., Malaisse-Lague, F., and Malaisse, W. T. (1972) *J. Clin. Invest.* 51: 232–241.

Broches, J. P., Berg, D. K., and Hall, Z. W. (1976) *Cold Spring Harbor Symp. Quant. Biol.* 40: 253–262.

Brooks, A. M., Johnson, L. R., and Grossman, M. I. (1970) *Gastroenterology* 58: 470–475.

Brostrom, C. O., Brostrom, M. A., and Wolff, D. J. (1977) *J. Biol. Chem.* 252: 5677–5685.

Brostrom, C. O., Hunkeler, F. L., and Krebs, E. G. (1971) *J. Biol. Chem.* 246: 1961–1967.

Brostrom, M. A., Brostrom, C. O., Breckenridge, B. M., and Wolff, D. J. (1975) *Proc. Natl. Acad. Sci. U S A* 72: 64–68.

Brostrom, M. A., Brostrom, C. O., Breckenridge, B. M., and Wolff, D. J. (1976) *J. Biol. Chem.* 251: 4744–4750.

Brostrom, M. A., Brostrom, C. O., Breckenridge, B. M., and Wolff, D. J. (1978) *Adv. Cyclic Nucl. Res.* 9: 85–99.

Brostrom, M. A., Brostrom, C. O., and Wolff, D. J. (1979) *J. Biol. Chem.* 254: 7548–7557.

Brunelli, M., Castellucci, V., and Kandel, E. R. (1976) *Science* 194: 1178–1181.

Bruns, D. E., Black, B., McDonald, J. M., and Jarrett, L. (1977) *In* Ca^{2+} Binding Proteins and Ca^{2+} Function. R. H. Wasserman, R. A. Corradino, E. Carofoli, R. H. Kretsinger, D. H. MacLennan, and F. L. Seigel, Eds., Elsevier, New York, p. 181.

Burgen, A. S. V. (1956) *J. Physiol. (London)* 132: 20–39.

Busis, N. A., Weight, F. F., and Smith, P. A. (1978) *Science* 200: 1079–1081.

Butcher, F. R. (1975) *Metabolism* 24: 409–418.

Butcher, F. R. (1978a) *Adv. Cyclic Nucl. Res.* 9: 707–712.

Butcher, F. R. (1978b) Biochemical Actions of Hormones. G. Litwack, Ed. Vol. V, Academic, New York, pp. 54–101.

Butcher, F. R. (1979) *Life Sci.* 24: 1979–1982.

Butcher, F. R. (1980) *Biochim. Biophys. Acta* 630: 254–260.

Butcher, F. R., Boldman, J. A., and Memerovski, M. (1975) *Biochim. Biophys. Acta* 392: 82–94.

Butcher, F. R., McBride, P. A., and Rudich, L. (1976) *Mol. Cell. Endocrinol.* 5: 243–254.

Butcher, F. R., and Putney, J. W. (1980) *Adv. Cyclic Nucl. Res.* 13: 215–250.

Bygrave, F. L. (1978) *Biol. Rev.* 53: 43–49.

Bygrave, F. L., and Tranter, C. J. (1978) *Biochem. J.* 174: 1021–1030.

Candia, O. A., Montoreano, R., and Podos, S. M. (1977) *Am. J. Physiol.* 233: F94–F101.

Carafoli, E. (1979) *FEBS Lett.* 104: 1–5.

Carafoli, E., and Crompton, M. (1976) *In* SEB Symposium XXX, Calcium in Biological Systems. Cambridge University Press, New York, pp. 90–115.

Carafoli, E., and Crompton, M. (1978) *Ann. N.Y. Acad. Sci.* 307: 269–284.

Carafoli, E., Rossi, C. S., and Lehninger, A. L. (1964) *J. Biol. Chem.* 239: 3055–3061.

Caravoris, C. P., Franki, N., Levine, S. D., and Hays, R. M. (1979) *J. Membr. Biol.* 49: 253–268.

Caron, M. G., Srinivasan, Y., Pitha, J., Kociolak, K., and Lefkowitz, R. J. (1979) *J. Biol. Chem.* 254: 2292–2927.

Carpentier, J.-L., Gorden, P., Amherdt, M., Van Obberghen, E., Kahn, C. R., and Orci, L. (1978) *J. Biol. Chem.* L53: 4900–4906.

Carsten, M. E. (1971) *Arch. Biochem. Biophys.* 147: 353–357.

Carstens, M., and Weller, M. (1979) *Biochim. Biophys. Acta* 551: 420–431.

Carter, D. C., Forrest, J. A. H., Werner, M., Heading, R. C., Park, J., and Shearman, J. C. (1974) *Br. Med. J.* 3: 554–556.

Case, R. M. (1973a) *Acta Hepatogastroenterol.* 20: 435–444.

Case, R. M. (1973b) *Digestion* 8: 269–288.

Case, R. M. (1978) *Biol. Rev.* 53: 211–354.

Case, R. M., and Clausen, T. (1973) *J. Physiol.* 235: 75–102.

Cassel, D., Levkowitz, H., and Selinger, A. (1977) *J. Cyclic Nucl. Res.* 3: 393–406.

Cassel, D., and Selinger, Z. (1977a) *Biochem. Biophys. Res. Commun.* 77: 868–673.

Cassel, D., and Selinger, Z. (1977b) *Biochim. Biophys. Acta* 452: 538–551.

Cassel, D., and Selinger, Z. (1977c) *Proc. Natl. Acad. Sci. USA* 74: 3307–3311.

Cassel, D., and Selinger, Z. (1978) *Proc. Natl. Acad. Sci. USA* 75: 4155–4159.

Cassidy, P., Hoar, P. E., and Kerrick, W. C. L. (1979) *J. Biol. Chem.* 254: 11148–11153.

Casteels, R., and Raeymaekers, L. (1979) *J. Physiol.* 294: 51–68.

Castellucci, V., and Kandel, E. R. (1976) *Science* 194: 1176–1178.

Castellucci, V., Pinsker, H., Kupfermann, I., and Kandel, E. R. (1970) *Science* 167: 1745–1748.

Catt, K. J., Harwood, J. P., Aguilera, G., and Dufau, M. L. (1979) *Nature* 280: 109–116.

Caveny, S. (1978) *Science* 199: 192–194.

Caveny, S., and Podgorski, C. (1975) *Tissue Cell* 7: 559–574.

Cereijido, M., Robbins, E. S., Dolan, W. J., Rotuanno, C. A., and Sabatini, D. D. (1976) *J. Cell. Biol.* 77: 853–880.

Chacko, S., Conti, M. S., and Adelstein, R. S. (1977) *Proc. Natl. Acad. Sci. USA* 74: 129–133.

Chan, T. M., and Exton, J. H. (1977) *J. Biol. Chem.* 252: 8645–8651.

Chan, T. M., and Exton, J. H. (1978) *J. Biol. Chem.* 253: 6393–6400.

Chance, B. (1965) *J. Biol. Chem.* 240: 2729–2748.

Chandler, D. E., and Williams, J. A. (1974) *J. Physiol.* 243: 831–846.

Chandler, D. E., and Williams, J. A. (1977) *J. Membr. Biol.* 32: 201–230.

Chang, H. W. (1974) *Proc. Natl. Acad. Sci. USA* 71: 2113–2117.

Changeux, J. P., Benedetti, L., Bourgeois, J. P., Brisson, A. D., Cartand, J., Devaux, P., and Grünhagen, H. H. (1976) *Cold Spring Harbor Symp. Quant. Biol.* 40: 211–230.

Changeux, J. P., Kasai, M., and Lee, C. Y. (1970) *Proc. Natl. Acad. Sci. U S A* 67: 1241–1247.

Changeux, J. P., Meunier, J. C., and Huchet, M. (1971) *Mol. Pharmacol.* 7: 538–553.

Changeux, J. P., Podleski, T. R., and Meunier, J. C. (1969) *J. Gen. Physiol.* 54: 225S–244S.

Changeux, J. P., Thiery, J., Tung, T., Kittel, C. (1967) *Proc. Natl. Acad. Sci. USA* 57: 335–341.

Chapman, R. A. (1979) *Prog. Biophys. Mol. Biol.* 35: 1–52.

Charles, M. A., Lawecki, J., Picket, R., and Grodsky, G. M. (1975) *J. Biol. Chem.* 240: 6134–6140.

Charo, I., Feinman, R. D., and Deturler, T. C. (1976) *Biochem. Biophys. Res. Commun.* 72: 1462–1467.

Charp, P. A., and Whitson, G. L. (1978) *Radiat. Res.* 74: 323–334.

Chase, L. R., and Aurbach, G. D. (1967) *Proc. Natl. Acad. Sci. USA* 58: 518–525.

Chassy, B. M. (1972) *Science* 175: 1016–1018.

Chen, J. J., Babcock, D. F., and Lardy, H. A. (1978) *Proc. Natl. Acad. Sci. USA* 75: 2234–2238.

Chen, T. L., and Feldman, D. (1978) *Endocrinology* 102: 589–596.

Cherrington, A. D., Assimacopoules, F. D., Harper, S. C., Corbin, J. D., Park, C. R., and Exton, J. H. (1976) *J. Biol. Chem.* 251: 5209–5218.

Cheung, W. Y. (1970) *Biochem. Biophys, Res. Commun.* 38: 533–545.

Cheung, W. Y. (1980) *Science* 207: 19–27.

Cheung, W. Y., Bradham, L. S., Lynch, T. J., Lin, V. M., and Tallant, E. A. (1975) *Biochem. Biophys. Res. Commun.* 66: 1055–1062.

Cheung, W. Y., Lynch, T. J., Wallace, R. W., and Tallant, E. A. (1981) *J. Biol. Chem.* 256: 4439–4443.

Chu, H. I., Franks, D. J., Rowe, R., and Malamud, D. (1976) *Biochim. Biophys. Acta* 551: 29–40.

Christophe, J., Deschodt-Lanckman, M., Adler, N., and Robberecht, P. (1977) *In* Hormonal Receptors in Digestive Tract Physiology. S. Bonfils, P. Fromageot, and G. Rosselin., Eds. North-Holland, Amsterdam, pp. 247–259.

Christophe, J. P., Frandsen, E. K., Conlon, T. P., Kirshna, G., and Gardner, J. D. (1976) *J. Biol. Chem.* 251: 4640–4645.

Claret-Berthon, B., Claret, M., and Mazet, J. L. (1977) *J. Physiol.* 272: 529–552.

Clark, M. G., and Jarrett, J. G. (1978) *Biochem. J.* 176: 805–816.

Clarke, M., and Spudich, J. A. (1974) *J. Mol. Biol.* 86: 209–222.

Clausen, T., Elbrink, J., and Dahl-Hansen, A. B. (1975) *Biochim. Biophys. Acta* 375: 292–308.

Clayberger, C., Goodman, D. B. P., and Rasmussen, H. (1981) *J. Membr. Biol.* 58: 191–201.

Clemente, F., and Meldolesi, J. (1975a) *Br. J. Pharmacol.* 55: 369–379.

Clemente, F., and Meldolesi, J. (1975b) *J. Cell. Biol.* 65: 88–102.

Clements, R. S., Jr., and Rhoten, W. (1976) *J. Clin. Invest.* 57: 684–691.

Cochrane, D. E., and Douglas, W. W. (1974) *Proc. Natl. Acad. Sci. USA* 71: 408–412.

Cockeroft, S., and Gomperts, B. D. (1979) *Biochem. J.* 178: 681–687.

Cohen, J. L., Weiss, K. R., and Kupfermann, I. (1978) *J. Neurophysiol.* 41: 157–180.

Cohen, P. (1973) *Eur. J. Biochem.* 34: 1–14.

Cohen, P. (1978) *Curr. Top. Cell. Reg.* 14: 117–186.

Cohen, P., Burchell, A., Foulkes, J. G., and Cohen, P. T. W. (1978) *FEBS* Lett. 92: 287–293.

Cohen, R. S., Blomberg, F., Berzins, K., and Siekevitz, P. (1977) *J. Cell. Biol.* 74: 181–203.

Cohn, D. V., and Forscher, B. K. (1962) *J. Biol. Chem.* 237: 615–618.

Cohn, D. V., and Wong, G. L. (1978) *In* Endocrinology of Calcium Metabolism. D. H. Copp, and R. V. Talmage, Eds. Excerpta Medica, Amsterdam/Oxford.

Collins, J. H. (1976a) *Nature* 259: 699–700.

Collins, J. H. (1976b) *In* SEB Symposium XXX, Calcium in Biological Systems. Cambridge University Press, New York, pp. 303–334.

Collins, J. H., Potter, J. D., Horn, M. J., Wilshire, G., and Jackson, N. (1973) *FEBS Lett.* 36: 268–272.

Condeelis, J. S., Taylor, D. L., Moore, P. L., and Allen, R. D. (1976) *Exp. Cell. Res.* 101: 134–142.

Conti, M. A., and Adelstein, R. S. (1980) *Fed. Proc.* 39: 1569–1573.

Cooke, A. R. (1970) *Gastroenterology* 58: 633–637.

Corbin, J. D., and Lincoln, T. M. (1978) *Adv. Cyclic Nucl. Res.* 9: 159–170.

Cori, G. T., Colowick, S. P., and Cori, C. F. (1938) *J. Biol. Chem.* 123: 381–389.

Cori, G. T., and Cori, C. F. (1945) *J. Biol. Chem.* 158: 321–332.

Constantin, L. L. (1970) *J. Gen. Physiol.* 55: 703–715.

Coupland, R. E. (1965) The Natural History of the Chromaffin Cell. Longmans Green and Co., London.

Crane, F. L., and Löw, H. (1978) *FEBS Lett.* 68: 153–156.

Crompton, M., Moser, R., Lüdi, H., and Carafoli, E. (1978) *Eur. J. Biochem.* 82: 25–31.

Crouch, T. H., and Klee, C. B. (1981) *Biochemistry* 19: 3692–3698.

Cubeddu, L., Barnes, X. E., and Weiner, N. (1974) *J. Pharmacol. Exp. Ther.* 193: 105–127.

Cullis, P. R., and DeKruijff, B. (1979) *Biochim. Biophys. Acta* 599: 399–420.

Curry, D. L., Bennett, L. L., and Grodsky, G. M. (1968) *Am. J. Physiol.* 214: 174–178.

Cuthbert, A. W., Painter, E., and Prince, W. T. (1969) *Br. J. Pharmacol.* 36: 97–106.

Cuthbert, A. W., and Wong, P. Y. D. (1974) *J. Physiol. (London)* 241: 407–422.

Dabrowska, R., Aramatorio, D., Sherry, J. M. F., and Hartshorne, D. J. (1978) *Biochemistry* 17: 253–257.

Dabrowska, R., and Hartshorne, D. J. (1978) *Biochem. Biophys. Res. Commun.* 85: 1352–1359.

Dambach, N. G., and Friedmann, N. (1974) *Biochim. Biophys. Acta* 332: 374–386.

Davis, J. P. (1961) *Rec. Prog. Horm. Res.* 17: 293–351.

Davis, W. L., Goodman, D. B. P., Jones, R. G., and Rasmussen, H. (1978) *Tissue Cell* 10: 451–462.

Davis, W. L., Goodman, D. B. P., Martin, J. H., Matthews, J. L., and Rasmussen, H. (1974) *J. Cell. Biol.* 61: 544–547.

Davis, W. L., Goodman, D. B. P., Schuster, R. J., Martin, J. H., and Rasmussen, H. (1974) *J. Cell. Biol.* 63: 986–997.

Dean, P. M., and Matthews, E. K. (1970a) *J. Physiol.* 210: 225–264.

Dean, P. M., and Matthews, E. K. (1970b) *J. Physiol.* 210: 265–275.

Dean, P. M., and Matthews, E. K. (1972) *Diabetologia* 8: 173–178.

Dedman, J. R., Brinkley, B. R., and Means, A. R. (1979) *In* Advances in Cyclic Nucleotide Research, Vol. 11. P. Greengard, and G. A. Robinson, Eds. Raven Press, New York, pp. 131–174.

Dedman, J. R., Jackson, R. L., Schreiber, W. E., and Means, A. R. (1978) *J. Biol. Chem.* 253: 343–346.

Dedman, J. R., Potter, J. D., Jackson, R. L., Johnson, J. D., and Means, M. R. (1977a) *J. Biol. Chem.* 252: 8415–8422.

Dedman, J. R., Potter, J. D., and Means, A. R. (1977b) *J. Biol. Chem.* 252: 2437–2440.

Dehtaan, R. L., and Sachs, H. G. (1972) *Curr. Top. Dev. Biol.* 7: 194–228.

Délèze, J., and Loewenstein, W. R. (1976) *J. Membr. Biol.* 28: 71–86.

DeLorenzo, R. J. (1976) *Biochem. Biophys. Res. Commun.* 71: 590–597.

DeLorenzo, R. J., and Freedman, S. D. (1977a) *Biochem. Biophys. Res. Commun.* 77: 1036–1043.

DeLorenzo, R. J., and Freedman, S. D. (1977b) *Epilepsia* 18: 357–365.

DeLorenzo, R. J., and Freedman, S. D. (1978) *Biochem. Biophys. Res. Commun.* 80: 183–192.

Delorenzo, R. J., Freedman, S. D., Yohe, W. B., and Maurer, S. D. (1979) *Proc. Natl. Acad. Sci. USA* 76: 1838–1842.

DeLorenzo, R. J., and Greengard, P. (1973) *Proc. Natl. Acad. Sci. USA* 70: 1831–1835.

DeLorenzo, R. J., Walton, K. G., Curran, P. F., and Greengard, P. (1973) *Proc. Natl. Acad. Sci. USA* 70: 880–884.

DeLuca, H. F., Engstrom, G. W., and Rasmussen, H. (1962) *Proc. Natl. Acad. Sci. USA* 48: 1604–1609.

DeMeyts, P., Bianco, A. R., and Roth, J. (1976) *J. Biol. Chem.* 251: 1877–1888.

Denton, R. M., Randle, P. J., and Martin, B. R. (1972) *Biochem. J.* 128: 161–169.

Denton, R. M., Richards, D. A., and Chin, J. G. (1978) *Biochem. J.* 176: 899–906.

DePaoli-Roach, A. A., Roach, P. J., and Larner, J. (1979) *J. Biol. Chem.* 254: 4212–4219.

DePont, J. H. M., Luyben, D., and Bonting, S. L. (1979) *Biochim. Biophys. Acta* 584: 33–42.

Deth, R., and Van Breeman, C. V. (1977) *J. Membr. Biol.* 30: 363–380.

DeTorrentegui, G., and Berthet, J. (1966) *Biochem. Biophys. Acta* 116: 467–476.

Detwiler, T. C. (1972) *Biochim. Biophys. Acta* 256: 163–174.

Detwiler, T. C., and Feinman, R. D. (1973) *Biochemistry* 12: 282–289.

Devis, G., Somers, G., Obberghen, E. V., and Malaisse, W. J. (1975) *Diabetes* 24: 546–551.

Diamond, J. M. (1962) *J. Physiol.* 161: 474–502.

Diamond, J. M. (1964) *J. Gen. Physiol.* 48: 1–14.

Dietschy, J. M. (1964) *Gastroenterology* 47: 395–408.

Dills, W. L., Beavo, J. A., Bechtel, P. J., Meyers, K. T., Sakai, J., and Krebs, E. G. (1976) *Biochemistry* 15: 3724–3731.

Dinbar, A., and Grossman, M. I. (1972) *Gastroenterology* 62: 242–246.

Dipolo, R., Requena, J., Brinley, F. J., Jr., Mullins, L. J., Scarpa, A., and Tiffert, T. (1976) *J. Gen. Physiol.* 67: 433–467.

Disalvo, J., Gruenstein, E., and Silver, P. (1978) *Proc. Soc. Exp. Biol. Med.* 158: 410–413.

Donatsch, P., Lowe, D. A., Richardson, B. P., and Taylor, P. (1977) *J. Physiol.* 267: 357–376.

Donnellan, J. F., and Beechey, R. B. (1969) *J. Insect Physiol.* 15: 367–375.

Douglas, J., Aguilera, G., Kondo, T., and Catt, K. J. (1978) *Endocrinology* 102: 685–696.

Douglas, W. W. (1966) *Pharmacol. Rev.* 18: 471–480.

Douglas, W. W. (1968) *Br. J. Pharmacol.* 34: 451–474.

Douglas, W. W., and Rubin, R. P. (1961) *J. Physiol.* 159: 40–57.

Douglas, W. W., and Veda, Y. J. (1973) *J. Physiol. (London)* 234: 97P.

Dousa, T. P., Sands, H., and Hechter, O. (1972) *Endocrinology* 91: 757–763.

Dozois, R. R., Wollin, A., Riettman, R. D., and Dousa, T. P. (1977) *Am. J. Physiol.* 232: E35–E38.

Drummond, A. H., Benson, J. A., and Leviten, I. B. (1980) *Proc. Natl. Acad. Sci. USA* 77: 5013–5017.

Dufau, M. L., Charreau, E. H., and Catt, K. J. (1973) *J. Biol. Chem.* 248: 6973–6982.

Dufau, M. L., Ryan, D. W., Baukal, A. J., and Catt, K. J. (1975) *J. Biol. Chem.* 240: 7885–7893.

Durham, J. P., Baserga, R., and Butcher, F. R. (1974) *Biochim. Biophys. Acta* 372: 196–217.

Durham, J. P., Galanti, N., and Revis, N. W. (1975) *Biochim. Biophys. Acta* 394: 388–405.

Dziak, R., and Stern, P. (1976) *Calcif. Tiss. Res.* 22: 137–147.

Ebashi, S. (1961) *Prog. Theoret. Phys. Suppl.* 17: 35–40.

Ebashi, S. (1976) *Ann. Rev. Physiol.* 38: 293–309.

Ebashi, S. (1979) *Adv. Pharmacol. Ther.* 3: 81–98.

Ebashi, S., and Endo, M. (1968) *Prog. Biophys. Med. Biol.* 18: 81–98.

Ebashi, S., Endo, M., and Ohtsuki, I. (1969a) *Q. Rev. Biophys.* 2: 351–384.

Ebashi, S., Endo, M., and Ohtsuki, I. (1969b) *Q. Rev. Biophys.* 5: 123–183.

Ebashi, S., Iwakura, H., Nakajima, H., Nakanura, R., and Ooi, Y. (1966) *Biochemistry* 345: 201–211.

Ebashi, S., Kodama, A., and Ebashi, F. (1968) *J. Biochem. Tokyo* 64: 465–477.

Ebashi, S., and Lipmann, F. (1962) *J. Cell. Biol.* 14: 389–400.

Ebashi, S., Mikawa, T., Hirata, M., and Nonomura, Y. (1978) *Ann. N.Y. Acad. Sci.* 307: 451–461.

Ebashi, S., Toyo-Oka, T., and Nonomura, Y. (1975) *J. Biochem. (Tokyo)* 78: 859–861.

Eccles, R. M. (1952) *J. Physiol.* 117: 196–209.

Eccles, R. M., and Libet, B. (1961) *J. Physiol.* 157: 484–503.

Eckert, R. (1972) *Science* 176: 473–481.

Edmonds, C. J., and Marriott, J. (1968) *J. Physiol. (London)* 194: 479–494.

Eldefrawi, M. E., Eldefrawi, A. T., and O'Brien, R. D. (1971) *Proc. Natl. Acad. Sci. USA* 68: 1047–1050.

Emmelin, N., and Gjörstrup, P. (1976) *Arch. Oral Biol.* 21: 27–32.

England, P. J. (1975) *FEBS Lett.* 50: 57–60.

England, P. J., Stull, J. T., Huang, T. S., and Krebs, E. G. (1973) *Metab. Interconvers. Enzymes* 3: 175–184.

England, P. J., Stull, J. T., and Krebs, E. G. (1972) *J. Biol. Chem.* 247: 5275–5277.

Entman, M. L., Bornet, E. P., Van Winkle, W. B., Goldstein, M. A., Schwartz, A., Garber, A. J., and Levey, G. S. (1978) *Adv. Cyclic Nucl. Res.* 9: 381–396.

Exton, J. H. (1979) *Biochem. Pharmacol.* 28: 2237–2244.

Exton, J. H., and Harper, S. C. (1975) *Adv. Cyclic Nucl. Res.* 5: 519–532.

Ezawa, I., and Ogata, E. (1977) *Eur. J. Biochem.* 77: 427–435.

Fabiato, A., and V. Fabiato, F. (1978) *Ann. N.Y. Acad. Sci.* 307: 491–522.

Fain, J. N., and Berridge, M. J. (1979) *Biochem. J.* 178: 45–58.

Fain, J. N., and Garcia-Sáinz, A. (1980) *Life Sci.* 26: 1183–1194.

Fakunding, J. L., and Catt, K. J. (1980) *Endocrinology* 107: 1345–1353.

Fakunding, J. L., Chow, R., and Catt, K. J. (1979) *Endocrinology* 105: 327–333.

Fambrough, D. M., and Hartzell, H. C. (1972) *Science* 176: 189–191.

Farese, R. V. (1971a) *Endocrinology* 89: 1057–1063.

Farese, R. V. (1971b) *Endocrinology* 89: 1064–1974.

Farese, R. V. (1971c) *Science* 173: 447–450.

Farese, R. V., and Sabir, A. M. (1980) *Endocrinology* 106: 1869–1879.

Farese, R. V., Sabir, A. M., and Larson, R. E. (1980) *J. Biol. Chem.* 255: 7232–7237.

Farese, R. V., Sabir, A. M., and Vandor, S. L. (1979) *J. Biol. Chem.* 254: 6842–6844.

Farese, R. V., Sabir, A. M., Vandor, S. L., and Larson, R. E. (1980) *J. Biol. Chem.* 255: 5728–5734.

Farley, J. M., and Miles, P. R. (1978) *J. Pharmacol. Exp. Ther.* 207: 340–346.

Farnham, C. J. M. (1975) *Exp. Cell. Res.* 91: 36–46.

Farrance, M. L., and Vincenzi, F. F. (1977a) *Biochim. Biophys. Acta* 471: 49–58.

Farrance, M. L., and Vincenzi, F. F. (1977b) *Biochim. Biophys. Acta* 471: 59–66.

Fast, D., and Tenenhouse, A. (1976) *Br. J. Pharmacol.* 58: 605–612.

Feinstein, M. B. (1978) *In* Calcium in Drug Action. G. B. Weiss, Ed. Plenum, New York, Chap. 9.

Feinstein, M. B., Fiekers, J., and Fraser, C. (1976) *J. Pharmacol. Exp. Ther.* 197: 215–223.

Feinstein, M. B., and Fraser, C. (1975) *J. Gen. Physiol.* 66: 561–581.

Feinstein, H., and Schramm, M. (1970) *Eur. J. Biochem.* 13: 158–163.

Ferguson, D. R., and Twite, B. R. (1974) *J. Endocrinol.* 61: 501–507.

Fertel, R. M., and Weiss, B. (1976) *Mol. Pharmacol.* 12: 678–687.

Field, M. (1971) *Am. J. Physiol.* 221: 992–997.

Field, M. (1974) *Gastroenterology* 65: 467–497.

Field, M., Fromm, D., Al-Awqati, Q., and Greenough, W. B. (1972) *J. Clin. Invest.* 51: 796–804.

Field, M., Karnaky, K. J., Smith, P. L., Bolton J. E., and Kinter, W. B. (1978) *J. Membr. Biol.* 141: 265–293.

Field, M., Plotkin, G. R., and Silen, W. (1968) *Nature* 217: 469–471.

Fine, R., Lehman, W., Head, J., and Blitz, A. (1975) *Nature* 258: 260–262.

Fischer, E. H., Heilmeyer, M. G., and Haschke, R. H. (1971) *Curr. Top. Cell. Reg.* 4: 211–251.

Fleckenstein, A. (1971) *In* Calcium and the Heart. P. Harris and L. Opie, Eds. Academic, New York, pp. 135–188.

Fleckenstein, A. (1974) *Adv. Cardiol.* 12: 183–197.

Fleckenstein, A. (1977) *Ann. Rev. Pharmacol. Toxicol.* 17: 148–166.

Floyd, J. J., Jr., Fajans, S. S., Conn, J. W., Knoff, R. F., and Rull, J. (1966) *J. Clin. Invest.* 45: 1487–1502.

Foden, S., and Randle, P. J. (1978) *Biochem. J.* 170: 615–625.

Foldes, M., and Barrett, G. J. (1977) *J. Biol. Chem.* 252: 5372–5380.

Foreman, J. C., and Garland, L. G. (1974) *J. Physiol. (London)* 239: 381–391.

Foreman, J. C., Garland, L. G., and Mongar, J. L. (1976) *In* SEB Symposium XXX Calcium in Biological Systems. Cambridge University Press, New York, pp. 193–218.

Foreman, J. C., Hallett, M. B., and Mongar, J. L. (1977) *J. Physiol.* 271: 193–214.

Foreman, J. C., and Mongar, J. L. (1975) *In* Calcium Transport in Contraction and Secretion. E. Carafoli, F. Clementi, W. Drabikowsky, and A. Margreth, Eds. North-Holland, Amsterdam, pp. 175–184.

Foreman, J. C., Mongar, J. L., and Gompertz, B. P. (1973) *Nature* 245: 249–251.

Foster, R., Lobo, M. V., Rasmussen, H., and Marusic, E. T. (1981) *Endocrinology* In Press.

Foulkes, J. G., and Cohen, P. (1979) *Eur. J. Biochem.* 97: 251–256.

Franzi-Armstrong, C., Landmesser, L., and Pilar, G. (1974) *J. Cell. Biol.* 64: 493–497.

Fredlund, P., Saltman, S., Kondo, T., Douglas, J., and Catt, K. J. (1977) *Endocrinology* 100: 481–486.

Friedmann, N., and Dambach, G. (1973) *Biochim. Biophys. Acta* 307: 339–403.

Friedmann, N., and Dambach, G. (1980) *Biochim. Biophys. Acta* 596: 180–185.

Friedmann, N., and Park, C. R. (1968) *Proc. Natl. Acad. Sci. USA* 61: 584–588.

Friedmann, N., and Rasmussen, H. (1970) *Biochim. Biophys. Acta* 222: 41–52.

Friedmann, N., Somlyo, A. V., and Somlyo, A. P. (1971) *Science* 171: 400–402.

Friedricks, D., and Schoner, W. (1973) *Biochim. Biophys. Acta* 304: 142–160.

Frizzel, R. A. (1977) *J. Membr. Biol.* 35: 164–187.

Frizzell, R. A., Dugas, M., and Schultz, S. G. (1975) *J. Gen. Physiol.* 65: 759–795.

Frizzell, R. A., Field, M., and Schultz, S. G. (1979) *Am. J. Physiol.* 236: F1–F8.

Frizzell, R. A., Koch, M. J., and Schultz, S. G. (1976) *J. Membr. Biol.* 27: 297–316.

Frizzell, R. A., and Schultz, S. G. (1972) *J. Gen. Physiol.* 59: 318–346.

Fujita, K. (1954) *Folia Pharmacol. Jpn.* 50: 183–192.

Fujita, K., Aguilera, G., and Catt, K. J. (1979) *J. Biol. Chem.* 254: 8567–8574.

Furshpan, E. J., and Potter, D. D. (1968) *Curr. Top. Dev. Biol.* 3: 95–127.

Gallagher, J. P., and Shinnick-Gallagher, P. (1977) *Science* 198: 851–852.

Ganong, W. F., Biglieri, E. F., and Mulrow, P. J. (1966) *Rec. Prog. Horm. Res.* 22: 381–430.

Garcia, A. G., Kirpekar, S. M., and Prat, J. C. (1975) *J. Physiol.* 244: 253–262.

Gardner, J. D., Christophe, J. P., Conlon, T. P., and Fransen, E. K. (1977) *In Hormonal Receptors in Digestive Tract Physiology.* S. Bonfils, P. Fromageot, G. Rosselin, Eds. North-Holland, Amsterdam, pp. 227–236.

Gardner, J. D., Conlon, T. P., Klaeveman, H. L., Adams, T. D., and Ondetti, M. A. (1975) *J. Clin. Invest.* 56: 366–375.

Gardner, J. D., Conlon, T. P., and Adams, T. D. (1976) *Gastroenterology* 70: 29–35.

Gardner, J. D., and Hahne, W. F. (1977) *Biochim. Biophys. Acta* 471: 466–476.

Gardner, J. D., and Jackson, M. J. (1977) *J. Physiol. (London)* 270: 439–454.

Gardner, J. D., and Rottman, A. J. (1979) *Biochim. Biophys. Acta* 585: 250–265.

Gardner, J. D., and Rottman, A. J. (1980) *Biochim. Biophys. Acta* 627: 230–243.

Gárdos, G. (1958) *Biochim. Biophys. Acta* 30: 653–654.

Garren, L. D., Gill, G. N., Masui, H., and Walton, G. M. (1971) *Rec. Prog. Horm. Res.* 27: 433–478.

Garren, L. D., Ney, R. L., and Davis, W. W. (1965) *Proc. Natl. Acad. Sci. USA* 53: 1443–1450.

Garrison, J. C. (1978) *J. Biol. Chem.* 253: 7091–7100.

Garrison, J. C., and Borland, M. K. (1979) *J. Biol. Chem.* 254: 1129–1133.

Garrison, J. C., Borland, K., Florio, V. A., and Twible, D. A. (1979) *J. Biol. Chem.* 254: 7147–7156.

Garrison, J. C., and Haynes, R. C. (1975) *J. Biol. Chem.* 250: 2769–2777.

Geahlen, R. L., and Krebs, E. G. (1980) *J. Biol. Chem.* 255: 1164–1169.

Gear, A. R. L., and Schneider, W. (1975) *Biochim. Biophys. Acta* 392: 111–120.

Gebauer, U., and Fleisch, H. (1978) *Calcif. Tiss. Res.* 25: 223–225.

Gerich, J. E., Charles, M. A., and Grodsky, G. M. (1976) *Ann. Rev. Physiol.* 38: 353–388.

Gerisch, G., Malchow, D., Huesgen, A., Nanjundiah, V., Roos, W., Wick, U., and Hülser, D. (1975) *In* Proceedings of the ICN–UCLA Symposium on Developmental Biology. D. McMahon and C. F. Fox, Eds. W. A. Benjamin, Menlo Park, Calif.

Gerisch, G., and Hess, B. (1975) *Proc. Natl. Acad. Sci. USA* 71: 2118–2122.

Gerisch, G., and Wick, U. (1975) *Biochem. Biophys. Res. Commun.* 65: 364–370.

Ghazarian, J. C., Jefcoate, C. R., Knutson, J. C., Orme-Johson, W. H., and DeLuca, H. F. (1974) *J. Biol. Chem.* 249: 3026–3033.

Gillard, R. D. (1970) *In* Calcium and Cell Function. A. W. Cuthbert, Ed. Macmillan, London, pp. 4–16.

Gillespie, I. E., and Grossman, M. J. (1964) *Gut* 5: 71–76.

Gillis, J. M., and O'Brien, E. J. (1975) *In* Calcium Transport in Contraction and Secretion. E. Carafoli, F. Clementi, W. Drabikowski, and A. Margreth, Eds. North-Holland, Amsterdam, pp. 497–500.

Gillis, J. M., and Gerday, C. C. (1977) *In* Ca^{2+} Binding Proteins and Ca^{2+} Function. R. H. Wasserman, R. A. Corradino, E. Carofoli, R. H. Kretsinger, D. H. MacLennan, and F. L. Seigel, Eds. Elsevier, New York. pp. 193–207.

Glossman, H., Baukal, A., and Catt, K. J. (1974) *J. Biol. Chem.* 249: 664–666.

Gnegy, M. E., Lau, Y. S., and Treisman, G. (1981) *Ann. N.Y. Acad. Sci.* 356: 304–318.

Gnegy, M. E., Nathanson, J. A., and Uzunov, P. (1977) *Biochem. Biophys. Acta* 497: 75–85.

Gnegy, M. E., Uzunov, P., and Costa, E. (1976) *Proc. Natl. Acad. Sci. USA* 73: 3887–3890.

Goebell, H. (1976) *Acta Hepato-Gastroenterol.* 23: 151–161.

Goldbeter, A., and Segal, L. A. (1977) *Proc. Natl. Acad. Sci. USA* 74: 1543–1547.

Goldenberg, H., Crane, F. L., and Morré, D. J. (1978) *Biochem. Biophys. Res. Commun.* 83: 234–240.

Goldfine, I. D., Smith, G. J., Wong, K. Y., and Jones, A. L. (1977) *Proc. Natl. Acad. Sci. USA* 74: 1368–1372.

Goldstein, I., Hoffstein, S., Gallin, J., and Weissmann, G. (1973) *Proc. Natl. Acad. Sci. USA* 70: 2916–2920.

Goodman, D. B. P., Bloom, F. E., Battenberg, E. R., Rasmussen, H., and Davis, W. L. (1975) *Science* 188: 1023–1025.

Gopinath, R. M., and Vincenzi, F. F. (1977) *Biochem. Biophys. Res. Commun.* 77: 1203–1209.

Gorden, P., Carpentier, J.-L., Freychet, P., LeCam, A., and Orci, L. (1978) *Science* 200: 782–784.

Gorecka, A., Aksoy, M. D., and Hartshorne, D. J. (1976) *Biochem. Biophys. Res. Commun.* 71: 325–331.

Gorman, R. R., Bundy, G. L., Peterson, D. C., Sun, F. F., Miller, O. V., and Fitzpatrick, F. A. (1977) *Proc. Natl. Acad. Sci. USA* 74: 4007–4011.

Goth, A., Adams, H. R., and Knoohuizen, M. (1971) *Science* 173: 1034–1035.

Grab, D. J., Berzins, K., Cohen, R. S., and Siekevitz, P. (1979) *J. Biol. Chem.* 243: 8690–8696.

Grahame-Smith, D. G., Butcher, R. W., New, R. L., and Sutherland, E. W. (1967) *J. Biol. Chem.* 242: 5535–5541.

Grand, R. J. A., Perry, S. V., and Weeks, R. A. (1979) *Biochem. J.* 177: 521–529.

Green, A. A., and Newell, P. G. (1975) *Cell* 6: 129–136.

Green, I. C., Howell, S. L., Montague, W., and Taylor, K. W. (1973) *Biochem. J.* 134: 481–487.

Greengard, P. (1974) *Fed. Proc.* 38: 2208–2217.

Greengard, P. (1976) *Nature* 260: 101–108.

Greengard, P. (1978) Cyclic Nucleotides, Phosphorylated Proteins and Neuronal Function. Raven Press, New York, pp. 124.

Greengard, P., and Kebabian, J. W. (1974) *Fed. Proc.* 33: 1059–1067.

Grill, V., and Cerasi, E. (1974) *J. Biol. Chem.* 249: 4196–4201.

Grinstein, S., and Erlij, D. (1978) *Proc. R. Soc. London B* 202: 353–360.

Grodsky, G. M. (1970) *Vitam. Horm.* 28: 37–78.

Grodsky, G. M. (1972) *Diabetes* 21 (Suppl. 2): 584–593.

Grodsky, G. M., and Bennett, L. L. (1966) *Diabetes* 15: 910–913.

Grodsky, G. M., Bennett, C. L., Smith, D. F., and Schimid, F. G. (1967) *Metabolism* 16: 222–233.

Grossman, M. I. (1967) *Handb. Physiol.* 2 (Sect. 6): 835–863.

Grossman, M. I. (1974) *Gastroenterology* 67: 1081–1082.

Grossman, M. I., and Konturek, S. J. (1974) *Gastroenterology* 66: 517–521.

Guder, W. G. (1979) *Biochim. Biophys. Acta* 584: 507–519.

Guder, W. G., and Rupprecht, A. (1975) *Eur. J. Biochem.* 52: 283–290.

Guidotti, D. M., Chuang, R., Hollenbeck, R., and Costa, E. (1978) *Adv. Cyclic Nucl. Res.* 9: 185–207.

Guidotti, A., Hanbauer, I., and Costa, E. (1975) *Adv. Cyclic Nucl. Res.* 5: 619–640.

Gutman, Y., Lichtenberg, D., Cohen, J., and Boonyaviro, P. (1979) *Biochem. Pharmacol.* 28: 1209–1211.

Haddas, R. A., Landis, C. A., and Putney, J. W., Jr. (1979) *J. Physiol. (London)* 291: 457–465.

Haga, T., Haga, K., and Gilman, A. G. (1977) *J. Biol. Chem.* 252: 5774–5782.

Hahn, H. J., Gylfe, E., and Hellman, B. (1979) *FEBS Lett.* 103: 348–351.

Hahn, H. J., Gylfe, E., and Hellman, B. (1980) *Biochim. Biophys. Acta* 630: 425–432.

Haksar, A., and Peron, F. G. (1972) *Biochem. Biophys. Res. Commun.* 47: 445–450.

Hales, C. N., and Milner, R. D. G. (1968) *J. Physiol.* 199: 177–187.

Hall, P. F. *Endocrinology* 78: 690–698.

Hall, P. F., Charpponnier, C., Nakamura, M., and Gabbianni, G. (1979) *J. Biol. Chem.* 254: 9080–9084.

Hall, P. F., and Koritz, S. B. (1965) *Biochemistry* 4: 1037–1943.

Hamilton, M. N., and Hamilton, R. T. (1979) *Nature* 279: 446–448.

Hanbauer, I., Pradhan, S., and Yang, H.-Y. T. (1981) *Ann. N.Y. Acad. Sci.* 356: 292–303.

Handler, J. S., Butcher, R. W., Sutherland, E. W., and Orloff, J. (1965) *J. Biol. Chem.* 240: 4524–4526.

Hanford, C. P. (1962) *Arch. Pathol.* 73: 161–168.

Hansen-Bay, C. M. (1978) *J. Physiol.* 274: 421–435.

Hansford, R. G., and Chappell, J. B. (1967) *Biochem. Biophys. Res. Commun.* 27, 6: 686–692.

Hanski, E., Rimon, G., and Levitzki, A. (1979) *Biochemistry* 18: 846–853.

Hardy, M. A. (1978) *J. Cell. Biol.* 76: 878–791.

Harper, J. F., and Brooker, G. (1977) *Mol. Pharmacol.* 13: 1048–1059.

Hasselbach, W., and Makinose, M. (1961) *Biochem. Z.* 333: 518–528.

Hasselbach, W., and Makinose, M. (1963) *Biochem. Z.* 339: 94–111.

Hathaway, D. R., and Adelstein, R. S. (1979) *Proc. Natl. Acad. Sci. USA* 76: 1653–1657.

Hawthorne, J. N., and White, D. A. (1975) *Vitam. Horm.* 33: 529–573.

Hayashi, K., Sala, G., Catt, K., and Dufau, M. L. (1979) *J. Biol. Chem.* 254: 6678–6683.

Haylett, D. G., and Jenkinson, D. H. (1969) *Nature* 224: 80–81.

Haymovits, A., and Scheele, G. A. (1976) *Proc. Natl. Acad. Sci. USA* 73: 156–160.

Haynes, R. C. (1958) *J. Biol. Chem.* 233: 1220–1222.

Haynes, R. C., and Berthet, L. (1957) *J. Biol. Chem.* 225: 115–124.

Hazelbauer, J., and Changeux, J. P. (1974) *Proc. Natl. Acad. Sci. USA* 71: 1479–1483.

Hechter, O. (1955) *Vitam. Horm.* 13: 293–346.

Heilbrunn, L. V. (1940) *Physiol. Zool.* 13: 88–94.

Heilbrunn, L. V., and Wiercinski, F. J. (1947) *J. Cell. Comp. Physiol.* 29: 15–32.

Heisler, S. (1974) *Br. J. Pharmacol.* 52: 387–392.

Heisler, S., Fast, D., and Tenenhouse, A. (1972) *Biochim. Biophys. Acta* 279: 561–572.

Heizmann, C. W., Haeuptle, M. T., and Eppenberger, H. M. (1977) *Eur. J. Biochem.* 80: 433–441.

Hellman, B. (1975a) *Endocrinology* 97: 392–398.

Hellman, B. (1975b) *Biochim. Biophys. Acta.* 399: 157–169.

Hellman, B., Sahlin, J., and Täljedal, I. B. (1976) *J. Physiol.* 254: 639–656.

Helmreich, E. J. M., Zenner, H. P., and Pfeuffer, T. (1977) *Curr. Top. Cell. Reg.* 10: 41–87.

Henderson, E. J. (1975) *J. Biol. Chem.* 250: 4730–4736.

Hendrix, T. R., and Paulk, H. T. (1977) *In* International Review of Physiology. Gastrointestinal Physiology II, Vol. 12. R. K. Crane, Ed. University Park Press, Baltimore.

Henkart, M., Landis, D. M. D., and Reese, T. S. (1976) *J. Cell. Biol.* 70: 338–347.

Henkart, M. P., and Nelson, P. G. (1979) *J. Gen. Physiol.* 73: 655–673.

Henquin, J. C. (1978a) *Nature* 271: 271–273.

Henquin, J. C. (1978b) *Nature (London)* 271: 271–273.

Henquin, J. (1980) *Biochem. J.* 186: 541–550.

Henquin, J. C., and Lambert, A. E. (1974) *Diabetologia* 10: 368–369.

Henquin, J. C., and Lambert, A. E. (1975) *Am. J. Physiol.* 228: 1669–1677.

Henry, H. L., and Norman, A. W. (1974) *J. Biol. Chem.* 249: 7529–7535.

Herman, G., and Rossignol, B. (1975) *Eur. J. Biochem.* 55: 103–110.

Herrmann-Erlee, M. P. M., Gaillard, P. J., Hekkelman, J. W., and Nijweide, P. J. (1977) *Eur. J. Pharmacol.* 46: 51–58.

Hermann-Erlee, M. P. M., Gaillard, P. J., and Hekkelman, J. W. (1978) *In* Endocrinology of Calcium Metabolism. D. H. Copp, and R. V. Talmage, Eds. Excerpta Medica, Amsterdam/Oxford.

Heslop, J. P., and Berridge, M. J. (1980) *Biochem. J.* 192: 247–255.

Hidaka, T. R., Yamaik, T., Totsuka, T., and Masahisa, A. (1979) *Mol. Pharmacol.* 15: 49–59.

Hinds, T. R., Larsen, F. L., and Vincenzi, F. F. (1978) *Biochem. Biophys. Res. Commun.* 81: 455–461.

Hinkle, P., and Mitchell, P. (1970) *Bioenergetics* 1: 45–60.

Hirata, F., and Axelrod, J. (1978) *Proc. Natl. Acad. Sci. USA* 75: 2348–2352.

Hirata, F., and Axelrod, J. (1980) *Science* 209: 1082–1090.

Hirata, F., Axelrod, J., and Crews, F. T. (1979) *Proc. Natl. Acad. Sci. USA* 76: 4813–4816.

Hirata, F., Strittmatter, W. J., and Axelrod, J. (1979) *Proc. Natl. Acad. Sci. USA* 76: 368–372.

Hirata, F., Toyoshimo, S., Axelrod, J., and Waxdal, M. J. (1980) *Proc. Natl. Acad. Sci. USA* 77: 862–865.

Hitchcock, S. E. (1977) *J. Cell. Biol.* 74: 1–15.

Hitchcock, S. E., Kendrick-Jones, J. (1975) *In* Calcium Transport in Contraction and Secretion. E. Carafoli, F. Clementi, W. Drabikowski, and A. Margreth, Eds. North-Holland, Amsterdam, pp. 447–458.

Ho, H. C., Desai, R., and Wang, J. H. (1975) *FEBS Lett.* 50: 374–377.

Ho, H. C., Teo, T. S., Desai, R., and Wang, J. H. (1976) *Biochim. Biophys. Acta* 429: 461–473.

Ho, H. C., Wirch, E., Stevens, F. C., and Wang, J. H. (1977) *J. Biol. Chem.* 252: 43–50.

Hoar, P. E., Kerrick, W. G. L., and Cassidy, P. S. (1979) *Science* 204: 503–506.

Hodgkin, A. L., and Keynes, R. D. (1957) *J. Physiol. (London)* 138: 253–281.

Hoffer, B. J., Siggins, G. R., and Bloom, F. E. (1971) *Brain Res.* 25: 523–534.

Hoffer, B. J., Siggins, G. R., and Bloom, F. E. (1973) *J. Pharmacol. Exp. Ther.* 184: 553–569.

Hofman, F., Beavo, J. A., Bechtel, P. J., and Krebs, E. G. (1975) *J. Biol. Chem.* 250: 7795–7801.

Hokin, L. E., and Hokin, M. R. (1955) *Biochim. Biophys. Acta* 18: 102–110.

Hokin, L. E., and Hokin, M. R. (1956) *J. Physiol. (London)* 132: 442–453.

Hollosay, J. P., and Narahara, H. T. (1965) *J. Biol. Chem.* 240: 3493–3500.

Holman, G. D., and Naftalin, R. J. (1975a) *Biochim. Biophys. Acta* 382: 230–245.

Holman, G. D., and Naftalin, R. J. (1975b) *Biochim. Biophys. Acta* 406: 386–407.

Holman, G. D., and Naftalin, R. J. (1976) *Biochim. Biophys. Acta* 433: 597–614.

Holman, G. D., and Naftalin, R. J. (1979) *J. Physiol.* 290: 351–366.

Holman, G. D., Naftalin, R. J., Simmons, N. L., and Walker, M. (1979) *J. Physiol.* 290: 367–388.

Holmgren, J., Lange, S., and Lönnroth, J. (1978) *Gastroenterology* 75: 1103–1108.

Holmsen, H. (1975) *In* Biochemistry and Pharmacology of Platelets. Ciba Foundation Symposium 35, Elsevier/Excerpta Medica/North-Holland, Amsterdam, pp. 175–205.

Holmsen, H., Day, H. J., and Stormorker, H. (1969) *Scand. J. Haematol. (Suppl.)* 8: 3–26.

Holryode, M. J., Potter, J. D., and Solaro, R. J. (1979) *J. Biol. Chem.* 254: 6478–6482.

Honn, K. V., and Chavin, W. (1977) *Acta Endocrinol.* 85: 823–831.

Horl, W. H., and Heilmeyer, L. M. G., Jr. (1978) *Biochemistry* 17: 776–772.

Horl, W. H., Jennissen, H. P., Broschel-Stewart, B., and Heilmeyer, L. M. G., Jr. (1975) *In* Calcium Transport in Contraction and Secretion. E. Carafoli, F. Clementi, W. Drabikowski, and A. Margreth, Eds. North-Holland, Amsterdam, pp. 535–546.

Horl, W. H., Jennissen, H. P., Broschel-Stewart, B., and Heilmeyer, L. M. G., Jr. (1978) *Biochemistry* 17: 776–772.

Horl, W. H., Jennissen, H. P., and Heilmeyer, L. M. G., Jr. (1978) *Biochemistry* 17: 759–776.

Houslay, M. D., Metcalfe, J. C., Warren, G. B., Hesheth, T. R., and Smith, G. A. (1976) *Biochim. Biophys. Acta* 436: 489–494.

Hovig, T. (1963) *Thromb. Diath. Haemmorrh.* 9: 264–278.

Howell, S. L., Green, I. C., and Montague, W. (1973) *Biochem. J.* 136: 343–349.

Howell, S. L., and Montague, W. (1973) *Biochim. Biophys. Acta* 320: 44–52.

Howell, S. L., and Montague, W. (1975) *FEBS Lett.* 1: 48–52.

Howell, S. L., Montague, W., and Tyhurst, M. (1975) *J. Cell. Sci.* 19: 395–409.

Huang, K. P., Lee, S. L., and Huang, F. L. (1979) *J. Biol. Chem.* 254: 9867–9870.

Huang, C. Y., Chau, V., Chock, P. B., Wang, J. H., and Sharma, R. K. (1981) *Proc. Natl. Acad. Sci. USA* 78: 871–874.

Hutson, N. J., Brumley, F. T., Assimacopoulos, F. D., Harper, S. C., and Exton, J. H. (1976) *J. Biol. Chem.* 251: 5200–5208.

Huttner, W., and Greengard, P. (1979) *Proc. Natl. Acad. Sci. USA* 76: 5402–5406

Huxley, A. F. (1971) *Proc. R. Soc. London B* 178: 1–27.

Huxley, A. F., and Taylor, R. E. (1958) *J. Physiol. (London)* 144: 426–441.

Huxley, H. E. (1964) *Nature* 202: 1067–1071.

Ignarro, L. J. (1977) *In* Cyclic 3',5'-Nucleotides: Mechanisms of Action. H. Cramer, and J. Schultz, Eds. Wiley, New York, pp. 189–206.

Ignarro, L. J., and George, W. J. (1974a) *Proc. Natl. Acad. Sci. USA* 71: 2027–2031.

Ignarro, L. J., and George, W. J. (1974b) *J. Exp. Med.* 140: 225–238.

Ignarro, L. J., Lint, T. F., and George, W. J. (1974) *J. Exp. Med.* 139: 1395–1414.

Ilundain, A., and Naflatin, R. J. (1979) *Nature* 279: 446–448.

Ishizaka, T., Foreman, J. C., Sterk, A. R., and Ishizaka, K. (1972) *Proc. Natl. Acad. Sci. USA* 76: 5858–5862.

Ishizaka, T., Hirata, F., Ishizaka, K., and Axelrod, J. (1980) *Proc. Natl. Acad. Sci. USA* 77: 1903–1906.

Ishizaka, T., Ishizaka, K., Orange, R. P., and Austen, K. F. (1970) *Fed. Proc.* 29: 575.

Itarte, E., and Huang, K. P. (1979) *J. Biol. Chem.* 254: 4052–4057.

Ito, N., and Holta, K. (1976) *J. Biochem.* 50: 401–403.

Iwatsuki, N., and Petersen, O. H. (1977a) *Nature* 268: 147–149.

Iwatsuki, N., and Petersen, O. H. (1977b) *J. Physiol.* 269: 735–751.

Iwatsuki, N., and Petersen, O. H. (1978) *J. Clin. Invest.* 61: 41–46.

Jaanus, S. D., Rosenstein, M. J., and Rubin, R. P. (1970) *J. Physiol. (London)* 209: 530–556.

Jeanus, S. D., Rosenstein, M. J., and Rubin, R. P. (1971) *J. Physiol. (London)* 213: 581–598.

Jackson, R. L., Dedman, J. R., Schreiber, W. E., Bhatnagar, P. K., Knapp, R. D., and Means, A. R. (1977) *Biochem. Biophys. Res. Commun.* 77: 723–729.

Jacobs, R. S., and McNiece, D. M. (1977) *J. Pharmacol. Exp. Ther.* 202: 404–410.

Jaffe, L. F., and Niccitelli, R. (1977) *Ann. Rev. Biophys. Bioeng.* 6: 445–476.

Jain, M. K., and White, H. B., III. (1977) *Adv. Lipid Res.* 15: 1–60.

Jakob, A., and Diem, S. (1975) *Biochim. Biophys. Acta* 404: 57–66.

Jarrett, H. W., and Kyte, J. (1979) *J. Biol. Chem.* 254: 8237–8244.

Jensen, P., and Rasmussen, H. (1977) *Biochim. Biophys. Acta* 468: 146–156.

Jett, M. F., and Soderling, T. R. (1979) *J. Biol. Chem.* 254: 6739–6745.

Johnson, A. R., and Moran, N. C. (1969) *Am. J. Physiol.* 216: 453–459.

Johnson, A. R., and Moran, N. C. (1970) *J. Pharmacol. Exp. Ther.* 175: 632–640.

Johnson, A. R., Moran, N. C., and Meyer, S. E. (1974) *J. Immunol.* 112: 511–519.

Johnson, L. R., and Grossman, M. I. (1969) *Gastroenterology* 56: 687–692.

Jolles, J., Zwiers, H., van Dongen, C. J., Schotman, P., Wirtz, K. W. A., and Gispen, W. H. (1980) *Nature* 286: 623–625.

Jones, L. M., and Michell, R. H. (1974) *Biochem. J.* 142: 583–590.

Jones, L. M., and Michell, R. H. (1975) *Biochem. J.* 148: 479–485.

Jones, L. M., and Michell, R. H. (1976) *Biochem. J.* 158: 505–507.

Jones, L. M., and Michell, R. H. (1978) *Biochem. Soc. Trans.* 6: 673–688.

Jungman, R. A., Hiestand, P. C., and Schweppe, J. S. (1974) *Endocrinology* 94: 168–183.

Juzu, H. A., and Holdsworth, E. S. (1980) *J. Membr. Biol.* 52: 185–186.

Kahn, C. R. (1976) *J. Cell. Biol.* 70: 261–286.

Kakiuchi, S., and Yamazaki, R. (1970) *Biochem. Biophys. Res. Commun.* 41: 1104–1110.

Kakiuchi, S., Yamazaki, R., and Teshima, H. (1971) *Biochem. Biophys. Res. Commun.* 42: 968–974.

Kakiuchi, S., Yamazaki, R., Teshima, H., and Menishi, K. (1973) *Proc. Natl. Acad. Sci. USA* 70: 3526–3530.

Kaliner, M., and Austen, K. F. (1974) *J. Immunol.* 112: 664–674.

Kalix, P., McAfee, D. A., Schorderet, M., and Greengard, P. (1974) *J. Pharmacol. Exp. Ther.* 88: 676–687.

Kamada, T., and Kinosita, H. (1943) *Jpn. J. Zool.* 10: 469–493.

Kaminsky, N. I., Ball, J. H., Broadus, A. E., Hardman, J. G., Sutherland, E. W., and Liddle, G. W. (1970) *Trans. Am. Assoc. Phys.* 33: 235–243.

Kanagasuntheram, P., and Randle, P. J. (1976) *Biochem. J.* 160: 547–564.

Kanno, T., Cochrane, D. E., and Douglas, W. W. (1973) *Can. J. Physiol. Pharmacol.* 51: 1001–1004.

Kaplan, N. M. (1965) *J. Clin. Invest.* 44: 2029–2039.

Karaboyas, G. C., and Koritz, S. B. (1965) *Biochemistry* 4: 462–468.

Karl, R. C., Zawalich, W. S., Ferrendelli, J. A., and Matschinsky, F. M. (1975) *J. Biol. Chem.* 250: 4575–4579.

Karlin, A. (1974) *Life Sci.* 14: 1385–1415.

Käser-Glanzmann, R. Jakábová, M., George, J. N., and Lüschea, E. F. (1977) *Biochim. Biophys. Acta* 466: 429–440.

Katz, A. M. (1979) *Adv. Cyclic Nucl. Res.* 11: 303–343.

Katz, A. M., Tada, M., and Kirchberger, M. (1975) *Adv. Cyclic Nucl. Res.* 5: 453–472.

Katz, B. (1950) *Proc. R. Soc. London B* 137: 45–47.

Katz, B. (1962) *Proc. R. Soc. London* 13B, 155: 455–477.

Katz, B. (1966) Nerve, Muscle and Synapse. McGraw-Hill, New York.

Katz, B., and Miledi, R. (1965) *Proc. R. Soc. London B* 161: 496–503.

Katz, B., and Miledi, R. (1967) *J. Physiol.* 189: 535–544.

Katz, B., and Miledi, R. (1968) *J. Physiol.* 195: 481–492.

Kazimierczak, W., and Diamant, B. (1978) *Prog. Allergy* 24: 295–365.

Kebabian, J. W., Bloom, F. E., Steiner, A. L., and Greengard, P. (1975) *Science* 190: 157–159.

Kebabian, J. W., and Greengard, P. (1971) *Science* 174: 1346–1349.

Keely, S. L., Corbin, J. D., and Park, C. R. (1975) *Proc. Natl. Acad. Sci. USA* 72: 1501–1504.

Kempen, H. J. M., DePont, J. J. H. H. M., and Bonting, S. L. (1974) *Biochim. Biophys. Acta* 370: 573–584.

Kempen, H. J. M., DePont, J. J. H. H. M., and Bonting, S. L. (1977a) *Biochim. Biophys. Acta* 496: 65–76.

Kempen, H. J. M., DePont, J. J. H. H. M., and Bonting, S. L. (1977b) *Biochim. Biophys. Acta* 496: 521–531.

Kempner, E. W., and Schiegel, W. (1979) *Analyst Biochim.* 92: 2–10.

Kendrick-Jones, J., Lehman, W., and Szent-Györgyi, A. G. (1970) *J. Mol. Biol.* 54: 313–326.

Kennerly, D., Sullivan, T. J., and Parker, C. W. (1979) *J. Immunol.* 122: 152–159.

Kentera, D., and Varagic, V. (1975) *Br. J. Pharmacol.* 54: 375–381.

Keppens, S., and de Wulf, H. (1976) *FEBS Lett.* 68: 279–282.

Keppens, S., and de Wulf, H. (1979) *Biochim. Biophys. Acta* 588: 63–69.

Keppens, S., Vandenhude, J. R., and de Wulf, H. (1977) *Biochem. Biophys. Acta* 496: 448–457.

Kerrick, W. G. L., Hoar, P. E., and Cassidy, P. S. (1980) *Fed. Proc.* 39: 1558–1563.

Keryer, G., Herman, G., and Rossignol, B. (1979) *FEBS Lett.* 102: 4–8.

Keryer, G., and Rossignol, B. (1976) *Am. J. Physiol.* 230: 99–104.

Kikuchi, M., Wollheim, C. B., Siegel, E. G., Renold, A. E., and Sharp, G. W. G. (1979) *Endocrinology* 105: 1013–1019.

Kilimann, M., and Heilmeyer, L. M. G. (1977) *Eur. J. Biochem.* 73: 191–197.

Kimberg, D. V., Field, M., Johnson, J., Henderson, A., and Gershon, E. (1971) *J. Clin. Invest.* 50: 1218–1230.

Kimura, S., and Rasmussen, H. (1977) *J. Biol. Chem.* 252: 1217–1225.

Kirchberger, M. A., Schwartz, I. L., and Walter, R. (1972) *Proc. Soc. Exp. Biol. Med.* 140: 657–660.

Kirchberger, M. A., and Tada, M. (1976) *J. Biol. Chem.* 251: 725–729.

Kirchberger, M. A., Tada, M., and Katz, A. M. (1974) *J. Biol. Chem.* 249: 6166–6173.

Kirchberger, M. A., Tada, M., Repke, D. I., and Katz, A. M. (1979) *J. Mol. Cell. Cardiol.* 4: 673–680.

Kirk, D. J., Verrinder, T. R., and Hems, D. A. (1977) *FEBS Lett.* 83: 267–271.

Kishimoto, A., Takai, H., and Nishizuka, H. (1977) *J. Biol. Chem.* 252: 7449–7452.

Klahr, S., Nawar, T., and Schoolwerth, A. C. (1973) *Biochim. Biophys. Acta* 304: 161–168.

Klausner, R. D., Kleinfeld, A. M., Hoover, R. L., and Karnovsky, M. J. (1980) *J. Biol. Chem.* 255: 1286–1295.

Klee, C. B. (1977) *Biochemistry* 16: 1017–1024.

Klee, C. B., Crouch, T. H., and Krinks, M. H. (1978) *Fed. Proc.* 37: 188–201.

Klein, M., and Kandel, E. R. (1978) *Proc. Natl. Acad. Sci. USA* 75: 3512–3516.

Klingenberg, M., and Buchholz, M. (1970) *Eur. J. Biochem.* 13: 247–252.

Kneer, N. M., Wagner, M. J., and Lardy, H. A. (1979) *J. Biol. Chem.* 254: 12160–12168.

Koefoed-Johnsen, V., and Ussing, H. H. (1953) *Acta Physiol. Scand.* 28: 60–76.

Kondo, S., and Schultz, I. (1976) *Biochim. Biophys. Acta* 419: 76–92.

Konijin, T. M., Van de Meener, J. G. F., Bonner, J. T., and Barkley, D. S. (1967) *Proc. Natl. Acad. Sci. USA* 58: 1152–1157.

Konturek, S. J., and Oleksy, J. (1967) *Gastroenterology* 53: 912–917.

Konturek, S. J., Oleksy, J., and Wysocki, A. (1968) *Am. J. Dig. Dis.* 13: 792–800.

Korenman, S. G., Bhalla, R. C., Sanborn, B. M., and Stevens, R. N. (1974) *Science* 183: 430–432.

Kornguth, S. E., and Sunderland, E. (1975) *Biochim. Biophys. Acta* 393: 100–114.

Kowalewski, K., and Kolodej, A. (1972) *Pharmacology (Basel)* 7: 357–365.

Kowaleski, K., and Saab, M. (1972) *Pharmacology (Basel)* 7: 225–236.

Krause, E.-G., and Wollenberger, A. (1977) *In* Cyclic 3′,5′-Nucleotides: Mechanism of Action. H. Cramer and J. Schultz, Eds. Wiley, New York, pp. 229–250.

Krebs, E. G. (1972) *Curr. Top. Cell Reg.* 5: 99–133.

Krebs, E. G., and Fischer, E. H. (1956) *Biochim. Biophys. Acta* 20: 150–157.

Krebs, H. A., Bennett, D. A. H., de Gasquet, P., Gascoyne, T., and Yoshida, T. (1963) *Biochem. J.* 86: 22–27.

Kretsinger, R. H. (1972) *Nature New Biol.* 240: 85–88.

Kretsinger, R. H. (1975) *In* Calcium Transport in Contraction and Secretion. E. Carafoli, F. Clementi, W. Drabikowski, and H. Margreth, Eds. North-Holland, Amsterdam, pp. 469–478.

Kretsinger, R. H. (1976) *Ann. Rev. Biochem.* 46: 239–258.

Kretsinger, R. H. (1979) *Adv. Cyclic Nucl. Res.* 11: 1–26.

Kretsinger, R. H. (1980) *Ann. N.Y. Acad. Sci.* 356: 14–19.

Kretsinger, R. H., and Nockolds, C. E. (1973) *J. Biol. Chem.* 248: 3313–3326.

Krnjevic, K. (1974) *Physiol. Rev.* 54: 418–540.

Krnjevic, K., and Miledi, R. (1958) *J. Physiol.* 141: 291–302.

Kumagi, H., and Nishida, E. (1979) *J. Biochem.* 85: 1267–1274.

Krueger, B. K., Forn, J., and Greengard, P. (1977) *J. Biol. Chem.* 252: 2764–2773.

Kuo, C.-H., Ichida, S., Matsuda, T., Kakuichi, S., and Yoshida, H. (1979) *Life Sci.* 25: 235–240.

Kuo, I. C. Y., and Coffee, C. J. (1976a) *J. Biol. Chem.* 251: 1603–1609.

Kuo, I. C. Y., and Coffee, C. J. (1976b) *J. Biol. Chem.* 251: 6315–6319.

Kuo, J. F., and Greengard, P. (1969) *Proc. Natl. Acad. Sci. USA* 64: 1349–1355.

Kuo, W. N., Hodgins, O. S., and Kuo, J. F. (1973) *J. Biol. Chem.* 248: 2705–2711.

Kupfermann, I., Cohen, J. L., Mandelbaum, D. E., Schonberg, M., Sussein, A. J., and Weiss, K. R. (1979) *Fed. Proc.* 38: 2095–2102.

Kurokawa, K., and Rasmussen, H. (1973a) *Biochim. Biophys. Acta* 313: 17–31.

Kurokawa, K., and Rasmussen, H. (1973b) *Biochim. Biophys. Acta* 313: 42–58.

Kurokawa, K., and Rasmussen, H. (1973c) *Biochim. Biophys. Acta* 313: 59–71.

Kurokawa, K., Ohno, T., and Rasmussen, H. (1973) *Biochim. Biophys. Acta* 313: 32–41.

Kury, P. G., Ramwell, P. W., and McConnell, H. M. (1974) *Biochem. Biophys. Res. Commun.* 56: 478–483.

Kusamran, K., Mattox, S. M., and Thompson, G. A., Jr. (1980) *Biochim. Biophys. Acta* 598: 16–26.

Lamb, J. F., and Lindsay, R. (1971) *J. Physiol.* 218: 691–708.

Lambert, A. (1976) *Rev. Physiol. Biochem. Pharmacol.* 75: 98–180.

Lambert, M., Camus, J., and Christophe, J. (1975) *Biochem. Pharmacol.* 24: 1755–1758.

Langer, S. Z. (1977) *Br. J. Pharmacol.* 60: 481–497.

LaRaia, P. J., and Morkin, E. (1974) *Circ. Res.* 35: 298–306.

Larsen, F. L., and Vincenzi, F. F. (1979) *Science* 204: 306–309.

Lawson, D., Fewtrell, C., and Raff, M. C. (1978) *J. Cell. Biol.* 79: 394–400.

Lawson, D., and Raff, M. C. (1979) *In* SEB Symposium XXXIII, Secretory Machanisms. Cambridge University Press, New York, pp. 337–348.

Leaf, A. (1965) *Ergebn. Physiol.* 56: 216–263.

Leaf, A. (1967) *Am. J. Med.* 42: 745–756.

LeBreton, G. C., and Dinerstein, R. J. (1977) *Thrombosis Res.* 10: 521–523.

LeBreton, G. C., Dinerstein, R. J., Roth, L. J., and Feinberg, H. (1976) *Biochem. Biophys. Res. Commun.* 71: 362–370.

LeCann, A., and Freychet, P. (1978) *Endocrinology* 102: 379–385.

Lefkowitz, R. J. (1975) *Biochem. Pharmacol.* 24: 1651–1658.

Lefkowitz, R. J., Limbird, L. E., Mukherjee, C., and Caron, M. G. (1976) *Biochim. Biophys. Acta* 457: 1–39.

Lefkowitz, R. J., Roth, J., and Pastan, I. (1971) *Ann. N.Y. Acad. Sci.* 185: 195–209.

Lefkowitz, R. J., and Williams, L. T. (1977) *Proc. Natl. Acad. Sci. USA* 74: 515–519.

Lefkowitz, R. J., and Williams, L. T. (1978) *Adv. Cyclic Nucl. Res.* 9: 1–17.

Lehman, W., and Szent Gyorgyi, A. G. (1972) *J. Gen. Physiol.* 59: 375–387.

Lehninger, A. L. (1970) *Biochem. J.* 119: 129–138.

Lehninger, A. L., Carafoli, E., and Rossi, C. S. (1967) *Adv. Enzymol.* 29: 259–320.

Lehninger, A. L., Vecces, A., and Bababonmi, E. A. (1978) *Proc. Natl. Acad. Sci. USA* 75: 1690–1697.

Lehninger, A. L., Reynafarge, B., Vercesi, A., and Tew, W. P. (1978) *Ann. N.Y. Acad. Sci.* 307: 160–176.

Leighton, J., Brada, Z., Estes, L. W., and Justh, G. (1969) *Science* 163: 472–473.

Leier, D. J., and Jungmann, R. A. (1973) *Biochim. Biophys. Acta* 329: 196–210.

LePeuch, C. J., Haiech, J., and Demaille, J. G. (1979) *Biochemistry* 18: 5150–5157.

Leslie, B. A., Putney, J. W., and Sherman, J. M. (1976) *J. Physiol.* 260: 351–370.

Levin, R. M., and Weiss, B. (1976) *Mol. Pharmacol.* 12: 581–589.

Levine, S., Frankl, N., and Hays, R. M. (1973) *J. Clin. Invest.* 52: 1435–1447.

Levine, S. D., Levine, R. D., Worthington, R. D., and Hays, R. M. (1976) *J. Clin. Invest.* 58: 980–988.

Levinson, S. L., and Blume, A. J. (1977) *J. Biol. Chem.* 252: 3766–3774.

Levitzki, A. (1978) *Rev. Physiol. Biochem. Pharmacol.* 82: 1–26.

Levitzki, A., Atlas, D., and Steer, M. L. (1974) *Proc. Natl. Acad. Sci. USA* 71: 2773–2776.

Libet, B. (1970) *Fed. Proc.* 29: 1945–1956.

Lichtenstein, L. M., and Margolis, S. (1968) *Science* 161: 902–903.

Limbird, L. D., and Lefkowitz, R. J. (1976) *Mol. Pharmacol.* 12: 559–567.

Limbird, L. E., and Lefkowitz, R. J. (1977) *J. Biol. Chem.* 252: 799–801.

Limbird, L. D., and Lefkowitz, R. J. (1978) *Proc. Natl. Acad. Sci. USA* 75: 228–232.

Lin, M. C., Nicosia, S., Lad, P. M., and Rodbell, M. (1977) *J. Biol. Chem.* 252: 2790–2791.

Lindl, T. (1979) *Biochem. Biophys. Res. Commun.* 86: 300–311.

Lipkin, D., Cook, W. H., and Markham, R. (1959) *J. Am. Chem. Soc.* 81: 6198–6203.

Liu, Y. P., and Cheung, W. Y. (1976) *J. Biol. Chem.* 251: 4193–4198.

Loewenstein, W. R. (1968) *Dev. Biol.* 19 (Suppl. 2): 151–183.

Loewenstein, W. R., Kanno, Y., and Socolar, S. J. (1978) *Fed. Proc.* 37: 2645–2650.

Loewenstein, W. R., and Rose, B. (1978) *Ann. N.Y. Acad. Sci.* 307: 283–307.

Loomis, W. F. (1979) *Dev. Biol.* 70: 1–12.

Löw, H., and Crane, F. L. (1976) *FEBS Lett.* 68: 157–159.

Löw, H., and Crane, F. L. (1978) *Biochim. Biophys. Acta* 515: 141–161.

Löw, H., Crane, F. L., Grebing, C., Tally, M., and Hall, K. (1978) *FEBS Lett.* 91: 166–168.

Luben, R. A., Goggins, J. F., and Raisz, L. G. (1974) *Endocrinology* 94: 737–746.

Luben, R. A., Wong, G. L., and Cohn, D. V. (1976) *Endocrinology* 99: 526–533.

Luben, R. A., Wong, G. L., and Cohn, D. V. (1977) *Nature* 265: 629–630.

MacDonald, D. W. R., and Saggerson, D. E. (1977) *Biochem. J.* 168: 33–42.

MacIntyre, J. D., and Green, J. W. (1978) *Biochim. Biophys. Acta* 510: 373–377.

Mackie, C. M., Simpson, E. R., Mee, M. S. R., Tait, S. A. S., and Tait, J. F. (1977) *Clin. Sci. Mol. Med.* 53: 289–296.

Maggi, A., U'Prichard, D. C., and Enna, S. J. (1980) *Science* 207: 645–647.

Maguire, M. E., and Erdos, J. J. (1980) *J. Biol. Chem.* 255: 1030–1035.

Maguire, M. E., Ross, E. M., and Gilman, A. G. (1977) *Adv. Cyclic Nucl. Res.* 8: 1–83.

Mahaffee, D., Reitz, R. C., and Ney, R. L. (1974) *J. Biol. Chem.* 249: 227–233.

Malchow, D., Fuchila, J., and Nanjundiah, U. (1975) *Biochim. Biophys. Acta* 385: 421–428.

Malchow, D., Nagele, B., Schwarz, H., and Gerisch, G. (1972) *Eur. J. Biochem.* 28: 136–142.

Malchow, D., Nanjundiah, U., Wurster, B., Eckstein, F., and Gerisch, G. (1978) *Biochim. Biophys. Acta* 538: 473–480.

Malaisse-Lague, F., and Malaisse, W. J. (1971) *Endocrinology* 88: 72–80.

Malaisse, W. J. (1973) *Diabetologia* 9: 167–173.

Malaisse, W. J., Boschero, A. C., Kawazu, S., and Hutton, C. (1978) *Pfluegers Arch.* 373: 237–242.

Malaisse, W. J., Brisson, G. R., and Baird, L. E. (1973) *Am. J. Physiol.* 224: 389–394.

Malaisse, W. J., Devis, G., Pipeleers, D. G., and Somers, G. (1976) *Diabetologia* 12: 77–81.

Malaisse, W. J., Devis, G., Pipeleers, D. G., Somers, G., and Obberghen, E. van. (1974) *Diabetologia* 10: 379.

Malaisse, W. J., Herchuelz, A., Devis, G., Somers, G., Boschero, A. C., Hutton, J. C., Kawazu, S., Sener, A., Atwater, I. J., Duncan, G., Ribalet, B., and Rojas, E. (1978) *Ann. N.Y. Acad. Sci.* 307: 562–582.

Malaisse, W. J., Herchuelz, A., Levy, J., Sener, A. (1977) *Biochem. Pharmacol.* 26: 735–740.

Malaisse, W. J., Hutton, J. C., Kawazu, S., Herchuelz, A., Valverde, I., and Sener, A. (1979) *Diabetologia* 16: 331–341.

Malaisse, W. J., Hutton, J. C., Kawazu, S., and Sener, A. (1978) *Eur. J. Biochem.* 87: 121–130.

Malaisse, W. J., Kawazu, S., Herchuelz, A., Hutton, J. C., Somers, G., Devis, G., and Sener, A. (1979) *Arch. Biochem. Biophys.* 194: 1–12.

Malaisse, W. J., Sener, A., Boschero, A. C., Kawazu, S., Devis, G., and Somers, G. (1978) *Eur. J. Biochem.* 87: 111–120.

Malaisse, W. J., Sener, A., Herchuelz, A., and Hutton, J. C. (1979) *Metabolism* 28: 373–386.

Mallorya, P., Tallman, J. F., Henneberry, R. C., Hirata, F., Strittmatter, W. J., and Axelrod, J. (1980) *Proc. Natl. Acad. Sci. USA* 77: 1341–1345.

Malström, K., and Carafoli, E. (1976) *Biochem. Biophys. Res. Commun.* 69: 658–664.

Marcum, J. M., Dedman, J. R., Brinkley, B. R., and Means, A. R. (1978) *Proc. Natl. Acad. Sci. USA* 75: 3771–3775.

Marier, S. H., Putney, J. W., Jr., and Van de Walle, C. M. (1978) *J. Physiol. (London)* 279: 141–151.

Marsh, B. B. (1952) *Biochim. Biophys. Acta* 9: 247–260.

Marshall, P. J., Dixon, J. F., and Hokin, L. E. (1980) *Proc. Natl. Acad. Sci. USA* 77: 3292–3296.

Martinez, J. R., Quissell, D. O., and Giles, M. (1976) *J. Pharmacol. Exp. Ther.* 198: 385–394.

Martinosi, A. N., Chyn, T. L., and Schibeci, A. (1978) *Ann. N.Y. Acad. Sci.* 307: 148–159.

Mason, J. W., Rasmussen, H., and DiBella, F. F. (1971) *Exp. Cell. Res.* 67: 158–160.

Mason, M. (1974) *Biochim. Biophys. Res. Commun.* 60: 64–69.

Massini, P., and Lüscher, E. F. (1972) *Thromb. Diath. Haemorrh.* 27: 121–133.

Massini, P., and Lüscher, E. F. (1974) *Biochim. Biophys. Acta* 372: 109–121.

Matchinsky, F. M., and Ellerman, J. (1973) *Biochem. Biophys. Res. Commun.* 50: 193–199.

Matchinsky, F. M., Ellerman, J. E., Kranowski, J., Kotler-Bratjburg, J., Landgraf, R., and Fertel, R. (1971) *J. Biol. Chem.* 246: 1007–1011.

Matthews, E. K. (1970) *Acta Diabet. Lat.* 7 (Suppl.): 83–88.

Matthews, E. K. (1975) *In* Calcium Transport in Contraction and Secretion. E. Carafoli, F. Clementi, W. Drabikowski, and A. Margreth, Eds. North-Holland, Amsterdam, pp. 203–210.

Matthews, E. K. (1979) *In* SEB Symposium XXXIII, Secretory Mechanisms. Cambridge University Press, New York, pp. 225–250.

Matthews, E. K., and Sakamoto, Y. (1975) *J. Physiol. (London)* 246: 421–437.

May, D. C., Levine, B. B., and Weissman, G. (1970) *Proc. Soc. Exp. Biol. Med.* 133: 758–763.

Mayer, S. E., Dobson, J. G., Jr., Ingebretsen, W. R., Jr., Becher, E., Brown, J. H., Friedman, W. F., and Ross, J., Jr. (1978) *Adv. Cyclic Nucl. Res.* 9: 305–314.

McAfee, D. A., and Greengard, P. C. (1972) *Science* 178: 310–312.

McAfee, D. A., Schorderet, M., and Greengard, P. (1971) *Science* 171: 1156–1158.

McIlhinney, J., and Schulster, D. (1975) *J. Endocrinol.* 64: 175–184.

McIntosh, E. N., Uzgiris, V. I., Alonso, C., and Salhanick, H. A. (1971) *Biochemistry* 10: 2909–2916.

Mears, D. C. (1971) *Endocrinology* 88: 1021–1028.

Meech, R. W. (1976) *In* SEB Symposium XXX, Calcium in Biological Systems. Cambridge University Press, New York, pp. 161–191.

Meech, R. W. (1978) *Ann. Rev. Biophys. Bioeng.* 7: 1–18.

Melson, G. L., Chase, L. R., and Aurbach, G. D. (1970) *Endocrinology* 86: 511–518.

Menez, A., Morgat, J.-L., Fromageot, P., Ronseray, A. M., Boquet, P., and Changeux, J.-P. (1971) *FEBS Lett.* 17: 333–335.

Meunier, J. C., Olsen, R., Sealock, R., and Changeux, J.-P. (1974) *Eur. J. Biochem.* 45: 371–394.

Meyer, W. L., Ficher, E. H., and Krebs, E. G. (1964) *Biochemistry* 3: 1033–1039.

Michaelson, D. M., and Raftery, M. A. (1974) *Proc. Natl. Acad. Sci. USA* 71: 4768–4772.

Micheli, R. H. (1975) *Biochim. Biophys. Acta* 415: 81–114.

Michell, R. H., Jafferji, S. S., and Jones, L. M. (1977) *Adv. Exp. Med. Biol.* 83: 447–464.

Mickey, J. V., Tate, R., Mullikin, D., and Lefkowitz, R. J. (1976) *Mol. Pharmacol.* 12: 409–419.

Miller, B. E., and Nelson, D. L. (1977) *J. Biol. Chem.* 252: 3629–3636.

Miller, J. L., Katz, A. J., and Feinstein, M. B. (1975) *Thromb. Diath. Haemorrh.* 33: 286–309.

Milner, R. D. G., and Hales, C. N. (1968) *Biochim. Biophys. Acta* 150: 165–167.

Milutinovic, S., Argent, B. E., Schulz, I., and Sachs, G. (1977) *J. Membr. Biol.* 36: 281–295.

Misfeldt, D. S., Hamamoto, S. T., and Pitelka, D. R. (1976) *Proc. Natl. Acad. Sci. USA* 73: 1212–1216.

Mitchell, P. (1969) *FEBS Symp.* 17: 219–232.

Mitchell, P. (1976) *J. Theor. Biol.* 62: 327–367.

Miyake, M., and Kakiuchi, S. (1978) *Brain Res.* 139: 378–380.

Miyamoto, M. D., and Breckenridge, B. M. (1974) *J. Gen. Physiol.* 63: 609–624.

Mockrin, S. C., and Spudich, J. A. (1976) *Proc. Natl. Acad. Sci. USA* 73: 2321–2325.

Moews, P. D., and Kretsinger, R. H. (1975) *J. Mol. Biol.* 91: 201–228.

Montague, W. (1977) *In* Cyclic 3',5'-Nucleotides: Mechanism of Action. H. Cramer, and J. Schulz, Eds. Wiley, New York. pp. 133–146.

Montague, W., and Cook, J. R. (1971) *Biochem. J.* 122: 115–120.

Montague, W., Green, I. C., and Howell, S. C. (1976) *In* Eukaryotic Cell Function and Growth. Dumont, J. E., Brown, B. L., and Marshall, N. J., Eds. Plenum, New York, pp. 609–632.

Montague, W., and Howell, S. L. (1973) *Biochem. J.* 134: 321–327.

Moore, L., Fitzpatrick, D. F., Chen, T. S., and Landon, E. J. (1974) *Biochim. Biophys. Acta* 345: 405–418.

Moore, L., and Landon, E. (1979) *Life Sci.* 25: 1029–1034.

Moore, L., and Pastan, I. (1978) *Ann. N.Y. Acad. Sci.* 307: 177–184.

Moore, L., and Pastan, I. (1976) *J. Cell. Physiol.* 91: 289–296.

Moore, R. Y., and Bloom, F. E. (1979) *Ann. Rev. Neurosci.* 2: 113–168.

Moreno, J. A. (1975) *J. Gen. Physiol.* 66: 97–115.

Morgenroth, V. H., Boadle-Berber, M. C., and Roth, R. H. (1975) *Mol. Pharmacol.* 11: 427–439.

Morse, E. E., Jackson, D. P., and Conley, C. L. (1965) *J. Clin. Invest.* 44: 809–816.

Moyle, W. R., Kong, Y. C., and Ramachandian, J. (1973) *J. Biol. Chem.* 248: 2409–2417.

Mrolek, J. J., and Hall, P. F. (1977a) *Biochem. Biophys. Res. Commun.* 64: 891–896.

Mrolek, J. J., and Hall, P. F. (1977b) *Biochemistry* 16: 3177–3181.

Mueller, E., and Van Breemen, C. (1979) *Nature* 281: 682–683.

Mulle., J. (1971) Regulation of Aldosterone Biosynthesis. Springer-Verlag, New York.

Munson, P. L., and Hirsch, P. F. (1967) *Am. J. Med.* 43: 678–683.

Mürer, E. H. (1972) *Biochim. Biophys. Acta* 261: 435–443.

Murphy, E., Catt, K., Rich, T. L., and Williamson, J. R. (1980) *J. Biol. Chem.* 255: 6600–6608.

Mustard, J. F., and Packham, M. A. (1970) *Pharmacol. Rev.* 22: 97–187.

Mutsuda, G., Maita, T., Suyama, Y., Setoguichi, M., and Klmegane, T. (1977) *J. Biochem.* 81: 809–811.

Naccache, P. H., Showell, H. J., Becker, E. L., and Sha'afi, R. I. (1977) *J. Cell. Biol.* 73: 428–444.

Naccache, P. H., Showell, H. J., Becker, E. L., and Sha'afi, R. I. (1979) *Biochem. Biophys. Res. Commun.* 89: 1224–1230.

Naccache, P. H., Volpi, M., Showell, H. J., Becker, E. L., and Sha'afi, R. I. (1979) *Science* 203: 461–463.

Naftalin, R., and Curran, P. F. (1974) *J. Membr. Biol.* 16: 257–278.

Naftalin, R., and Holman, G. D. (1974) *Biochim. Biophys. Acta* 373: 453–470.

Naftalin, R. J., and Simmons, N. L. (1979) *J. Physiol.* 290: 331–350.

Nagata, N., Ono, Y., and Kimura, N. (1977) *Biochem. Biophys. Res. Commun.* 78: 19–826.

Nagata, N., and Rasmussen, H. (1968) *Biochemistry* 7: 3788–3733.

Nagata, N., and Rasmussen, H. (1970) *Proc. Natl. Acad. Sci. USA* 65: 368–374.

Nakamura, M., Ide, M., Okabayashi, T., and Tanaka, A. (1972) *Endocrinol. Japan.* 19: 443–449.

Namm, D. H., and Mayer, S. F. (1968) *Mol. Pharmacol.* 4: 61–69.

Nandini-Kishore, S. G., and Thompson, G. A., Jr. (1979) *Proc. Natl. Acad. Sci. USA* 76: 2708–2711.

Nathan, D., and Beeler, G. W., Jr. (1975) *J. Mol. Cell. Cardiol.* 7: 1–15.

Nellans, H. N., Frizzell, R. A., and Schultz, S. G. (1973) *Am. J. Physiol.* 225: 467–475.

Nellans, H. N., Frizzell, R. A., and Schultz, S. G. (1974) *Am. J. Physiol.* 226: 1131–1141.

Nelson, M. J., and Huestis, W. H. (1980) *Biochim. Biophys. Acta* 600: 398–405.

Nelson, P. G., and Peacock, J. H. (1972) *Science* 177: 1005–1007.

Newell, P. C. (1978) *J. Gen. Microbiol.* 104: 1–13.

Nichel, E., and Potter, L. T. (1973) *Brain Res.* 57: 508–517.

Nicholls, D. G. (1978a) *Biochem. J.* 179: 511–522.

Nicholls, D. G. (1978b) *Biochem. J.* 176: 463–474.

Nicholls, D. G., and Scott, L. D. (1980) *Biochem. J.* 186: 833–839.

Nickersen, M. (1956) *Nature* 178: 697–698.

Niggli, V., Ronner, P., Carafoli, E., and Penniston, J. T. (1979) *Arch. Biochem. Biophys.* 198: 124–130.

Nisbet, J. A., Helliwell, S., and Nordin, B. E. C. (1970) *Clin. Orthoped. Rel. Res.* 28: 220–230.

Nishida, E., Kumagai, H., Ohtsuki, I., and Sakai, H. (1979) *J. Biochem.* 85: 1257–1266.

Nishida, E., and Saki, H. (1977) *J. Biochem.* 82: 303–306.

Nishikori, K., and Maeno, H. (1979) *J. Biol. Chem.* 254: 6099–6106.

Nishizuka, Y., Takai, G., Hashimoto, E., Kishimoto, A., Kuroda, Y., Sakai, K., and Yamamura, H. (1979) *Mol. Cell. Biochem.* 23: 153–165.

Nishizuka, Y., Takai, Y., Kishimoto, A., Hashimoto, E., Inoue, M., Yamamoto, M., Criss, W., and Kuroda, Y. (1978) *Adv. Cyclic Nucl. Res.* 9: 209–220.

Nuccitelli, R., Poo, M., and Jaffe, L. F. (1977) *J. Gen. Physiol.* 69: 743–763.

O'Doherty, J., Youmars, S. J., Armstrong, W. McD., and Stark, R. J. (1980) *Science* 209: 510–513.

Ohashi, T., Uchida, S., Nagai, K., and Yoshida, H. (1970) *J. Biochem.* 67: 635–641.

O'Lague, P., Dalen, H., Rubin, H., and Tobias, C. (1970) *Science* 170: 464–466.

Oota, I., and Nagai, T. (1977) *Jpn. J. Physiol.* 27: 195–213.

Orloff, J., and Handler, J. S. (1962) *J. Clin. Invest.* 41: 702–709.

Orloff, J., and Handler, J. S. (1967) *Am. J. Med.* 42: 757–768.

Orly, J., and Schramm, M. (1976) *Proc. Natl. Acad. Sci. USA* 73: 4410–4414.

Oron, Y., Lowe, M., and Selinger, Z. (1975) *Mol. Pharmacol.* 11: 79–86.

Os, C. H., van, and Sleegers, J. F. G. (1971) *Biochim. Biophys. Acta* 24: 89–96.

Otto, D. A., and Ontko, J. A. (1978) *J. Biol. Chem.* 253: 789–799.

Ozawa, E., Itosoi, K., and Ebashi, S. (1967) *J. Biochem. (Tokyo)* 61: 531–535.

Pace, C. S., and Price, S. (1972) *Biochem. Biophys. Res. Commun.* 46: 1557–1563.

Packham, M. A., Guiccione, M. A., Chang, L.-L., and Mustard, J. F. (1973) *Am. J. Physiol.* 225: 38–47.

Pagliara, A. S., and Goodman, A. D. (1969) *J. Clin. Invest.* 48: 1408–1412.

Palmer, W. K., Castagna, M., and Walsh, D. A. (1974) *Biochem. J.* 143: 469–471.

Pannbacher, R. G., and Bravard, L. J. (1972) *Science* 175: 1014–1015.

Parisa, M. W., Butcher, F. R., Becker, J. E., and Potter, V. R. (1977) *Proc. Natl. Acad. Sci. USA* 74: 234–237.

Parod, R. J., and Putney, J. W., Jr. (1978) *J. Physiol. (London)* 281: 371–381.

Parsons, J. A., and Robinson, C. J. (1971) *Nature* 230: 581–582.

Pastan, I., Anderson, W. B., Carchman, R. A., Wellingham, M. C., Russel, T. R., and Johnson, G. S. (1974) Cold Spring Harbor Conf. Cell Prolif. pp. 563–570.

Patrick, J., and Lindstrom, J. (1973) *Proc. Natl. Acad. Sci. USA* 70: 3334–3337.

Peach, M. J. (1972) *Proc. Natl. Acad. Sci. USA* 69: 834–836.

Peach, M. J. (1977) *Physiol. Rev.* 57: 313–370.

Peachey, L. D., and Adrian, R. H. (1973) *In* Structure and Function of Muscle, Vol. 3. G. Bourne, Ed. Academic, New York, pp. 1–30.

Peachey, L. D., and Rasmussen, H. (1961) *J. Biochem. Biophys. Cytol.* 10: 529–553.

Peachey, L. D., and Schild, R. F. (1968) *J. Physiol. (London)* 194: 249–258.

Pechere, J.-F., Demaille, J., Dutruge, E., Capony, J.-P., Baron, G., and Pina, C. (1975) *In* Ca^{2+} Transport in Contraction and Secretion. E. Carafoli, F. Clementi, W. Drabikowski, and A. Margreth, Eds. Elsevier, New York, pp. 459–468.

Peck, W. A., Burks, J. K., Wilkins, J., Rodan, S. B., and Rodan, G. A. (1977) *Endocrinology* 100: 1357–1364.

Perchellet, J.-P., Shanker, G., and Sharma, R. K. (1978) *Science* 203: 1259–1261.

Perchellet, J.-P., Shanker, G., and Sharma, R. K. (1978) *Science* 199: 311–312.

Perry, S. V., Amphlett, G. A., Grand, R. J. A., Jackson, P., Syska, H. and Wilkinson, J. M. (1975) *In* Calcium Transport in Contraction and Secretion. E. Carafoli, W. Drabikowski, and A. Margreth, Eds. North-Holland, Amsterdam, pp. 431–440.

Perry, S. V., and Cole, H. A. (1974) *Biochem. J.* 141: 733–743.

Peterson, C. (1974) *Acta Physiol. Scand. Suppl.* 413: 1–34.

Petersen, M. J., and Edelman, I. S. (1964) *J. Clin. Invest.* 43: 583–594.

Petersen, O. H. (1976) *Physiol. Rev.* 56: 535–577.

Petersen, O. H. (1978) *Proc. Physiol. Soc.* 30P–31P.

Petersen, O. H., and Iwatsuki, N. (1978) *Ann. N. Y. Acad. Sci.* 307: 599–615.

Petersen, O. H., and Pedersen, G. L. (1974) *J. Membr. Biol.* 16: 353–362.

Petersen, O. H., Veda, N., Hall, R. A., and Gray, T. A. (1977) *Pfluegers Arch.* 372: 231–237.

Pershadsingh, H. A., and McDonald, J. M. (1979) *Nature* 281: 495–498.

Pfeuffer, T. (1977) *J. Biol. Chem.* 252: 7224–7234.

Pfeuffer, T. (1979) *FEBS Lett.* 101: 85–89.

Phillips, S. F. (1969) *Gastroenterology* 56: 966–971.

Piascik, M. T., Wisler, P. L., Johnson, C. L., and Potter, J. D. (1980) *J. Biol. Chem.* 255: 4176–4181.

Pickett, W. C., Jesse, R. L., and Cohen, P. (1977) *Biochem. Biophys. Acta* 486: 209–213.

Pinsker, H. M., Hening, W. A., Carew, T. J., and Kandel, E. R. (1973) *Science* 182: 1039–1042.

Pogglioli, J., Berton, B., and Claret, M. (1980) *FEBS Lett.* 115: 243–246.

Potter, J. D., Johnson, J. D., Dedman, J. R., Schreiber, F. M., Jackson, R. L., and Means, A. R. (1977) *In* Ca^{2+} Binding Proteins and Ca^{2+} Function. R. H. Wasserman, R. A. Corradino, E. Carofoli, R. H. Kretsinger, D. H. MacLennan, and F. L. Seigel, Eds. Elsevier, New York, pp. 239–247.

Poulsen, J. H., and Williams, J. A. (1977) *J. Physiol.* 27: 323–339.

Powell, D. W. (1974) *Am. J. Physiol.* 227: 1436–1444.

Powell, D. W., Binder, H. J., and Curran, P. F. (1972) *Am. J. Physiol.* 223: 531–537.

Powell, D. W., Binder, H. J., and Curran, P. F. (1973) *Am. J. Physiol.* 225: 781–787.

Pratje, E., and Heilmeyer, L. M. G. (1972) *FEBS Lett.* 27: 89–93.

Pratje, E., and Heilmeyer, L. M. G. (1973) *Metabl. Interconvers. Enzymes* 3: 185–195.

Prince, W. M., and Berridge, M. J. (1973) *J. Exp. Biol.* 58: 367–384.

Prince, W. T., Berridge, M. J., and Rasmussen, H. (1972) *Proc. Natl. Acad. Sci. USA* 69: 553–557.

Prince, W. T., Rasmussen, H., and Berridge, M. J. (1973) *Biochim. Biophys. Acta* 329: 98–107.

Puchwein, G., Pfeuffer, T., and Helmreich, J. M. (1974) *J. Biol. Chem.* 249: 3232–3240.

Puskin, J. S., Gunter, T. E., Gunter, K. K., and Bussell, P. R. (1976) *Biochemistry* 15: 3834–3842.

Putney, J. W., Jr. (1976) *J. Pharmacol. Exp. Ther.* 198: 375–384.

Putney, J. W. (1977) *J. Physiol.* 268: 139–149.

Putney, J. W. (1979) *Pharmacol Rev.* 30: 209–245.

Putney, J. W., Jr., and Parod, R. J. (1978) *J. Pharmacol. Exp. Ther.* 205: 449–458.

Putney, J. W., Jr., Van de Walle, C. M., and Leslie, B. A. (1978) *Mol. Pharmacol.* 14: 1046–1053.

Putney, J. W., Weiss, S. J., Leslie, B. A., and Marier, S. H. (1977) *J. Pharmacol. Exp. Ther.* 203: 144–155.

Puzas, J. E., Vignery, A., and Rasmussen, H. (1979) *Calcif. Tiss. Intl.* 27: 263–268.

Radich, L., and Butcher, F. R. (1976) *Biochim. Biophys. Acta* 444: 704–711.

Raisz, L. G., Trummel, C. L., Holick, M. F., and DeLuca, H. F. (1972) *Science* 175: 867–769.

Rall, T. W., Sutherland, E. W., and Berthet, J. (1957) *J. Biol. Chem.* 224: 463–475.

Randle, P. J., Foden, S., and Kanagasuntheram, P. (1979) *In* Symposium Society for Experimental Biology XXXIII, Secretory Mechanisms pp. 199–221.

Rasmussen, H. (1966) *Fed. Proc.* 25: 903–910.

Rasmussen, H. (1970) *Science* 170: 404–412.

Rasmussen, H., and Bikle, D. D. (1975) *In* Ca^{2+} Transport in Contraction and Secretion. E. Carafoli, F. Clementi, W. Drabikowski, and A. Margreth, Eds. North-Holland, Amsterdam, pp. 111–122.

Rasmussen, H., and Bordier, P. (1974) The Physiological and Cellular Basis of Metabolic Bone Disease. Williams and Wilkins, Baltimore.

Rasmussen, H., and Clayberger, C. (1979) *In* Membrane Transduction Mechanisms. R. A. Cone, and J. E. Downling, Eds. Soc. General Physiologists Series Vol. 33. Raven Press, New York. pp. 139–159.

Rasmussen, H., Clayberger, C., and Gustin, M. C. (1979) *In* SEB Symposium XXXIII, Secretory Mechanisms. Cambridge University Press, New York, pp. 161–199.

Rasmussen, H., and Feinblatt, J. (1971) *Cal. Tiss. Res.* 6: 265–279.

Rasmussen, H., and Goodman, D. B. P. (1977) *Physiol. Rev.* 57: 421–509.

Rasmussen, H., Goodman, D. B. P., and Tenenhouse, A. (1972) *CRC Crit. Rev. Biochem.* 1: 95–148.

Rasmussen, H., and Gustin, M. (1978) *Ann. N. Y. Acad. Sci.* 307: 391–401.

Rasmussen, H., Jensen, P., Lake, W., and Goodman, D. B. P. (1976) *Clin. Endocrinol.* 5(Suppl.) 11s–27s.

Rasmussen, H., Lake, W., and Allen, J. E. (1975) *Biochim. Biophys. Acta* 411: 63–73.

Rasmussen, H., Pechet, M., and Fast, D. (1968) *J. Clin. Invest.* 47: 1843–1850.

Rasmussen, H., and Tenenhouse, A. (1968) *Proc. Natl. Acad. Sci. USA* 59: 1364–1470.

Rasmussen, H., Wong, M., Bikle, D., and Goodman, D. B. P. (1972) *J. Clin. Invest.* 51: 2502–2505.

Reaven, E. P., and Axline, S. G. (1973) *J. Cell. Biol.* 59: 12–27.

Rebhun, L. I. (1977) *Int. Rev. Cytol.* 49: 1–54.

Reed, K. C., and Bygrave, F. L. (1975) *Eur. J. Biochem.* 55: 497–504.

Reed, K., Vandlen, R., Bode, J., Duguid, J., and Raftery, M. A. (1975) *Arch. Biochem. Biophys.* 167: 138–144.

Reed, P. W., and Lardy, H. A. (1972) *J. Biol. Chem.* 247: 6970–6977.

Reimers, H. J., Packham, M. A., Kenlough-Rathbone, R. L., and Mustard, J. F. (1973) *Br. J. Haematol.* 25: 675–689.

Reinhart, P. H., Taylor, W. M., and Bygrave, F. L. (1980) *FEBS Lett.* 120: 71–74.

Renchens, B. A. M., Schrijen, J. J., Swarts, H. G. P., DePont, J. J. H. H. M., and Bonting, S. L. (1978) *Biochim. Biophys. Acta* 544: 338–350.

Reuter, H. (1973) *Pro. Biophys.* 26: 1–43.

Reuter, H., and Scholz, H. (1976) *J. Physiol. (London)* 264: 17–47.

Ridgway, E. B., Gilhey, J.C., and Jaffe, L. F. (1977) *Proc. Natl. Acad. Sci. USA* 74: 623–627.

Reidel, V., Malchow, D., Gerisch, G., and Nägele, B. (1972) *Biochem. Biophys. Res. Commun.* 46: 279–287.

Rindler, M. J., Chuman, L. M., Shaffer, L., and Saier, M. H., Jr. (1979) *J. Cell. Biol.* 81: 635–648.

Rindler, M. J., Taub, M., and Salier, M. H. (1979) *J. Biol. Chem.* 254: 11431–11439.

Rink, T. J., and Baker, P. F. (1974) *In* Calcium Transport in Contraction and Secretion. E. Carofoli, F. Clement, W. Drabikowski, and A. Margreth, Eds., North-Holland, Amsterdam, pp. 235–242.

Rittenhouse-Simmons, S. (1979) *J. Clin. Invest.* 63: 580–587.

Rittenhouse-Simmons, S., and Deykin, D. (1978) *Biochim. Biophys. Acta* 543: 409–422.

Roach, P. J., DePaoli-Roach, A. A., and Lerners, J. (1978) *J. Cyclic Nucl. Res.* 4: 245–257.

Robberecht, P., Deschodt-Lanckman, M., DeNeef, P., Borgeat, P., and Christophe, J. (1974) *FEBS Lett.* 43: 139–143.

Robblee, L. S., Sherpro, D., and Belamarich, F. A. (1973) *J. Gen. Physiol.* 61: 462–481.

Roberts, M. L., and Petersen, O. H. (1978) *J. Membr. Biol.* 39: 297–312.

Robison, G. A., Butcher, R. W., and Sutherland, E. W. (1971) Cyclic AMP. Academic, New York.

Rodan, S. B., and Rodan, G. A. (1974) *J. Biol. Chem.* 249: 3068–3074.

Rodbell, M. (1980) *Nature* 284: 17–22.

Rodbell, M., Birnbaumer, L., Pohl, S. L., and Krans, H. M. J. (1971) *J. Biol. Chem.* 246: 1877–1882.

Rodbell, M., Krans, H. M. J., Pohl, S. L., and Birnbaumer, L. (1971) *J. Biol. Chem.* 246: 1872–1876.

Rodbell, M., Liu, M. C., Salomon, Y., Louclos, C., Harwood, J. P., Martin, B. R., Rendell, M., and Berman, M. (1975) *Adv. Cyclic Nucl. Res.* 5: 23–29.

Rona, G., Chappel, C. I., Balazs, T., and Gaudry, R. (1959) *A.M.A. Arch. Pathol.* 67: 443–449.

Roohol, A., and Alleyene, G. A. O. (1973) *Biochem. J.* 134: 157–165.

Roos, W., Sheidegger, C., and Gerisch, G. (1977) *Nature* 266: 259–261.

Rose, B., and Loewenstein, W. R. (1975) *Science* 190: 1204–1206.

Rose, B., and Loewenstein, W. R. (1976) *J. Membr. Biol.* 28: 87–119.

Rose, B., and Rick, R. (1978) *J. Membr. Biol.* 44: 377–415.

Rose, B., Simpson, I., and Loewenstein, W. R. (1977) *Nature* 267: 625–627.

Rosen, O. M., and Erlichman, J. (1975) *J. Biol. Chem.* 250: 7788–7794.

Rosenkrantz, H. (1959) *Endocrinology* 64: 355–362.

Ross, E. M., and Gilman, A. G. (1977) *Proc. Natl. Acad. Sci. USA* 74: 3715–3719.

Ross, E. M., and Gilman, A. G. (1980) *Ann. Rev. Biochem.* 49: 533–564.

Ross, E. M., Howlett, A. C., Ferguson, K. M., and Gilman, A. G. (1978) *J. Biol. Chem.* 253: 6401–6412.

Rossignol, B., Keryer, G., Herman, G., Chanbaut-Guerin, A. M., and Cahoreau, C. (1977) *In* Hormone Receptors in Digestive Tract Physiology. S. Bonfils, P. Fromageot, and G. Rosselin, Eds. North-Holland, Amsterdam, pp. 311–320.

Rossomando, E. S., and Sussman, M. (1973) *Biochem. Biophys. Res. Commun.* 47: 604–610.

Roth, J. (1973) *Metabolism* 22: 1059–1073.

Rottenberg, H., and Scarpa, A. (1974) *Biochemistry* 13: 4811–4817.

Rubin, R. P. (1970) *Pharmacol. Rev.* 22: 389–428.

Rubin, R. P., and Laychock, S. G. (1978) *In* Calcium in Drug Action, G. B. Weiss, Ed. Plenum, New York, Chap. 6.

Russell, T. R., Terasaki, W. L., and Appleman, M. M. (1973) *J. Biol. Chem.* 248: 1334–1340.

Saermark, T., and Vilhardt, H. (1979) *Biochem. J.* 181: 321–330.

Saez, J. M., Evans, D., and Gallet, D. (1978) *J. Cyclic Ncul. Res.* 4: 311–321.

Sala, G. B., Hayashi, K., Catt, K. J., and Dufau, M. L. (1979) *J. Biol. Chem.* 254: 3861–3865.

Salganicoff, L., Hebda, P. A., Handrasitz, H., and Fukami, M. H. (1975) *Biophys. Acta* 385: 294–304.

Salomon, Y., and Schramm, M. (1970) *Biochem. Biophys. Res. Commun.* 38: 106–111.

Salzman, E. W. (1972) *N. Engl. J. Med.* 286: 358–363.

Sampson, J. (1977) *Cell* 11: 173–180.

Sandermann, H. (1978) *Biochim. Biophys. Acta* 515: 209–237.

Sandow, A. (1952) *Yale J. Biol. Med.* 25: 176–201.

Saruta, T., Cook, R., and Kaplan, N. M. (1972) *J. Clin. Invest.* 51: 2239–2245.

Sayers, G., Beall, R. J., and Seelig, S. (1972) *Science* 175: 1131–1133.

Sawyer, W. H. (1958) *Endocrinology* 63: 694–698.

Scarpa, A. (1979) *In* Membrane Transport in Biology. G. Briebisch, D. C. Tosteson, and H. H. Ussing, Eds. Springer-Verlag, Berlin, Chap. 7, p. 263.

Scarpa, A., Brinley, F. J., Jr., and Dubyak, G. (1978) *Biochemistry* 17: 1378–1386.

Scarpa, A., Malmstrom, K., Chiesi, M., and Carafoli, E. (1976) *J. Membr. Biol.* 29: 205–206.

Schanne, F. A. X., Kane, A. B., Young, E. E., and Farber, J. L. (1979) *Science* 206: 700–702.

Scharff, P. (1981) Cell Calcium 2: 1–28.

Schatzmann, H. J., and Bürgin, H. (1978) *Ann. N.Y. Acad. Sci.* 307: 125–147.

Schatzmann, H. J., and Vincenzi, F. F. (1969) *J. Physiol.* 201: 369–395.

Scheele, G., and Haymovits, A. (1979) *J. Biol. Chem.* 254: 10346–10353.

Scheid, C. R., Honeyman, T. W., and Fay, F. S. (1979) *Nature* 277: 32–36.

Schlegel, W., Kempner, E. S., and Rodbell, M. J. (1979) *J. Biol. Chem.* 254: 5168–5176.

Schlessinger, J., Shechter, Y., Wittingham, M. C., and Pastan, I. (1978) *Proc. Natl. Acad. Sci. USA* 75: 2659–2663.

Schmidt, J., and Raftery, M. A. (1973) *Biochemistry* 12: 852–856.

Schneyer, C. A., Sucanthapree, C., and Schneyer, I. H. (1977) *Proc. Soc. Exp. Biol. Med.* 156: 132–135.

Schneyer, I. H. (1976) *Am. J. Physiol.* 230: 341–345.

Schramm, M. (1979) *Proc. Natl. Acad. Sci. USA* 76: 1174–1178.

Schramm, M., Orly, J., Eimerl, S., and Korner, M. (1977) *Nature* 268: 310–313.

Schramm, M., and Selinger, Z. (1974) *In* Advances in Cytopharmacology, Vol. 2. B. Ceccarelli, F. Clementi, and J. Meldolesi, Eds. Raven Press, New York, pp. 29–32.

Schramm, M., and Selinger, Z. (1975a) *In* Hormonal Receptors in Digestive Tract Physiology. S. Bonfils, P. Fromageot, and G. Rosselin, Eds. North-Holland, Amsterdam.

Schramm, M., and Selinger, Z. (1975a) *J. Cyclic Nucl. Res.* 1: 181–192.

Scheurs, V. V. A. M., Swarts, H. G. P., DePont, J. J. H. H. M., and Bonting, S. L. (1976) *Biochem. Biophys. Acta* 436: 664–674.

Schrey, M. P., and Rubin, R. P. (1979) *J. Biol. Chem.* 254: 11234–11241.

Schudt, C., Gaertner, U., and Pette, D. (1976) *Eur. J. Biochem.* 68: 103–111.

Schulman, H., and Greengard, P. (1978a) *Proc. Natl. Acad. Sci. USA* 75: 5432–5436.

Schulman, H., and Greengard, P. (1978b) *Nature* 271: 478–479.

Schultz, S. G. (1979) *Am. J. Physiol.* 233: E249–E254.

Schultz, S. G., and Curran, P. F. (1970) *Physiol. Rev.* 50: 637–715.

Schultz, S. G., Frizzell, R. A., and Nellans, H. N. (1977) *J. Membr. Biol.* 33: 351–384.

Schultz, S. G., and Zalusky, R. (1964a) *J. Gen. Physiol.* 47: 567–584.

Schultz, S. G., and Zalusky, R. (1964b) *J. Gen. Physiol.* 47: 1043–1059.

Schulz, I. (1975) *Pfluegers Arch. Eur. J. Physiol.* 360: 165–181.

Schulz, I. (1980) *Am. J. Physiol.* 239: 6335–6347.

Schulz, I., and Heil, K. (1975) *J. Membr. Biol.* 46: 41–70.

Schwartz, C. J., Kimberg, D. V., Sheerin, H. E., Field, M., and Said, S. I. (1974) *J. Clin. Invest.* 54: 536–544.

Schwartz, I. L., Huang, C.-J., Reisman, L., Scalettar, E., Wyssbrod, H. R., Cort, J. H., Roth, L. B., Li, H.-C., and Ripoche, P. A. (1979) *In* Hormonal Control of Epithelial Transport, INSERM SYMPOSIUM 85: 71–84.

Schwartz, I. L., Schlatz, L. J., Kinne-Saffran, E., and Kinne, R. (1974) *Proc. Natl. Acad. Sci. U S A* 71: 2595–2599.

Schwartz, I. L., and Walter, R. (1969) *In* Protein and Polypeptide Hormones. M. Margoulies, Ed. Excerpta Medica Foundation, Amsterdam, pp. 264–269.

Scott, R. E. (1970) *Blood* 35: 514–516.

Scratcherd, T., and Case, R. M. (1973) *In* Pharmacology of Gastrointestinal Motility and Secretion, Vol. 2. Pergamon, New York, pp. 547–612.

Sehlin, J., and Taljedal, I. B. (1975) *Nature* 253: 635–636.

Selinger, Z., Batzri, S., Eimerl, S., and Schramm, M. (1973) *J. Biol. Chem.* 248: 369–372.

Selinger, Z., Eimerl, S., and Schramm, M. (1974) *Proc. Natl. Acad. Sci. USA* 71: 128–131.

Sen, K. K., Azhar, S., and Menon, K. M. J. (1979) *J. Biol. Chem.* 254: 5664–5671.

Sener, A., Hutton, J. C., Kawazu, S., Boschero, A. C., Somers, G., Herchuelz, A., and Malaisse, W. I. (1978) *J. Clin. Invest.* 62: 868–878.

Sener, A., and Malaisse, W. J. (1979) *Eur. J. Biochem.* 98: 141–147.

Severin, E. S., Sashchenko, L. P., Kockelkov, S. M., and Kurochkin, S. M. (1978) *Adv. Cyclic Nucl. Res.* 9: 171–184.

Sharma, R. K., Ahmed, N. K., and Shanker, G. (1976) *Eur. J. Biochem.* 70: 427–433.

Sharma, R. K., and Sawhney, R. S. (1978) *Biochemistry* 17: 316–321.

Sharma, R. K., Desai, R., Waisman, D. M., and Wang, J. H. (1979) *J. Biol. Chem.* 254: 4276–4282.

Sharma, R. K., Wirch, E., and Wang, J. H. (1978) *J. Biol. Chem.* 253: 3575–3580.

Sharp, G. W. G., Wollheim, C., Muller, W. A., Gutzeit, A., Trueheart, P. A., Blondel, B., Orci, L., and Renold, A. E. (1975) *Fed. Proc.* 34: 1537–1548.

Shapiro, E., Castellucci, V. F., and Kandel, E. R. (1980) *Proc. Natl. Acad. Sci. USA* 77: 629–633.

Sheppard, H., and Burghardt, C. R. (1969) *Biochem. Pharmacol.* 18: 2576–2578.

Sherline, P., Lynch, A., and Glinsman, E. (1972) *Endocrinology* 91: 680–690.

Sherrington, C. S. (1947) The Integrative Action of the Nervous System. Yale University Press, New Haven.

Sherry, J. M. F., Gorecka, A., Oksay, M. O., Dabroska, R., and Hartshorne, D. J. (1978) *Biochemistry* 17: 4411–4418.

Shibata, S., and Briggs, A. H. (1977) *J. Pharmacol. Exp. Ther.* 153: 466–470.

Shima, S., Kawashima, Y., and Harai, M. (1978) *Endocrinology* 103: 1361–1369.

Shimahara, T., and Tauc, L. (1976) *Brain Res.* 118: 142–146.

Shimazu, T., and Amakawa, A. (1975) *Biochim. Biophys. Acta* 385: 242–256.

Sieghart, W., Forn, J., and Greengard, P. (1979) *Proc. Natl. Acad. Sci. USA* 76: 2475–2477.

Siggins, G. R., Hoffer, B. J., and Bloom, F. E. (1969) *Science* 165: 1018–1020.

Siggins, G. R., Hoffer, B. J., and Bloom, F. E. (1971) *Brain Res.* 25: 535–553.

Siggins, G. R., Hoffer, B. J. Oliver, A. P., and Bloom, F. E. (1971) *Nature (London)* 233: 481–483.

Siggins, G. R., Oliver, A. P., Hoffer, B. J., and Bloom, F. E. (1976) *Science* 171: 192–194.

Silver, P. J., and DiSalvo, J. (1979) *J. Biol. Chem.* 254: 9951–9954.

Simmons, N. L., and Naftalin, R. J. (1976a) *Biochem. Biophys. Acta* 448: 411–425.

Simmons, N. L., and Naftalin, R. J. (1976b) *Biochim. Biophys. Acta* 448: 426–450.

Simon, T. J. B. (1976) *J. Physiol.* 256: 209–244.

Simpson, E. R., and Boyd, G. S. (1967) *Eur. J. Biochem.* 2: 275–285.

Simpson, E. R., McCarthy, J. L., and Peterson, J. A. (1978) *J. Biol. Chem.* 253: 3135–3139.

Singer, S. J., and Nicolson, G. L. (1972) *Science* 175: 720–731.

Skaer, R. J., Peters, P. D., and Emmines, J. P. (1974) *J. Cell. Sci.* 15: 679–692.

Smith, D. M., and Johnston, C. C. (1973) *Cal. Tiss. Res.* 11: 56–69.

Smith, D. M., and Johnston, C. C. (1974) *Endocrinology* 95: 130–139.

Smith, J. B., Ingerman, C. M., and Silver, M. J. (1976) *J. Lab. Clin. Med.* 88: 167–172.

Smith, S. B., White, H. D., Siegel, J. B., and Krebs, E. G. (1981) Proc. Natl. Acad. Sci. USA 78: 1591–1595.

Smoake, J. A., Song, S. Y., and Cheung, W. T. (1974) *Biochim. Biophys. Acta* 341: 402–411.

Sneddon, J. M. (1972) *Nature New Biol.* 236: 103–106.

Sobieszek, A. (1977) *Eur. J. Biochem.* 73: 477–483.

Soderling, T. R., Hickenbottom, J. P., Reimann, E. M., Hunkeler, F. L., Walsh, D. A., and Krebs, E. G. (1970a) *J. Biol. Chem.* 245: 6317–6328.

Soderling, T. R., Hickinbottom, J. P., Reimann, E. M., Hunkeler, F. L., Walsh, D. A., and Krebs. E. G. (1970b) *J. Biol. Chem.* 245: 6617–6628.

Solaro, R. J., Moir, A. J. G., and Perry, S. V. (1976) *Nature (London)* 262: 615–617.

Soll, A. H. (1978a) *J. Clin. Invest.* 61: 70–380.

Soll, A. H. (1978b) *J. Clin. Invest.* 61: 381–389.

Soll, A. H. (1980a) *Am. J. Physiol.* 238: 6366–6375.

Soll, A. H. (1980b) *J. Clin. Invest.* 65: 1222–1229.

Soll, A. H. (1981) *J. Clin. Invest.* In Press.

Soll, A. H., and Wollin, A. (1979) *Am. J. Physiol.* 237: E444–E450.

Somers, G., Devis, G., van Obeerhen, E., and Malaisse, W. J. (1976) *Pfluegers Arch.* 365: 21–28.

Somlyo, A. P., and Somlyo, A. V. (1968) *Pharmacol. Rev.* 20: 197–272.

Spudich, J. A. (1974) *J. Biol. Chem.* 249: 6013–6020.

Spudich, J. A., and Clarke, M. (1974) *J. Supramol. Structure* 2: 150–162.

Spudich, J. A., and Cooke, R. (1975) *J. Biol. Chem.* 250: 7485–7491.

Stadel, J. M., and Goodman, D. B. P. (1978) *J. Cyclic Nucl. Res.* 4: 35–43.

Standaert, F. G., and Dretchen, K. L. (1979) *Fed. Proc.* 38: 2183–2192.

Steer, M. L., Atlas, D., and Levitzki, A. (1975) New Engl. J. Med. 292: 409–414.

Steer, M. L., and Wood, A. (1979) *J. Biol. Chem.* 254: 10791–10797.

Steiner, K. E., Chan, T. M., Claus, T. H., Exton, J. H., and Pilkis, S. (1980) *Biochim. Biophys. Acta* 632: 366–374.

Steiner, M., and Tateiski, T. (1974) *Biochim. Biophys. Acta* 367: 232–246.

Stephenson, E. W., and Podolsky, R. J. (1978) *Ann. N.Y. Acad. Sci.* 307: 462–476.

Stern, P. H., Trummel, C. L., Schnoes, H. K., and DeLuca, H. F. (1975) *Endocrinology* 97: 1552–1558.

Stevens, F. C., Walsh, M., Ho, H.-C., Teo, T. S., and Wang, J. H. (1976) *J. Biol. Chem.* 251: 4495–4500.

Stifel, F. B., Taunton, O. D., Greene, H. L., and Herman, R. H. (1974) *J. Biol. Chem.* 249: 7240–7244.

Stone, D., and Hechter, O. (1954) *Arch. Biochem. Biophys.* 51: 457–469.

Strittmatter, W. J., Davis, J. N., and Lefkowitz, R. J. (1977) *J. Biol. Chem.* 252: 5478–5482.

Strittmatter, W. J., Hirata, F., and Axelrod, J. (1979) *Science* 204: 1205–1207.

Strittmatter, W. J., Hirata, F., Axelrod, J., Mallorga, P., Tallman, J. F., and Henneberry, R. C. (1979) *Nature* 282: 857–859.

Study, R. E., Breakfield, X. O., Bartfai, T., and Greengard, P. (1978) *Proc. Natl. Acad. Sci. USA* 75: 6295–6299.

Stull, J. T., Brostrom, C. O., and Krebs, E. G. (1972) *J. Biol. Chem.* 247: 5272–7274.

Stull, J. T., Manning, D. R., Hoh, C. W., and Blumenthal, D. K. (1980) *Fed. Proc.* 39: 1552–1557.

Sugden, M. C., and Ashcroft, S. J. H. (1978) *Diabetologia* 15: 173–180.

Sugden, M. C., Christh, M. R., and Ashcroft, S. J. H. (1979) *FEBS Lett.* 105: 95–100.

Sulimouici, S., and Boyd, G. S. (1969) *Steroids* 12: 127–149.

Sullivan, T. J., Parker, K. L., Eisen, S. A., and Parker, C. W. (1975) *J. Immunol.* 114: 1480–1485.

Sutherland, E. W. (1950) *Rec. Prog. Horm. Res.* 5: 441–463.

Sutherland, E. W., and Rall, T. W. (1958) *J. Biol. Chem.* 232: 1065–1076.

Sutherland, E. W., and Rall, T. W. (1960) *Pharmacol. Rev.* 12: 265–299.

Sutherland, E. W., Robison, G. S., and Butcher, R. W. (1968) *Circulation* 37: 279–306.

Svoboda, M., Robberecht, P., Camus, J., Deschodt-Lanckman, M., and Christophe, J. (1976) *Eur. J. Biochem.* 69: 185–193.

Swillins, S., Van Cauter, E., Paiva, M., and Dumont, J. E. (1976) *In* Eukaryotic Cell Function and Growth. J. E. Dumont, B. L. Brown, and N. J. Marshall, Eds. Plenum, New York, pp. 203–230.

Szent-Györgyi, A. G. (1976) *In* SEB Symposium XXX, Calcium in Biological Systems. Cambridge University Press, New York, pp. 335–347.

Takai, Y., Kishimoto, A., Kikkawa, U., Mori, Mori, T., and Nishizuka, Y. (1979) *Biochem. Biophys. Res. Commun.* 91: 1218–1224.

Tait, J. F., and Tait, S. A. S. (1976) *J. Steroid Biochem.* 7: 687–690.

Täljedal, I. B. (1978) *J. Cell. Biol.* 76: 652–674.

Talmage, R. V., Anderson, J. J. B., and Cooper, C. W. (1972) *Endocrinology* 90: 1185–1191.

Talmage, R. V., Grubb, S. A., Norimatsu, H., and Vander Weil, C. J. (1980) *Proc. Natl. Acad. Sci. U S A* 77: 609–613.

Tateson, J. E., Moncada, S., and Vane, J. R. (1977) *Prostaglandins* 13: 389–397.

Taunton, O. D., Stifel, F. B., Greene, H. L., and Herman, R. H. (1974) *J. Biol. Chem.* 249: 7228–7239.

Taylor, D. L., Condeelis, J. S., Moore, P. L., and Allen, R. D. (1973) *J. Cell. Biol.* 59: 378–394.

Taylor, D. L., Moore, P. L., Condeelis, J. S., and Allen, R. D. (1976) *Exp. Cell Res.* 101: 127–131.

Teo, T. S., Wang, T. H., and Wang, J. H. (1973) *J. Biol. Chem.* 248: 588–595.

Terris, S., and Steiner, D. F. (1975) *J. Biol. Chem.* 250: 8389–8396.

Thomasset, M., Cuisinier-Gleizes, P., and Mathieu, H. (1979) *FEBS Lett.* 107: 91–94.

Theoharides, T. C., Sieghart, W., Greengard, P., and Doublas, W. W. (1980) *Science* 207: 80–81.

Thompson, W. J., and Appleman, M. M. (1971) *Biochemistry* 10: 311–316.

Tolbert, M. E. M., Butcher, F. R., and Fain, J. N. (1973) *J. Biol. Chem.* 248: 5686–5692.

Tolbert, M. E. M., and Fain, J. N. (1974) *J. Biol. Chem.* 249: 1162–1166.

Tolbert, M. E. M., White, A. C., Aspry, K., Cutts, J., and Fain, J. N. (1980) *J. Biol. Chem.* 255: 1938–1944.

Tolkovsky, A. M., and Levitzki, A. (1978a) *Biochemistry* 17: 3795–3810.

Tolkovsky, A. M., and Levitzki, A. (1978b) *Biochemistry* 17: 3811–3817.

Tsien, R. W. (1977) *Adv. Cyclic Nucl. Res.* 8: 363–420.

Tufty, R. M., and Kretsinger, R. H. (1975) *Science* 187: 167–169.

Turnberg, L. A. (1970) *Gut* 11: 1049–1054.

Uchikawa, T., and Borle, A. B. (1978) *Am. J. Physiol.* 234: R34–R38.

Ulbricht, W. (1977) *Ann. Rev. Biophys. Bioeng.* 6: 7–31.

Unger, R. H., Keherer, H., Dupre, J., and Eisentraut, A. M. (1967) *J. Clin. Invest.* 46: 630–645.

Ussing, H. H., and Zerahm, K. (1951) *Acta Pyhsiol. Scand.* 23: 110–127.

Valentish, J. D., Tchao, R., and Leighton, J. (1976) *J. Cell. Biol.* 70: 33a.

Valverde, I., Vandermeers, A., Anjaneyulu, R., and Malaisse, W. J. (1979a) *Science* 206: 225–227.

Valverde, I., Vandermeers, A., Anjaneyulu, R., and Malaisse, W. J. (1979b) *Science* 206: 925–927.

Vanaman T. C., Shariel, F., and Watterson, D. M. (1977) *In* Ca^{2+} Binding Proteins and Ca^{2+} Function. R. H. Wasserman, R. A. Corradino, G. Carofoli, R. H. Kretsinger, D. H. MacLennan, and F. L. Seigel, Eds. Elsevier, New York. p. 107.

Van Breeman, C. V., Farinas, B. R., Casteels, R., Gerba, P., Wuytack, F., and Deth, R. (1973) *Phil. Trans. R. Soc. London B* 265: 57–71.

Van Breeman, C. V., Farinas, B. R., Gerba, P., and McNaughton, E. D. (1972) *Circ. Res.* 30: 44–45.

Van den Bosch, H. (1980) *Biochim. Biophys. Acta* 604: 191–246.

Van de Werve, G., Hue, L., and Hers, H. (1977) *Biochem. J.* 162: 135–142.

Varagic̀, V., and Kentera, D. (1970) *Arch. Pharmacol.* 303: 47–53.

Varagic̀, V., Prostram, M., and Kentera, D. (1979) *J. Pharmacol.* 55: 1–9.

Vasington, F. D., and Murphy, J. U. (1962) *J. Biol. Chem.* 237: 2670–2677.

Venter, J. C., Roos, J., and Kaplan, N. O. (1975) *Proc. Natl. Acad. Sci. U S A* 72: 824–828.

Verna, M. J., Dabrowska, R., Hartshorne, D. J., and Goldman, R. C. (1979) *Proc. Natl. Acad. Sci. USA* 76: 184–188.

Vreugdenhil, A. P., and Roukema, P. A. (1975) *Biochim. Biophys. Acta* 413: 79–95.

Vulliet, P. R., Langan, T. A., and Weiner, N. (1980) *Proc. Natl. Acad. Sci. USA* 77: 92–96.

Waisman, D. M. (1979) A Ubiquitous Ca^{2+} Binding Protein and Its Possible Physiological Functions. Ph.D. thesis, University of Manitoba, Winnipeg, Manitoba, Canada.

Waisman, D. M., Gimble, J., Goodman, D. B. P., and Rasmussen, H. (1981) *J. Biol. Chem.* 256: 409–414.

Waisman, D. M., Singh, T. J., and Wang, J. H. (1978) *J. Biol. Chem.* 253: 3387–3390.

Waisman, D. M., Stevens, F. C., and Wang, J. H. (1975) *Biochem. Biophys. Res. Commun.* 65: 975–982.

Waisman, D. M., Stevens, F. C., and Wang, J. H. (1978) *J. Biol. Chem.* 253: 1106–1113.

Walaas, O., Walaas, E., Lystad, E., Alertsen, A. R., and Horn, R. S. (1979) *Mol. Cell. Endocrinol.* 16: 45–55.

Walkenbach, R. J., Hazen, R., and Larner, J. (1978) *Mol. Cell. Biochem.* 19: 31–41.

Walkenbach, R. J., Hazen, R., and Larner, J. (1980) Biochim. Biophys. Acta 629: 421–430.

Wallace, R. W., Lynch, T. J., Tallant, E. A., Maclead, R. M., and Cheung, W. Y. (1978) *Fed. Proc.* 37: 1302.

Walsh, D. A., Perkins, J. P., and Krebs, E. G. (1968) *J. Biol. Chem.* 243: 3763–3765.

Walsh, F. X., Milliken, D. M., Schlender, K. K., and Reimann, E. M. (1979) *J. Biol. Chem.* 254: 6611–6616.

Walsh, M. and Stevens, F. C. (1977) *Biochemistry* 16: 2742–2749.

Walsh, P. N. (1974) *In* Platelets and Thrombosis. S. Sherry, and A. Scriabine. Eds. University Park Press, Baltimore, pp. 23–43.

Waltenbaugh, A.-M. A. and Friedmann, N. (1978) *Biochem. Biophys. Res. Commun.* 82: 603–608.

Waltenbaugh, A., Kimura, S., Wood, J., Divakaray, P., and Friedmann, N. (1978) *Life Sci.* 23: 2437–2444.

Walton, K. G., DeLorenzo, R. J., Curran, P. F., and Greengard, P. (1975) *J. Gen. Physiol.* 65: 153–177.

Wang, J. H. (1976) *Ann. Rev. Biochem.* 45: 239–266.

Wang, J. H. (1977) 3',5'-Nucleotides: Mechanisms of Action. H. Cramer, and J. Schultz, Eds. Wiley, New York, pp. 37–56.

Wang, J. H., Stull, J. T., Huang, T. S., and Krebs, E. G. (1976) *J. Biol. Chem.* 251: 5421–5527.

Wang, J. H., Teo, T. S., Ho, H.-C., and Stevens, F. C. (1975) *Adv. Cyclic Nucl. Res.* 5: 179–194.

Wang, J. H., and Waisman, D. M. (1979) *Curr. Top. Cell. Reg.* 15: 47–107.

Warner, A. E., and Lawrence, P. A. (1973) *Nature* 245: 47–48.

Watanabe, A. M. (1978) *J. Biol. Chem.* 253: 4833–4836.

Watson, E. L., Williams, J. A., and Siegel, J. A. (1979) *Am. J. Physiol.* 236: C233–C237.

Watterson, D. M., and Vanaman, T.-C. (1976) *Biochem. Biophys. Res. Commun.* 73: 40–46.

Webb, R. C., and Bhalla, R. K. (1976) *J. Mol. Cell. Cardiol.* 8: 145–157.

Weber, A. (1959) *J. Biol. Chem.* 234: 2764–2769.

Weber, A., and Herz, R. (1962) *Biochem. Biophys. Res. Commun.* 6: 364–368.

Weber, A., and Murray, J. M. (1973) *Physiol. Rev.* 53: 612–673.

Weber, A., and Winicur, S. (1961) *J. Biol. Chem.* 236: 3198–3202.

Weeds, A., and McLachlan, A. (1974) *Nature* 252: 646–649.

Weeds, A., Wagner, P., Jakes, R., and Kendrick-Jones, J. (1977) *In* Ca^{2+} Binding Proteins and Ca^{2+} Function. R. H. Wasserman, R. A. Corradino, E. Carofoli, R. H. Kretsinger, D. H. MacLennan, and F. L. Seigel, Eds. Elsevier, New York. pp. 222–231.

Weill, C. L., McNamee, M. G., and Karlin, A. (1974) *Biochem. Biophys. Res. Commun.* 61: 997–1003.

Weiner, N. (1979) *Fed. Proc.* 38: 2193–2202.

Weiner, N., Lee, F. L., Barnes, E., and Dreyer, E. (1978) *Life Sci.* 22: 1197–1216.

Weiss, B., Fertel, R., Figlin, R., and Uzunov, P. (1974) *Mol. Pharmacol.* 10: 615–625.

Weiss, B., and Levin, R. M. (1978) *Adv. Cyclic Nucl. Res.* 9: 285–303.

Weiss, K. R., Cohen, J. L., and Kupfermann, I. (1975) *Brain Res.* 99: 381–386.

Weiss, K. R., Cohen, J. L., and Kupfermann, I. (1978) *J. Neurophysiol.* 41: 181–203.

Weiss, K. R., and Kupfermann, I. (1977) *Soc. Neurosci. Symp.* 3: 66–89.

Weiss, K. R., Mandelbaum, D. E., Schonberg, M., and Kupfermann, I. (1979) *J. Neurophysiol.* 42: 791–803.

Weiss, S. J., and Putney, J. W., Jr. (1978) *J. Pharmacol. Exp. Ther.* 207: 669–676.

Weissmann, G., Duker, P., and Zuerier, R. (1971) *Nature New Biol.* 231: 131–135.

Weissmann, G., Goldstein, I., Hoffstein, S., and Tsung, P. K. *Ann. N.Y. Acad. Sci.* 253: 750–762.

Welsh, M. J., Dedman, J. R., Brinkley, B. R., and Means, A. R. (1978) *Proc. Natl. Acad. Sci. USA* 75: 1867–1871.

Welsh, M. J., Dedman, J. R., Brinkley, B. R., and Means, A. R. (1979) *J. Cell. Biol.* 81: 624–634.

Westcott, K. R. LaPoute, D. C., and Storm, D. R. (1979) *Proc. Natl. Acad. Sci. USA* 76: 204–208.

Wheeler, H. D. (1963) *Am. J. Physiol.* 205: 427–438.

White, J. G., Rao, G. H. R., and Gerrand, J. M. (1974) *Am. J. Pathol.* 77: 135–149.

Whitfield, J. F., Rixon, R. H., MacManus, J. P., and Balk, S. D. (1973) *In Vitro* 8: 257–278.

Whitin, J. C., Chapman, C. E., Simon, E. R., Chovaniec, M. E., and Cohen, H. J. (1980) *J. Biol. Chem.* 255: 1874–1878.

Whittam, R. (1968) *Nature (London)* 219: 610.

Wick, U., Malchow, D., and Gerisch, G. (1978) *Cell. Biol. Int. Rep.* 2: 71–79.

Wiesmann, W., Sinha, S., and Klahr, S. (1977) *J. Clin. Invest.* 59: 418–475.

Williams, G. H., and Dluhy, R. G. (1972) *Am. J. Med.* 53: 595–605.

Williams, J. A., Cary, P., and Moffat, B. (1976) *Am. J. Physiol.* 231: 1562–1567.

Williams, J. A., and Lee, M. (1974) *Biochem. Biophys. Res. Commun.* 60: 542–548.

Wills, H., Schupke, B., and Wollenburger, A. (1976) *Acta Biol. Med. (Germany)* 35: 529–541.

Wilson, D. F. (1974) *J. Pharmacol. Exp. Ther.* 188: 447–452.

Wilson, L. D., and Harding, B. W. (1970) *Biochemistry* 9: 1621–1625.

Wolfe, S., and Shulman, N. R. (1970) *Biochem. Biophys. Res. Commun.* 41: 128–134.

Wolff, D. J., and Brostrom, C. O. (1979) *In* Advances in Cyclic Nucleotide Research, Vol. 11, P. Greengard, and G. A. Robison, Eds. Raven Press, New York.

Wolff, D. J., Poirer, P. G., Brostrom, C. O., and Brostrom, M. A. (1977) *J. Biol. Chem.* 252: 4108–4117.

Wolfsen, A. R., McIntyre, H. B., and Odell, W. D. (1972) *J. Clin. Endocrinol. Metab.* 34: 684–689.

Wollheim, C. B., Kikuchi, M., Renold, A. E., and Sharp, G. W. G. (1978) *J. Clin. Invest.* 62: 451–458.

Wollin, A., Soll, A. H., and Samloff, I. M. (1979) *Am. J. Physiol.* 237: E437–E443.

Wolpert, L. (1971) *Curr. Top. Dev. Biol.* 6: 183–224.

Wong, G. L., Luben, R., and Cohn, D. V. (1977) *Science* 197: 663–665.

Wong, P. Y. K., and Cheung, W. Y. (1979) *Biochem. Biophys. Res. Commun.* 90: 473–480.

Wray, H. L., and Gray, R. R. (1977) *Biochim. Biophys. Acta* 461: 441–459.

Wurster, B., Pan, P., Tyan, G. G., and Bonner, J. T. (1976) *Proc. Natl. Acad. Sci. U S A* 73: 795–799.

Wurster, B., Shubiber, K., Wick, U., and Gerisch, G. (1977) *FEBS Lett.* 76: 141–144.

Yagi, K., Yazawa, M., Kakiuchi, S., Ohshima, M., and Uenishi, K. (1978) *J. Biol. Chem.* 253: 1338–1340.

Yamaki, T., and Hidaka, H. (1980) *Biochem. Biophys. Res. Commun.* 94: 727–733.

Yamauchi, T., and Fujisawa, H. (1979) *Biochem. Biophys. Res. Commun.* 90: 28–35.

Yanagibashi, I. (1979) *Endocrinol. Jpn.* 26: 227–234.

Yanagibashi, K., Kaiya, N., Lin, G., and Matsuba, M. (1978) *Endocrinol. Jpn.* 25: 545–558.

Yin, H. L., and Stossel, T. P. (1979) *Nature* 281: 583–586.

Yong, J. A. (1979) *In* International Review of Physiology, Gastrointestinal Physiology III, Vol. 19, R. K. Crane, Ed. University Park Press, Baltimore, pp. 1–58.

Zawalich, W. S., Rognstod, R., Pagliara, A. S., and Matschinsky, F. M. (1977) *J. Biol. Chem.* 252: 8519–8523.

Ziegelhoffer, A., Anad-Srivastava, A., Khandelwal, R. L., and Dhalla, N. S. (1979) *Biochem. Biophys. Res. Commun.* 89: 1073–1081.

Index